The CORAIL® Hip System

Jean-Pierre Vidalain • Tarik Aït Si Selmi
David Beverland • Steve Young • Tim Board
Jens Boldt • Scott Brumby
(Editors)

The CORAIL® Hip System

A Practical Approach Based on 25 Years
of Experience

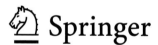 Springer

Editors

Dr. Jean-Pierre Vidalain
"La Boiserie"
Rue du Pont de Thé 8
74940 Annecy le Vieux, France
vidalain@nwc.fr

Dr. Tarik Aït Si Selmi
Centre Orthopédique Santy
Av. Paul Santy 24
69008 Lyon, France
tarik.aitsiselmi@gmail.com

Mr. David Beverland
Musgrave Park Hospital
Stockman's Lane
BT9 7JB Belfast
UK
david.beverland@belfasttrust.hscni.net

Mr. Steve Young
Warwick Hospital
Lakin Road
CV34 5BW Warwick
UK
skyoung@ukconsultants.co.uk

Mr. Tim Board
The Centre for Hip Surgery
Wrightington Hospital
Appley Bridge
Wigan WN6 9EP
UK
tim@timboard.co.uk

Dr. Jens Boldt
Department of Orthopaedics
Siloah Privat Hospital
Worbstreet 324
3073 Guemligen
Switzerland
bol@me.com

Dr. Scott Brumby
Wakefield Orthopaedic Clinic
270 Wakefield Street
Adelaide, South Australia, 5000
Australia
scottbrumby@woc.com.au

ISBN 978-3-642-18395-9   e-ISBN 978-3-642-18396-6
DOI 10.1007/978-3-642-18396-6
Springer Heidelberg Dordrecht London New York

Library of Congress Control Number: 2011921944

Cover design: eStudioCalamar, Figueres/Berlin

Printed on acid-free paper

Springer is part of Springer Science+Business Media (www.springer.com)

Foreword

I was honoured and delighted to be asked by Jean-Pierre Vidalain to write the forward to the book documenting the astonishing journey of the Corail® Hip – from its conception and humble beginnings to becoming the most widely used – and copied! – uncemented hip in the world.

It was only really in the early 1960s that total hip replacement became a routine surgical treatment for patients crippled with end-stage arthritis. In those early years, the procedure was virtually reserved for the elderly and markedly disabled. The increasing prevalence of osteolysis was erroneously identified as being due to "cement disease" and this led to many surgeons abandoning cemented stems in favour of uncemented fixation.

These early uncemented stems were usually large and often obtained fixation in the diaphysis. This led to a high incidence of thigh pain and proximal stress protection osteopenia. In the early 1980s, the question challenging the orthopaedic community was how to achieve predictable fixation with a reproducibly simple technique, while avoiding thigh pain and stress protection.

The Corail® was conceived in this era of uncertainty, not by the machinations of a contrived design and development team, but by the passion of the shared beliefs of a dedicated team of arthroplasty surgeons, the ARTRO Group. No scientific or design consideration was too small to warrant a robust debate to achieve consensus as to the best solution.

Bioactive coatings were being developed in the early 1980s. Early problems included rapid resorption if the coating was too thin and debonding if the coating was too thick. However, optimisation of the hydroxyapatite (HA) coating provided the adjacent cancellous bone with a willing partner in pursuit of rapid, reproducible, and durable osseointegration.

This book faithfully records the evolution of the philosophy in those early years.

The marriage of a stem design which impacted and preserved bone, was sympathetic to flexural matching in the proximal femur and with an optimised bioactive coating, has been one of the most successful and enduring in the history of hip arthroplasty. As it attains its 25th year, the Corail® Hip System celebrates unsurpassed long-term results in hip registries around the world. It has a very wide clinical application and its unqualified success in both the young and the old are reported in this book.

The success of the Corail® owes much to the teaching and training, which has formed the cornerstone of its global acceptance. Some 40 training courses have been held in Annecy and Lyon. This book is a treasure trove of the techniques, tips and tricks, which allow the Corail® to be reproducibly inserted with predictably favourable outcomes. The Corail® Hip is a complete hip system and its contribution to revision surgery – especially conservative revision – cannot be overstated.

The ARTRO Group – bonded by trust, friendship and loyalty – are to be congratulated on the vision and perseverance they displayed in developing and believing in the Corail® System. How the long-term results have justified their belief! They are to be admired for the undiminished passion and enthusiasm they sustain for the philosophy and concept of the Corail® Hip System. Underpinned by science, it is this passion that shines through the book and makes it such a pleasure to read.

Bristol, UK   Ian D. Learmonth

Preface

Twenty-five years already! In the history of the Corail® prosthesis, this quarter century is certainly an appropriate period of time after which to stand back and take a look at the decisive stages and high points in this fantastic and incredible odyssey. We do this without nostalgia, but with the greatest pleasure. We should keep in mind the main events, but also and above all, those who have contributed to the worldwide success of this prosthetic system, which, at the beginning and for many years, was subject to intense controversy and caustic criticism. These events are now ancient history, but deserve to be remembered, if only, briefly.

Everything started during the late 1970s, when a group of seven young surgeons of the same age, including myself, having developed a strong friendship and having trained at the same university (Medical University of Lyon), decided to leave the Department of Orthopaedic Surgery at the end of their training period and to start a private practice in the Rhône-Alpes region of France. At the same time, we decided to create our own association: The Association for Research in Traumatology and Orthopaedics. And so the ARTRO Group was born! We could not anticipate that we were at the beginning of an incredible saga. Actually, the group was not predisposed to play a key role within the international orthopaedic community. At that time, our sole ambition was to meet each other, sometimes over a few drinks, to talk about professional concerns and to discuss difficult clinical and radiological cases. These debates mainly focused on hip replacement and to broaden our knowledge acquired during our training with Prof. Georges de Mourgues, we undertook numerous educational trips to internationally renowned experts. We were at the beginning of our private practice and, of course, had minimal experience. We achieved some success, but also suffered some disappointment. We attempted to imagine the ideal hip prosthesis, perfectly suited to the majority of the patients and clinical cases encountered in our practice, but also easy to insert, reliable and reproducible by the majority of orthopaedic surgeons. This dream became a reality, when in 1982 we began collaborating with Landos, a new French orthopaedic company based in the Champagne region of France, and subsequently in 1985 with a small 'start-up company' called Bioland located in Toulouse. At that time, Bioland was the world leader in calcium phosphate ceramics and plasma-sprayed hydroxyapatite (HA) coatings. Only a few in the field knew about the behaviour of biomaterials and the extraordinary and promising osteo-conductive properties of calcium phosphates. There were even fewer who were prepared to trust this new technique for the fixation of implants in host bone. It is through this collaboration that the ARTRO Group joined the exclusive circle of pioneers, which included such famous figures as Ronald Furlong, Freidrich Osborn, and Rudolph Geesink. This is all ancient history, but in fact the path was long and laborious. Do not forget that in those days hydroxyapatite was considered, at best, as a short-term solution, but was also cautioned, at worst, as a dangerous constituent with disastrous consequences!

The history of the Corail® prosthesis can also be seen as a great human adventure. First, the ARTRO Group and its founding members continue to be very good friends and still share the same common values: honesty, loyalty and devotion towards each other and their colleagues. Gradually, the group expanded by including talented and energetic young people, who were driven by the same values and dynamism as the original group. The adventure has gradually exceeded the group. Let's pay a very sincere tribute to our friends, the French and foreign orthopaedic surgeons who committed themselves early to our basic principles, which were based upon the complementary nature of mechanical (material, technology, geometry) and biological requirements (integration, bone stock, remodelling) and who were able to resist the many criticisms of the system, most of which were without a strong scientific basis.

Thank you to our courageous friends in Belgium, Norway, Portugal, Spain and Israel who joined the adventure at the very beginning. Thank you to our American friends who joined us in the mid 1990s and helped us enter the New World market. And thank you to our UK friends who joined our cause in the 2000s: they have greatly contributed to the peaceful conquest of the Anglo-Saxon world, typically a traditional cement market.

The remarks and comments from renowned objective and independent experts have confirmed the validity of our initial choices. Over the last two decades, an abundant literature has enriched and confirmed our convictions. The fact that the concept and design of the intramedullary segment of the Corail® prosthesis has remained unchanged over the past 25 years demonstrates the excellence of the basic concepts. Improvements being made on the extramedullary part of the prosthesis do not compromise the founding principles. The Corail® prosthesis has, still, a future and each day more and more surgeons discover the incredible performance of the bioactive fixation and its adaptability to all types of patient situations and morphologies, both in primary and revision hip surgery.

Other individuals have also played a decisive role in this long adventure and we would like to extend our warmest thanks to the collaborative teams working at DePuy France and DePuy International Ltd. including senior management, sales and marketing, communications, administrative and regulatory affairs teams. A special thanks to the Research and Development engineers who successively worked on our projects. Their assistance and support made this project possible. The worldwide dissemination of our philosophy and concepts would never have been possible without the time spent by each of you, without your expertise and skills and without the whole educational program. We deeply appreciate and acknowledge your valuable contributions and we thank you for your efforts! We would like to thank our publishing editor, Mrs Gabriele M. Schröder and her team, from Springer, for her valuable cooperation, which was crucial to the completion of this project.

Certainly, we have a strong feeling of nostalgia for this quarter-century, but our feeling of pride is even stronger. However, we need to look forward as well as remember the past. This book not only describes the history, development and clinical results of this unique hip prosthesis system, but it also gives practical, everyday advice. So we are totally convinced that it will not just be a book that sits on the bookshelf! Hip arthroplasty is constantly evolving and implants and surgical techniques are constantly improving. We sincerely hope that in the future this book will help many surgeons improve their daily practice of hip replacement. Our sincerest wish is to keep on contributing to the improvement of the quality of life of patients, wherever they may be.

Once again, many thanks to all of you!

Annecy le vieux, France   Jean-Pierre Vidalain

Book Editors

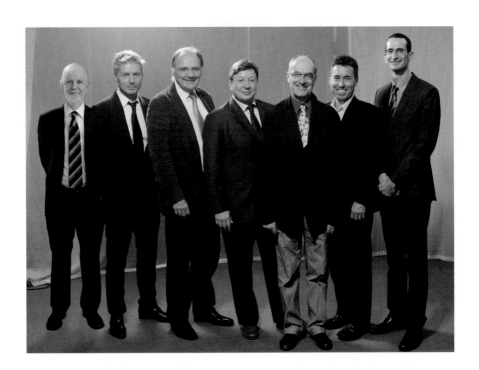

Jean-Pierre Vidalain
ARTRO Group

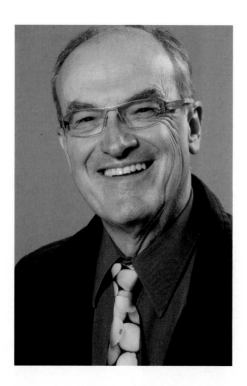

Jean-Pierre Vidalain is one of the original ARTRO Group members and has helped to forge what the team is today. He received his orthopaedic training in Lyon with Prof. Georges de Mourgues, one of the French pioneers in Total Hip Replacement. He also spent some time, in the early 1970s, with Sir John Charnley in Wrightington (UK) and with Prof. GK MacKee in Norwich (UK). Therefore, his major interest is surgery of the hip, with a special mention to hip biomechanics. His passion for bone biology led him to consider a more biological approach for implant fixation and to participate, as co-designer, in the development of the Corail® Hip System.

Jean-Pierre Vidalain routinely presents on the history, research and development, as well as the long-term clinical results associated with the Corail® stem. He is frequently invited as a guest speaker by many institutions and hip associations worldwide. He also acts as a chairperson at numerous international meetings.

As a practicing orthopaedic surgeon, he was based, since 1976, at the Clinique d'Argonay, Annecy, France, which was established as a Corail® Surgeon Visitation Centre in 1995. Although now officially retired from practice he remains an active founding member of the ARTRO Group with ongoing interests in research, education and training. Among many other responsibilities, he is an honorary member of several national and international orthopaedic societies and he is a reviewer for different orthopaedic publications.

Tarik Aït Si Selmi
ARTRO Group

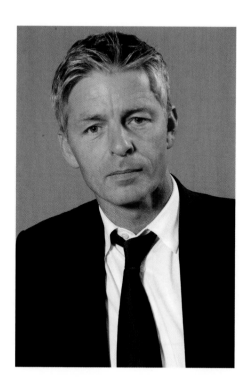

One of the latest ARTRO Group members, Tarik Aït Si Selmi excelled under the tutelage of Jean-Claude Cartillier. It was through this early education and training that Tarik Aït Si Selmi formed his own passionate belief in the Corail® Stem. He was gratified when Cartillier offered him a place within the ARTRO Group in 2004.

After a year vocation in Australia in 2008, Tarik Aït Si Selmi returned to his beloved Lyon to establish a thriving orthopaedic practice as part of the Centre Orthopédique Santy. Tarik Aït Si Selmi continues to be an active member of the ARTRO Group by assisting with research and development as well as the worldwide professional education programmes. He remains particularly interested in orthopaedic innovation.

As a part of his practice, Tarik Aït Si Selmi has a well-established Corail® surgeon visitation centre and regularly hosts international visitors. He is fluent in French and English languages.

David Beverland
Musgrave Park Hospital
Belfast, Northern Ireland

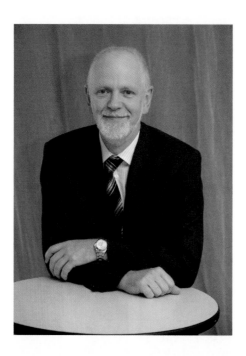

David Beverland is the lead consultant for primary joints at Musgrave Park Hospital, Belfast, Northern Ireland, where he has been an orthopaedic surgeon for the past 20 years. During this time, David Beverland has been instrumental in driving positive change. One notable accomplishment has been the creation and development of the Belfast Orthopaedic Information System (BOIS). David Beverland also established the BART Charity in 2001 which provides funding for a variety of research projects within his primary joint unit.

In 1988, David Beverland undertook the Sir John Charnley Hip Revision Fellowship at Wrightington Hospital in Manchester, UK. He also completed an orthopaedic trauma fellowship with special interest in pelvic and acetabular surgery in 1989 at Sunnybrook Hospital, Toronto, Canada. This training and education was the beginning of future interests specifically in relation to correct cup placement and conservative surgery.

At present, there are over 1,200 primary joints performed annually at Musgrave Park Hospital under the care of David Beverland. In order to manage this capacity, David Beverland has formed a skilled orthopaedic care team which is the largest single consultant primary joint unit in the UK. David Beverland has also been the senior author in over 60 publications with 26 of those published from 2005. He is also an accomplished presenter having given several hundred presentations on different aspects of hip and knee replacement.

Tim Board
Wrightington Hospital
Manchester, United Kingdom

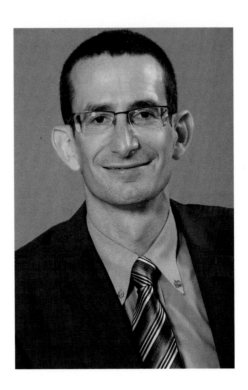

Tim Board specialises in the treatment of complex hip problems and reconstructions. He commonly performs both arthroplasty and arthroscopy of the hip and uses a range of techniques for revision hip surgery including the use of bone graft and cemented components as well as the Corail® Hip System.

He has a strong research interest and currently supervises a number of Ph.D. and M.D. students in collaborations with the University of Manchester's Bioengineering Department and the Tissue Regeneration Lab, where he holds an Honorary Senior Lecturer Position. He has presented over 110 papers at National and International Scientific meetings and published over 65 papers in scientific journals and written numerous book chapters. He is also a Research Advisor to the National Bone Bank and a Member of Editorial panel for the *Journal of Bone and Joint Surgery*.

Tim regularly lectures at international courses and meetings and is involved as a member of faculty on two M.Sc. courses. Throughout his training he received numerous awards and scholarships including ARC grant (1992), Peter Mallimson Bursary (2003), Treloars/Gauvain Fellowship (2004), Sir Harry Platt Fellowship (2005), AO Fellowship (2006) and the British Hip Society European Fellowship (2007).

Jens Boldt
Berne, Switzerland

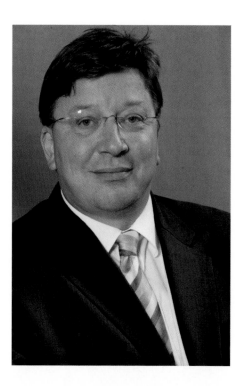

With a background in biomedical engineering, Jens Boldt has been actively involved in scientific research since before establishing himself as an orthopaedic consultant in 2004. As a result, Jens Boldt has published and presented many scientific papers over the last 10 years. One particularly significant study was the radiographic analysis of 206 consecutive Corail® patient x-rays and the resulting published paper. These results remain significant to this day.

Having recently established an orthopaedic department in Berne, Switzerland, Jens Boldt continues to pursue his interests in radiographic analysis and other scientific work on joint reconstruction. As an active member of the Corail® International Faculty, his contribution in research and publication of clinical papers as well as books is invaluable.

Scott Brumby
Wakefield Orthopaedic Clinic
Adelaide, Australia

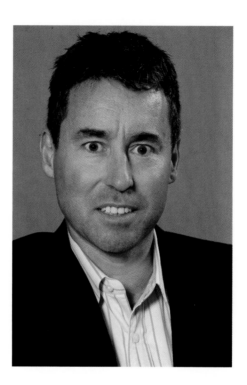

Scott Brumby is an orthopaedic surgeon at Wakefield Orthopaedic Clinic and operates at both Calvary Wakefield Hospital and Stirling District Hospital. He specialises in primary and revision hip and knee joint arthroplasty. Scott Brumby obtained his orthopaedic fellowship in 1999 after having completed a Ph.D. in joint replacement research in 1997. Awarded the Marjorie Hopper Travelling Fellowship, the Mark Jolly Travelling Fellowship and the Johnson and Johnson Joint Replacement Fellowship he worked at several centres excelling in the treatment of arthritic disorders of the hip and knee in Switzerland, Sweden, UK, and Harvard Medical School, USA.

He is currently a board member of the Stirling District Hospital and a Clinical Lecturer at The University of Adelaide. Scott Brumby has a strong interest in evidence based medicine and he is actively involved in reviewing data from the Australian Orthopaedic Association National Joint Replacement Registry and has been a member of the Arthroplasty Society of Australia surgeon review panel for the last 3 years. He is actively involved in arthroplasty education and surgical training within Asia Pacific and Internationally. Scott Brumby is a member of the Corail® International Faculty.

Steve Young
Warwick Hospital
Warwick, United Kingdom

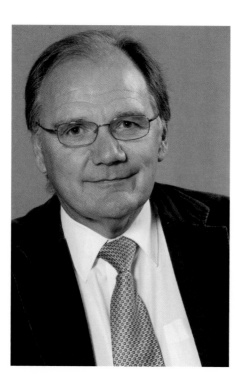

Steve Young has been an orthopaedic consultant at Warwick Hospital since 1988. He specialised in hip and knee arthroplasty but over the years he has developed an almost exclusive hip practice. Steve Young performs primary and revision hip arthroplasties. On average, he carries out over 300 primary joints and 30 revision hip arthroplasties each year.

Since 2002, Steve Young has been using the Corail® stem as his first choice hip implant. He embraces the Corail® surgical philosophy of conservative Total Hip Arthroplasty and will use the Corail® stem for all patient pathologies including complex primaries and revisions. He actively encourages the use of a patient algorithm to determine the best bearing combination dependent on age, morphology and activity level.

Over the years, Steve Young has regularly presented on hip arthroplasty at various meetings and congresses. He has a specific interest in hospital management solutions. He has worked with other clinical staff and Managers at Warwick Hospital to implement an effective programme that allows the safe early discharge of post hip replacement patients. This not only has reduced the length of stay for patients but also has reduced hospital costs dramatically.

Steve Young has also been instrumental in establishing the foremost cementless stem education and training programme in the UK for Orthopaedic Registrars.

Contents

Part IV   The Next 25 Years

Contributors

Pooler Archbold Primary Joint Unit, Musgrave Park Hospital, Belfast, UK

Bruno Balaÿ ARTRO Group, Saint Bernard, France

Valéry Barbour DePuy France, Saint Priest, France

Danielle Berberian DePuy Orthopaedics, Inc., USA

David Beverland Primary Joint Unit, Musgrave Park Hospital, Belfast, UK

Nicolas Bishop Institute of Biomechanics, TUHH Hamburg University of Technology, Hamburg, Germany

Tim Board The Centre for Hip Surgery Wrightington Hospital, Wigan, Lancashire, UK

Jens Boldt Department of Orthopaedic, Siloah Privat Hospital, Worbstreet 324 3073 Guemligen, Switzerland

Michel Bonnin ARTRO Group, Centre Orthopédique Santy, Lyon, France

Scott Brumby Wakefield Orthopaedic Clinic, Adelaide SA, Australia

James T. Caillouette Newport Orthopedic Institute, Newport Beach, California, USA

Jean-Claude Cartillier ARTRO Group, Lyon, France

Claude Charlet ARTRO Group, Saint Didier au Mont d'Or, France

Jean-Christophe Chatelet ARTRO Group, Polyclinique du Beaujolais, Arnas Villefranche, France

Charles R. Clark Department of Orthopaedics and Rehabilitation, University of Iowa Health Center, Iowa City, IA, USA

Vladimir V. Danilyak Russian Federation, 150040, Yaroslavl, Lenin's Prospect, Russia

Guillaume Demey Centre LIVET, Lyon, France

Rüdiger von Eisenhart-Rothe Department for Orthopaedic Surgery and Traumatology, Klinikum Rechts der Isar der TU München, München, Germany

Camdon Fary Department of Orthopaedics, The Royal Melbourne Hospital, Parkville, Australia

Michel-Henri Fessy ARTRO Group, Centre Hospitalier Lyon-Sud, Chemin du Petit Revoyet, Pierre-Bénite, France

John Fisher Institute of Medical & Biological Engineering, School of Mechanical Engineering, University of Leeds, Leeds, UK

Mark I. Froimson Department of Orthopaedic Surgery, Cleveland Clinic Foundation, Cleveland, OH, USA

Jonathan Garino School of Medicine, University of Pennsylvania, Philadelphia, PA, USA

Dirk Ghadamgahi DePuy International Ltd, Leeds, England, UK

Dominique C.R.J. Hardy Orthopaedic Department, Moliere Longchamps Hospital, Brussels, Belgium

Hans-Erik Henkus HAGAziekenhuis, The Hague, The Netherlands

Tom Hogervorst HAGAziekenhuis, The Hague, The Netherlands

Eileen Ingham Institute of Medical & Biological Engineering, School of Mechanical Engineering, University of Leeds, Leeds, UK

Laurent Jacquot ARTRO Group, Clinique d'Argonay, Argonay, France

Louise Jennings Institute of Medical & Biological Engineering, School of Mechanical Engineering, University of Leeds, Leeds, UK

Zhongmin Jin Institute of Medical & Biological Engineering, School of Mechanical Engineering, University of Leeds, Leeds, UK

Henry Wynn Jones The Centre for Hip Surgery, Wrightington Hospital, Appley Bridge, Lancashire, England

Thomas Kalteis OCM, Department for Orthopedic Surgery, Steinerstr. 6, D-81369 Muenchen

Robert Kipping OrthoPraxis, Bahnhofstraße 5, Gräfelfing, München, Deutschland

Sebastien Lustig Centre Albert Trillat, Lyon Croix Rousse University Hospital, Lyon, France

Alain Machenaud ARTRO Group, La Balme de Sillingy, France

Joel M. Matta Hip and Pelvis Institute, Saint John's Health Center, 2001 Santa Monica Blvd., #1090, Santa Monica, CA 90404, USA

Markus C. Michel Orthopaedic Center Münsingen OZM, Münsingen, Switzerland

Michael M. Morlock Institute of Biomechanics, TUHH Hamburg University of Technology, Hamburg, Germany

Rémi Philippot Hopital nord, CHU, Saint Etienne, France

Martyn L. Porter The Centre for Hip Surgery, Wrightington Hospital, Appley Bridge, Lancashire, England

Carole Reignier DePuy France, Saint Priest, France

Gurion Rivkin Cleveland Clinic, Cleveland, OH, USA

Jean-Charles Rollier ARTRO Group, Saint Martin Bellevue, France, Clinique d'Argonay, Argonay, France

Emilio Romanini Casa di Cura San Feliciano, Rome, Italy

Attilio Santucci Casa di Cura Villa Stuart, Rome, Italy

Tarik Aït Si Selmi ARTRO Group, Centre Orthopédique Santy, Lyon, France

Jean-Marc Semay ARTRO Group, Saint Priest en Jarez, France

Louis Setiey ARTRO Group, Lyon, France

Andrew G. Sloan Blackburn Royal Infirmary, Lancashire, England

Sam Sydney St. Agnes Hospital, Baltimone, Maryland, USA

Joanne Tipper Institute of Medical & Biological Engineering, School of Mechanical Engineering, University of Leeds, Leeds, UK

Jean-Pierre Vidalain ARTRO Group, Annecy le Vieux, France

Helge Wangen Orthopedic Department, Sykehuset Innlandet Hospital Trust, Elverum, Norway

Sophie Williams Institute of Medical & Biological Engineering, School of Mechanical Engineering, University of Leeds, Leeds, UK

Steve Young Specialist in Hip and Knee Surgery, Warwick Hospital, Warwick Warwickshire, England UK

History

Jean-Pierre Vidalain

1

Content

J.-P. Vidalain et al. (eds.), *The CORAIL® Hip System*,
DOI: 10.1007/978-3-642-18396-6_1, © Springer-Verlag Berlin Heidelberg 2011

1.1 The Corail® Birth: A Shared Parenthood

Louis Setiey

The Corail® prosthesis was born in 1986 from the collaboration of the ARTRO Group with Landos, a young French orthopaedic company. Three years before, we had developed the Titan cemented stem. This prosthesis provided excellent stability during trialling and the clinical results obtained confirmed our first impressions. We were convinced that changing the surface finish of the stem by combining a macro surface aspect with hydroxyapatite coating could lead to a high-performance uncemented stem. After 25 years of experience, our choices in terms of stem design, material and coating have proven to be successful.

Introduction

The ARTRO Group was founded in 1981 in Lyon. We were seven young orthopaedic surgeons with 4–5 years of private clinical practice. During our residency and fellowship training, we became familiar with the technique of cemented hip prosthesis implantation in the departments of Prof. de Mourgues and Prof. Dejour. The McKee hip prosthesis was widely used in Prof. de Mourgues' Department. Our chief had also performed hip replacements using the cementless Judet prosthesis, which had a porous metal coating. Implantation of this prosthesis proved challenging with a high rate of early failures.

Newly entered into private practice, we had chosen a more secure option by implanting the Charnley–Muller cemented stem and later the self-locking Muller stem. However, the self-locking prosthesis had the disadvantage of being stable only in the frontal plane, whereas it featured an identical thickness from proximal to distal in the sagittal plane. Stability was therefore ensured by cementation [18]. We then developed the Titan prosthesis in 1982, derived from the Muller stem but featuring a frontal and sagittal tulip flare in its metaphyseal portion. It was the first straight prosthesis with metaphyseal filling in the three planes and the clinical performance of this prosthesis was good. Due to the proximal filling it became known as the 'stereo-stability concept' stem.

Only a thin mantle of cement was necessary to ensure the reliable fixation of this straight quadrangular stem made of forged titanium alloy (Ti6Al4V). Since it demonstrated a high primary stability, we implanted a few hydroxyapatite (HA)-coated Titan stems. Sharing these observations, several Portuguese orthopaedic surgeons conducted an extensive study on the cementless Titan but without HA. Results were favourable in the first year, but soon after, the appearance of radiolucent lines indicated the absence of fixation between the stem and the bone.

At this point we were not sure which direction to take. We had good results with the cemented Titan stem, but with short-term clinical results. In the literature, cemented stems were associated with a high incidence of early failures along with aseptic loosening rates of more than 50% at 10 years [8]. The poor results with cemented fixation were attributed to cement ageing and to its lack of fatigue strength. This phenomenon was referred to as 'cement disease' by Hungerford and Jones [10]. Facing controversy over cemented femoral fixation, Harris suggested in 1970 a second-generation cementing technique in which the cement was pressure-injected in a retrograde fashion [8].

The use of a cementless stem was another direction in which we were heading. But at that time, the available cementless hip stems with different shapes and coatings were giving poor results. Many patients with cementless hips had thigh pain and early occurrence of radiolucent lines. Some surgeons even made a point to warn their patients before surgery of possible post-operative thigh pain. Despite these failures, we chose cementless fixation. We believed the cement acted as an additional foreign body within the femur and would have a negative effect on bone trophicity. We realised that the Titan stem gave satisfactory primary stability and we were convinced that only minor modifications were necessary to convert this stem into a reliable cementless prosthesis. Therefore, we defined the specifications regarding material, design, macrostructure and surface coating.

Material and Design

Good bone remodelling around the implant is a prerequisite for long-term survival of a cementless prosthesis. This is what emerges from the research work of Roux [15] on adaptive bone remodelling published in 1881 and taken on by Wolff, who made a mathematical law out of it [20].

The implant metallic structure and design of the implant transmit a mechanical signal to the bone. Repetitive dynamic loads on bone trigger remodelling, whereas decreased mechanical usage and acute disuse result in bone resorption. Regarding the metallic structure of the device, we chose titanium alloy (Ti6Al4V) as already mentioned for the Titan stem, since its modulus of elasticity more closely matches that of cortical bone. The Young's modulus of bone is 20 MPa and that of titanium alloy is 110 MPa, whereas the Young's modulus of CrCo and stainless steel is 210 MPa.

In 1982, when the Titan was developed, we had great difficulties in finding a manufacturer who was willing to make a forged titanium alloy femoral stem. The stiffness and flexibility of a femoral stem depend not only on the modulus of elasticity of the component, but also on its design and size as shown by Bobyn et al. [2, 3]. It is acknowledged that stem stiffness increases the potential for bone resorption. In 1984, we performed a series of total hip arthroplasties using the HA Titan. The results were highly satisfactory, since no thigh pain and excellent radiographic bone ingrowth were observed. The tulip-flared design provided optimum metaphyseal stability. This stem had a straight quadrangular design, since we were opposed to the development of an anatomically shaped stem. We were convinced that satisfactory filling of the dual curvature of the femoral canal could not be systematically achieved.

During this phase of the development of the Corail® stem, we decided to reduce the size of the middle and distal sections of the Titan to avoid any distal locking and to prevent the risk of stress-shielding due to the decreasing stiffness gradient. Moreover, our objective was not to achieve a 'fit and fill' of the stem as did the Anglo-Saxon since we believed that this approach destroys the endosteal vascularisation process. By destroying this process, bone is prevented from reacting to mechanical stress and so cannot form neoformed bone tissue, which is needed for implant osseointegration.

A flexible stem reduces the risk of stress-shielding, but increases the amount of stress at the bone-implant interface. Therefore, two different types of macrostructures were designed to reinforce stability without increasing stiffness: horizontal macrostructures to prevent stem subsidence and vertical ones to resist torsional loosening

forces. Moreover, these macrostructures increase by 15% the bone-implant contact surface.

The Corail® prosthesis design was born: a straight quadrangular Ti6Al4V femoral stem featuring a metaphyseal tulip flare in combination with horizontal and vertical grooves. Torsional and compressive strength tests had still to be carried out by engineers to validate the mechanical resistance of the stem. Moreover, the stem coating had to be selected.

HA Coating

While the Corail® stem was under development in 1984–1985, it was widely recognised that integrating inert bodies into living organisms was a real challenge. We became acquainted with the work of JF Osborn who achieved optimum bone regeneration in comminuted fractures of the jawbone by implanting hydroxyapatite ceramic (HAC) granules of porous consistency. These findings were later confirmed by the research work of Block and Kent published in 1984–1985 [1].

But at this time, little experimental data was available on the integration of HA-coated implants. Therefore, we performed a small experimental study in animals. Titanium blocks with a 150 μm thick HA coating applied on one face were implanted into the pelvis of Beagle dogs and removed after a period of 3 weeks and 2, 4 and 6 months. On the HA-coated face, trabecular bone tissue in close contact with the ceramic layer was observed, whereas on the sand-blasted titanium surfaces, a 200–300 μm thick fibrous tissue layer had formed.

The clinical results of the HA Titan prosthesis, the research work of Osborn and the findings from our experimental study enabled us to choose a 150 μm thick HA coating to cover the roughened, alumina-blasted surface of our implant, taking into consideration the fact that HA coatings maintain their mechanical properties up to a thickness of 200 μm.

By choosing a full coating, we aimed to achieve homogeneous and complete fixation of our implant through osteogenesis, since it is accepted that bone-implant contact does not exceed 60% of the whole surface.

Later on, the extensive work of Frayssinet [4, 5], Geesink [6, 7], Soballe [16, 17], Manley [13] and Kobayaski [12] confirmed the superiority of HA-coated implants over porous-coated ones, due to the osteoconductive properties of HAC [9], its excellent biocompatibility [11] and the absence of inflammatory response even to HA particles [14].

Since its creation and the first implantations performed in 1986 [19], the intramedullary portion of the Corail® stem has remained unchanged. Only its extramedullary section has been modified to reduce the risk of impingement, to improve the neck taper design and to better adapt the shape of this section to the patient's anatomical offset.

Key Points

> The Corail® prosthesis was developed in 1985 by the ARTRO Group and was first implanted in 1986.

> The choice of the stem material, the stem design and the coating were guided by the experience acquired with the Titan-cemented prosthesis and by experimental work, which was done at the time.

> The intramedullary portion of the stem has remained unchanged since 1986.

> Modifications were made to the neck and taper design to improve the range of motion, to reduce the risk of impingement and to more precisely match the patient's anatomical offset.

> After 25 years of experience, our choices have been validated by the clinical and radiographic results, which have been obtained.

References

1. Block MS, Kent JN (1985) Healing of mandibular ridge augmentations using HA with and without autogenous bone in dogs. J Oral Maxillofac Surg 43:3
2. Bobyn JD, Engh CA (1984) Human histology of the bone-porous metal implant interface. Orthopaedics 7:1410
3. Bobyn JD, Mortiomer ES, Glassman AH et al (1992) Producing and avoiding stress shielding: laboratory and observations of non-cemented total hip arthoplasty. J Clin Ortho 274:79
4. Frayssinet P, Vidalain JP (1991) Réponses d'un histologiste aux questions d'un chirurgien à propos d'un revêtement d'implants orthopédiques par l'hydroxyapatite de calcium. Rev Chir Orthop Reparatrice App Mot 77(6) Suppl 1:19
5. Frayssinet P, Hardy D, Rouquet N et al (1992) New observations on middle term hydroxyapatite coated titanium alloy hip prostheses. Biomaterials 13(10):668–674
6. Geesink RGT (1989) Experimental and clinical experience with hydroxyapatite coated hip implants. J Clin Orthop 12(9):1239–1242
7. Geesink RGT (1990) Hydroxyapatite coated total hip prostheses. Two-year clinical and roentgenographic results of 100 cases. J Clin Orthop 261:39–58
8. Harris WH, McCarthy JC, O'Neil DA (1982) Femoral component loosening using contemporary techniques of femoral cement fixation. J Bone Joint Surg Am 64(67):1063–1067
9. Hoogendoorn HA, Renooij W, Akkermans LMA et al (1987) Long term study of large ceramic implants (porous hydroxyapatite) in dog femora. Clin Orthop Relat Res 187:281–288
10. Hungerford DS, Jones LC (1988) The rationale for cementless revision of cemented arthroplasty failures. J Clin Orthop 235:12–24
11. Klein CPAT, Driessen AA, de Groot K et al (1983) Biodegradation behaviour of various calcium phosphate materials in bone tissue. J Biomed Mater Res 17:769–784
12. Kobayaski A, Donnelli WJ, Scott G et al (1997) Early radiological observations may predict the long term-survival of femoral hip prothesis. J Bone Joint Surg Br 79(4):583–589
13. Manley MT, Kay JF, Yoshiya S et al (1987) Accelerated fixation of weight bearing implants by hydroxyapatite coatings. Trans 33rd Annual Meeting. Orthop Res Soc 112:214
14. Ricci JL, Spivak JM, Alexender H et al (1989) Hydroxyapatite ceramics and the nature of the bone-ceramic interface. Bull Hosp Jt Dis Orthop Inst 49(2):178–191
15. Roux W (1881) Der züchtende Kampf der Teile, oder die Teilauslese im Organismus. Theorie der funktionellen Ampassung. Wilhem Engelmann, Leibzig
16. Søballe K, Hansen ES, B-Rasmussen H et al (1990) Hydroxyapatite coating enhances fixation of porous coated implants comparison between press fit and non-interference fit. Acta Orthop Scand 61(4):299–306
17. Søballe K, Hansen ES, B-Rasmussen H et al (1992) Tissue ingrowth into titanium and hydroxyapatite coated implants during stable and unstable mechanical conditions. J Orthop Res 10:285–299
18. Sutherland CJ, Wilde AM, Borden LS et al (1982) A ten year follow-up of one hundred consecutive curved-stem total hip-replacement arthroplasties. J Bone Joint Surg Am 64:970–982
19. Vidalain JP (1991) The Corail® prothesis: biodynamic implant. Advantages of the hydroxyapatite coating. ARTRO Group experience with 4 years follow-up. In: Küsswetter W (ed) Non-cemented total hip replacement. International symposium, 1990. Georg Thieme Verlag, Stuttgart, New-York
20. Wolff J (1982) Das Gesetz der Transformation der knochen. Kirchwald Berlin. English edition: (1986) The Law of Bone Remodeling (trans: Maquet P, Furlong R). Springer, Berlin

Basic Science

2

Tarik Aït Si Selmi

Contents

J.-P. Vidalain et al. (eds.), *The CORAIL® Hip System*,
DOI: 10.1007/978-3-642-18396-6_2, © Springer-Verlag Berlin Heidelberg 2011

2.1 Stem Design

2.1.1 Intramedullary Design: Squaring the Circle

Jean-Marc Semay and Valéry Barbour

The design requirements for an ideal hip stem are contradictory. The implant should be stiff enough to provide the necessary mechanical stability for bone ingrowth. At the same time, the flexibility of the stem should encourage homogeneous stress and strain distribution to avoid the risk of stress-shielding. The Corail® stem complies with these requirements, since its dual metaphyseal flare reinforces mechanical stability and its implantation in cancellous bone allows for a gradual load transfer along the length of the whole femur. Finite element analyses confirm that the stem design gives stem stability combined with axial and rotational load transfer.

Introduction

Various techniques are available to achieve good bone implant fixation. In cemented implants, the use of polymethylmethacrylate (PMMA) cement results in an extensive interconnected network between the cement and surrounding bone, whereas in cementless implants with bioactive coatings, fixation is provided by direct and intimate bonding to the adjacent bone without interposition of a fibrous tissue (osseointegration). To achieve successful osseointegration and bone ingrowth after stem implantation, a very strict mechanical requirement must be met, namely primary mechanical stability. High stiffness of the composite stem–femur construct is essential to achieve primary mechanical stability. However, such stiffness has a bad long-term effect, since it promotes stress-shielding associated with bone resorption, which may lead to stem failure. In order to prevent stress-shielding, the composite stem–femur construct should ideally have the same modulus of elasticity as the bone and should provide gradual load transfer to the bone.

Specifications: 'Squaring the Circle'

In the Short Term: Primary Mechanical Stability

Primary mechanical stability is of utmost importance to achieve osseointegration. This has been shown to be the case in many in vivo studies, particularly in canine models [6], which have demonstrated that when motion at the bone–implant interface was higher than $20\,\mu m$, bone ingrowth was compromised and replaced by a fibrous membrane between the bone and the implant.

There are two factors which contribute to the relative motion at the bone–implant interface:

- Implant migration due to insufficient press-fit and a coefficient of friction, which is too low to resist motion
- Micromotion related to cyclic movements induced by physiological weight bearing (walking, stair climbing) [1]

The mechanical stability of a cementless implant is dependent not only on the implant design, but also on the mechanical quality of the host bone, the nature of the bone–implant contact, the patient's weight and the size of the selected implant [7].

According to various cadaveric and finite element studies, the use of a solid, stiff implant providing optimal filling of the femoral cavity (the 'fit and fill' concept) should increase the initial press-fit effect of the femoral stem and should improve the primary mechanical stability of the implant.

In the Long Term: Gradual Stress and Strain Distribution

Even if a solid, stiff femoral stem provides initial mechanical stability by increasing the bone–stem interface coefficient of friction, it may also have mid- and long-term disastrous consequences. Such a rigid composite system reduces considerably the amount of mechanical stress transmitted to the adjacent bone by redistributing the stress more distally. According to Wolff's law, when bone is subjected to stresses substantially below its normal level, it responds by remodelling according to the new low stresses applied, and so the bone mass diminishes, leading to osteoporosis (internal remodelling) and cortex thinning (external remodelling). This phenomenon, often referred to as stress-shielding, has been observed for a long time by means of radiographic and densitometric analyses (dual-emission x-ray absorptiometry [DEXA] analysis).

An old study conducted by Huiskes et al. [4] using three-dimensional (3D) finite element analysis was performed to investigate the effects of implant stiffness, bone elasticity and bone response on bone remodelling around non-cemented femoral stems. This study clearly pointed out that low-stiffness femoral stems significantly reduce the risk of stress-shielding (advantage), but also increase the interface coefficient of friction and the risk of implant loosening (disadvantage). Therefore, a compromise has to be found (squaring the circle!) to reconcile these two contradictory requirements.

The Suggested Solution: The Corail® Stem

According to the above considerations, the objective of the ARTRO Group was to develop a femoral stem with sufficient stiffness to prevent harmful micromotion at the bone–implant interface.

The shape of this femoral stem should ensure initial mechanical stability by means of intra-femoral press-fit. As already mentioned this stability is considered to be a necessary prerequisite for successful biological osseointegration.

However, in order to avoid neutralization of mechanical stresses transmitted to the host bone, this relatively stiff stem was designed to be implanted in compacted cancellous bone. Therefore, the necessity to have a relatively flexible composite hip stem to reduce the risk of stress-shielding was respected, since persistent or neoformed bone trabeculae create a strong bond between the stem and the femur and provide sufficient elasticity to promote favourable bone remodelling.

The Corail® stem has the following features:

- It is manufactured from forged titanium alloy (Ti 6Al 4V ELI). Even though the stiffness of this titanium material is higher than that of cortical bone, its modulus of elasticity is closer to that of human bone than is the modulus of elasticity of CoCrMo alloy or stainless steel. In another study,

Huiskes [3] demonstrated that the stiffness of a titanium alloy stem is only 50% of that of an otherwise identical CoCrMo alloy stem, thus ensuring a better stress and strain distribution in bone.

- It is a straight and symmetrical stem featuring a metaphyseal flare both in the frontal and sagittal planes. This dual flare is intended to reinforce mechanical fixation in the metaphyseal region and to resist both axial and torsional loosening forces (walking, standing position, stair climbing). This feature is known as the 'stereostability concept'.
- Its quadrangular section enhances rotational stability, preserves trabecular bone in front of and behind the implant and stimulates osteogenesis in the four corners (this osteogenesis is clearly visible in histological cross sections of explanted stems studied by D. Hardy – Sect. 2.1.3.3).
- Its thin conical distal tip, with reduced canal filling, was designed to prevent stem-locking in the diaphyseal cortical bone and to provide the composite construct with sufficient distal flexibility without compromising the excellent biological fixation. These design features account for the absence of postoperative thigh pain.
- Its surface is macrostructured. This consists of horizontal grooves in the metaphyseal region and vertical grooves in the diaphyseal section. These groves have a dual objective:
- The mechanical objective is to resist axial forces in the metaphysis, while enabling easy stem removal (the rack principle) in the event of stem revision, and to resist torsional loosening forces in the diaphyseal section.
- The biological objective is to increase by 20% the contact and fixation surface with adjacent bone.
- The macrostructures on the medial aspect of the stem act as multiple support micro-collars, thus resulting in pressure micro-peaks, which enhance osteogenesis. Such a reaction has been observed in finite element studies and confirmed by histological analyses of explanted stems (Sect. 2.1.3.3).

The Corail® stem also features an optional collar, which acts as a support. The biomechanical usefulness

Fig. 2.1 Anterolateral view of the stem (Copyright DePuyInternational Limited)

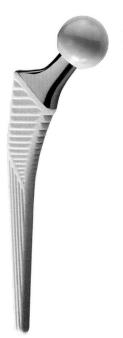

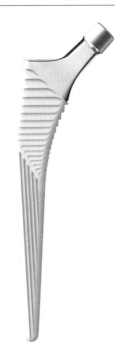

Fig. 2.3 Posterolateral view of the stem (Copyright DePuyInternational Limited)

Validation of Design Features

Through Clinical and Radiographic Results

The Corail® stem was developed in the 1980s from the experience acquired with other available prostheses such as the MÜLLER cemented self-locking stem. Cadaveric implantations were performed to assess implant stereostability. The bioactive properties of the hydroxyapatite (HA) coating were evaluated during in vivo implantations in canine models.

Since the results of these trials were promising, human implantations were started in 1986. These implantations gave encouraging preliminary clinical and radiographic outcomes. Long-term satisfactory results have been achieved as shown in an analysis, which is described in detail in another section of this book (Sect. 4.2.1).

During the following years no design-related defects were reported and the intramedullary features of the Corail® stem have remained unchanged over the past 25 years.

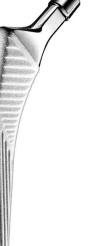

Fig. 2.2 Anteroposterior view of the stem (Copyright DePuyInternational Limited)

and function of this optional collar is described in detail in another section of this book (Sect. 2.1.2.3) (Figs. 2.1–2.3).

Through Finite Element Analysis

Finite element analyses have confirmed the success of the following chosen design features.

1. Material and Method

Two cementless stems were compared in this study: the Corail® stem whose design has been described in the previous section and a self-locking sabre-like stem featuring a thin section. These stems where implanted in the same bone block from which the intramedullary shape of each stem without macrostructure was substracted. Meshing was done under Ansys 11.0 Workbench using 10-node tetrahedral elements (Solid 147). The bone block was made of 197,922 elements and 300,707 nodes. Cancellous bone properties were considered to be isotropic and linear. An elastic modulus of 553 MPa and a Poisson's ratio of 0.3 were assigned. Stems were meshed from the 3D model using 20-node hexahedra.

The Corail® stem model was made of 47,605 tetrahedra (82,976 nodes). The material properties of the stem elements were assumed to be those of an isotropic titanium alloy with Young's Modulus = 105,000 MPa and Poisson's ratio of 0.27.

The sabre-like stem model was made of 40,615 tetrahedra (67,681 nodes). The material properties of the stem elements were assumed to be those of an isotropic stainless steel with Young's Modulus = 200,000 MPa and Poisson's Ratio = 0.3.

Boundary conditions were applied to the bone block and at the bone–implant interface depending on the applied force. Frictional contact was modelled at the bone–implant interface by means of asymmetric face-to-face contact elements. These are most accurate when compared to experimental measurements and allow a large amount of sliding [2, 5, 8]. The coefficient of friction was set at 0.3 [8].

2. Axial stability

For the study of axial stability, the external faces of the bone block were bonded and the implant was loaded with a force applied to the centre of the prosthetic head. The force direction was vertical and the magnitude was the same for the two stems.

A static calculation was conducted under Ansys 11.0 Workbench. A vertical 5,500 N ramped load was applied to study the axial stability.

3. Rotational stability

For study of rotational stability, a torque was applied to the external faces of the bone block and the implant was bonded on the neck area. The torque magnitude was the same for the two stems.

A static calculation was conducted under Ansys 11.0 Workbench. A ramped torque of 100 Nm was applied to study the rotational stability.

Results and Discussion

1. Axial stability

When a 5,500 N axial load was applied to the Corail® stem, the von Mises stress in the bony structure decreased by 20% (Fig. 2.4). The distribution is homogeneous for the Corail® stem (Fig. 2.4b). For the sabre-like stem, on the other hand, three hot points occurred (Fig. 2.4a). Moreover, the sliding distance decreased by 60% for the Corail® thanks to its fluted shape and its horizontal macrostructures (Fig. 2.5a, b). These macrostructures resist the load as stress riser (Fig. 2.4c) and allow better bone ingrowth under the macrostructures as evident in the histological studies (Sect. 2.1.3.3).

As a result, the proximal envelop of the Corail® stem is shaped to resist axial forces. In the frontal plane, the stem's fluted shape provides axial stability in combination with the horizontal grooves around the circumference of the stem.

2. Rotational stability

When 100 Nm torque was applied to the stem, the maximal principal stress induced by the Corail® stem is decreased by 20% (Fig. 2.6) compared to a sabre stem. However, the sliding at the bone interface is generally 25% higher on the Corail® stem (Fig. 2.7). This would suggest that the Corail® design is less accurate. But when looking at the first and second proximal sections (Fig. 2.6a, b), the interpretation is different. Even if the Corail® can slide more rotationally, the induced stress on the bone is more homogeneous. On the first proximal section, two hot points

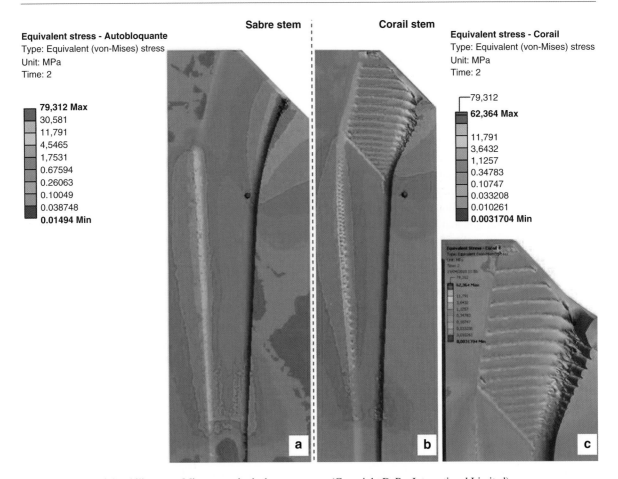

Fig. 2.4 (**a–c**) Axial stability – von Mises stress in the bony structure (Copyright DePuyInternational Limited)

appear diagonally (Fig. 2.6a). The ones on Corail® are located on the entire medial and lateral sides, whereas for the sabre-like stem, the stress is concentrated on the two respective corners (Fig. 2.6b). On the second proximal section, the sabre-like stem shows two hot points diagonally as on the first proximal section (Fig. 2.6a). On the other hand, the Corail® stem induces stress at the four corners thanks to its cross section (Fig. 2.6b).

As a result, the trapezoidal cross section avoids the occurrence of peak stresses in the bone, but creates a homogeneous stress distribution in the bony structure. This tends to prevent bone fracture during impaction or immediate postoperative weight bearing. Moreover, bone ingrowth will be activated around the stem allowing better fixation postoperatively.

To conclude, the proximal envelop of the Corail® stem is shaped to resist both axial and torsional loosening forces. In the frontal plane, the stem's pronounced lateral flare and medial curve provide axial and rotational stability. In the lateral plane a progressive anterior to posterior tulip flare fills the metaphysis and, in combination with horizontal grooves around the circumference of the stem, further reinforces axial stability. The well-defined rectangular section and vertical grooves provide rotational stability.

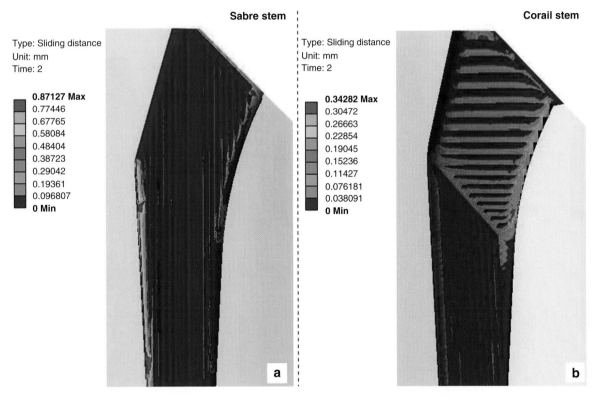

Fig. 2.5 (**a**, **b**) Axial stability – sliding distance (Copyright DePuyInternational Limited)

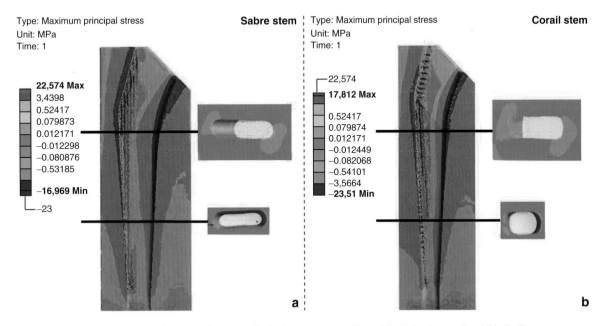

Fig. 2.6 (**a**, **b**) Rotational stability – von Mises stress in the bony structure (Copyright DePuyInternational Limited)

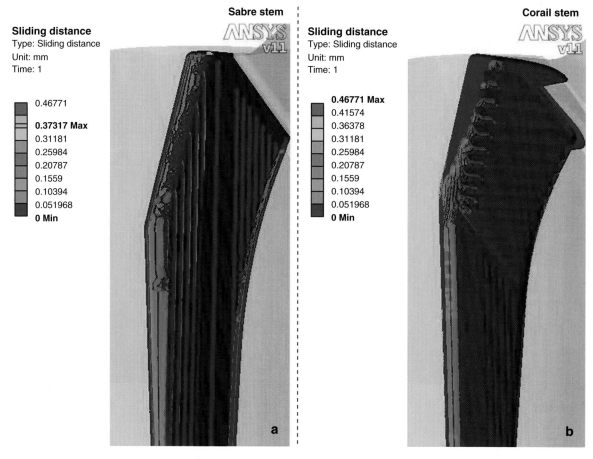

Fig. 2.7 (**a**, **b**) Rotational stability – sliding distance (Copyright DePuyInternational Limited)

Conclusion

Implantation of a femoral prosthetic stem considerably disrupts natural bone physiology and no ideal prosthesis exists up to now. To ensure a successful integration of the inert stem within the living bone, the properties of the stem should be as close as possible to those of the bone, both mechanically and biologically. Can it be said that the Corail® stem has fully satisfied this dual challenge? After 25 years of experience, long-term successful clinical and radiographic results have been reported; however, further improvements in 'squaring the circle' may still be achieved.

Key Learning Points

> The Corail® stem features dual metaphyseal flares, which provide primary mechanical stability. Its implantation in cancellous bone allows satisfactory biological fixation with the gradual transfer of the applied load to the whole femur.

> Finite element analyses have proven the superiority of these design features over those found in a self-locking stem with no metaphyseal flare.

> The intramedullary design of the Corail® stem has remained unchanged since it was developed, 25 years ago.

References

1. Clift SE (2009) Finite element modelling of uncemented implants: challenges in the representation of the press-fit conditions. In Lim CT, Goh JCH (eds) Proceedings of the 13th international conference on biomedical engineering, Singapore, 3–6 Dec 2008. Springer, Berlin/Heidelberg, pp 1608–1610

2. Hefzy MS, Singh SP (1997) Comparison between two techniques for modelling interface conditions in a porous coated hip endoprosthesis. Med Eng Phys 19:50–62

3. Huiskes R (1990) The various stress patterns of press-fit, ingrown, and cemented femoral stems. Clin Orthop Relat Res 261:27–37

4. Huiskes R, Weinans H, Van Rietbergen B (1992) The relationship between stress shielding and bone resorption around total hip stems and the effects of flexible materials. Clin Orthop Relat Res 274:124–134

5. Mann K, Bartel D, Wright T et al (1995) Coulomb frictional interfaces in modelling cemented total hip replacements: a more realistic model. J Biomech 28:1067–1078

6. Ramamunti BS, Orr TE, Bragdon CR et al (1998) Factors influencing stability at the interface between a porous surface and cancellous bone: a finite element analysis of a canine in vivo micromotion experiment. J Biomed Mater Res 36(2):274–280

7. Viceconti M, Brusi G, Pancati A et al (2006) Primary stability of an anatomical cementless hip stem: a statistical analysis. J Biomech 39:1169–1179

8. Viceconti M, Muccini R, Bernakiewicz M et al (2000) Large-sliding contact elements accurately predict levels of bone–implant micromotion relevant to osseointegration. J Biomech 33:1611–1618

2.1.2 Extramedullary Design: Custom-Made for All

2.1.2.1 Femoral Offset: Lateral Thinking

Michel-Henri Fessy and Michel Bonnin

Correct femoral component selection must reproduce the normal hip anatomy and restore the abductor muscle lever arm in addition to the femoral offset. To allow accurate restoration of hip joint biomechanics the ARTRO Group has designed two lateralized versions of the Corail® stem in addition to the standard offset range. Our objective in this chapter is to review the literature on femoral offset and biomechanics following total hip arthroplasty and describe the design rationale of the development and range of Corail® stems now available.

Introduction

The recent literature dedicated to hip arthroplasty highlights the need to restore the lever arm of the abductor muscles while preserving femoral lateralization. By definition, femoral offset, is the distance between the centre of the head and the anatomical axis of the femur.

Insufficient Lateralization Is Detrimental

Insufficient lateralization leads to hip abductor weakness [1] and increases polyethylene (PE) wear as noted by Devane and Horne [2], who demonstrated a negative correlation between polyethylene wear and lateralization. Sakalkal et al. [6] has been able to confirm this observation from other clinical series. The ARTRO Group has noticed this anecdotally. Harris provides an explanation for this phenomenon: based on Pauwels theory, increased lateralization reduces the articular resultant line. Because of this accelerated wear of the polyethylene, Amstutz states that insufficient lateralization causes loosening. Finally, the respect of the lateralization contributes significantly to the stability of the prosthesis [7].

Excessive Lateralization Is Detrimental

However, some authors warn against excessive lateralization. Lateralization values in excess of 52 mm [7] promote the loosening of the cemented stem through the increase of rotational constraints. Excessive lateralization could promote pseudo-inequalities on the one hand and tendinopathy of the gluteus medius on the other hand.

The Hip Biomechanical Architecture
Must Be Respected

The notion of lateralization is different from that of lever arm. Indeed, Pauwels [4] likened the hip to a balance composed of two arms, the abductor muscle lever arm and the weight lever arm. During arthroplasty, the restoration of the abductor lever arm (ALA) necessitates undoubtedly the restoration of the lateralization. Hence this notion of lateralization seems to be a key parameter to be implemented if the biomechanical characteristics of the hip joint are to be respected.

Corail® Lateralized Stems

Initially the Corail® stem was only designed and manufactured with only one range of stems with progressive variable offset. The ARTRO Group designed the Corail® stem with a non-homothetic neck; that is, the stem lateralization increases with the size of the stem through the increase of the medio-lateral width of the stem. Over time, the ARTRO Group found that the standard range of stems did not restore the femoral anatomy in all cases. A study was performed to assess the anatomical basis of femoral component offset and lateralisation.

Methods

We performed a plain radiographic-based anatomical study using an anteroposterior (AP) pelvis radiograph, the patient standing up with the lower limb in internal rotation so that the patella is in the frontal plane. The cohort comprised 150 patients, mean age 67, with one arthroplasty hip and one contralateral healthy, pathologically free hip.

On this AP pelvis radiograph we measured the lateralization; the distance between the centre of the femoral head and the anatomical axis of the proximal femur, as well as other extramedullary parameters; the cervicodiaphyseal (CD) angle, the abductor muscle lever arm, and the position of the head centre versus the apex of the lesser trochanter. We also measured intramedullary parameters, the width of the proximal and distal femur canal, in order to determine the femoral flaring index as per Noble (Fig. 2.8).

Finally, we measured the gluteus medius action angle (GMAA); the angle formed by a vertical line that passes on the extreme point of the anterosuperior iliac crest, and a line that passes over this point and the most extreme point of the greater trochanter (Fig. 2.9).

Results

Lateralization was plotted and found to represent a Gaussian distribution of the population. On average, lateralization was 39.75 mm (SD = 5.7) with a range between 25 and 60 mm.

The characteristics of the other parameters measured are as follows:

CD angle: 129°(SD = 6)
Height (H) of centre (C): 58.8 cm (SD = 8.6)
Abductor muscle lever arm: 7.8 cm
Width of proximal femur: 45.4 mm (SD = 5.7)
Distal femoral width: 13.5 mm (SD = 2.6)
Femoral flaring: 3.45 (SD = 0.61)
Gluteus medius action angle: 6° (SD = 1)

In our study, lateralization was independent of the endomedullary characteristics (width of proximal femoral canal, femoral flaring). The height of the head centre relative to the lesser trochanter and the lateralization are independent parameters. The ALA is poorly correlated with lateralization but highly correlated with the GMAA ($p < 0.001$).

The Corail® Range and Its Nomenclature

The Corail® range comprises a range of non-homothetic stems with a standard offset range and a high offset (lateralized) range (Fig. 2.10). Two CD angles are available: 135° and 125°. These two parameters characterize the extramedullary feature

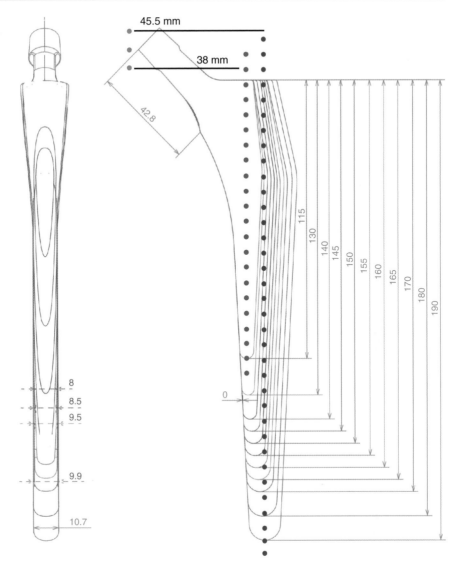

Fig. 2.8 Lateralization and the endo- and extramedullary parameters

of the stem. There is a standard Corail® with a 135° angle, with and without collar. The High Offset Corail® has a 135° CD angle and lateralises the head centre over more than 7 mm compared to the standard implant of the same size. Initially this implant had no collar and the ARTRO Group considers that it can be used with or without collar. The Coxa Vara implant has a 125° CD angle and lateralises the head centre over 7 mm and also lowers the head centre by 5 mm compared to a standard implant of the same size. This implant always comes with a collar which is positioned to increase the neck resistance to fracture.

The Corail® hip system consists of a range of cementless, fully hydroxyapatite (HA)-coated stems with various parameters (Fig. 2.11):

1. The CD angle (135° or 125°)
2. The offset (low, standard, high)
3. The size (from 6 to 20)
4. The collar option (collar, collarless)

Discussion

Our findings and philosophy match the data from the literature [3]. However, it appears that anatomical

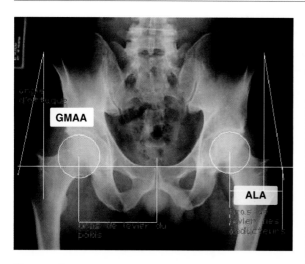

Fig. 2.9 Gluteus medius action angle (GMAA) and abductor lever arm (ALA)

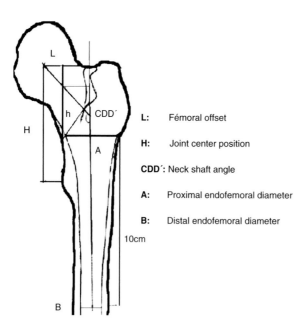

L:	Fémoral offset
H:	Joint center position
CDD´:	Neck shaft angle
A:	Proximal endofemoral diameter
B:	Distal endofemoral diameter

Fig. 2.10 Non-homothetic neck on a stem of increasing size (Copyright DePuyInternational Limited)

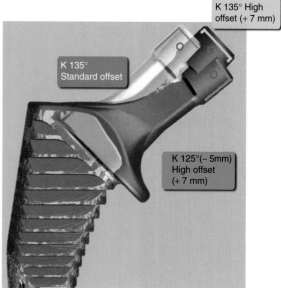

Fig. 2.11 The Corail® range of femoral stems (Copyright DePuyInternational Limited)

Table 2.1 Femoral offset: anatomical study/radiological study

Authors	Year	Number	3
Noble	1986	158	42.4 mm
Noble	1988	200	43 mm
Rubin	1989	10	43 mm
Aubagnac	1992	32	47 mm
Lindgren	1992	20	44 mm
Fessy	1992	30	41.8 mm
Fuku	1994	50	42 mm
McGrory	1995	86	39 mm
Rubin	1997	300	40.5 mm
Massin	2000	200	41 mm
Fessy	2002	147	39.75 mm

studies tend to increase lateralization compared to radiological studies (Table 2.1), possibly because of a better control of the rotation; yet the difference is not significant on comparable populations.

As described by Rubin et al. [5], it is accepted that horizontal dimensional parameters are influenced by femoral rotation, and lateralization is no exception to the rule. For example, external rotation reduces the real value of lateralization. It is thus important to perform the preoperative radiography in proper conditions, with the lower limb in internal rotation and the patella in the frontal plane to achieve maximum exposure of the neck. The value of the lateralization can be determined to plus/minus a few millimetres, which is negligible in clinical practice during the planning of the arthroplasty.

Statistical data show that lateralization is independent of endomedullary parameters since the former is not affected by the width of the medullary canal and by the femoral flaring.

Hence, lateralization is the same, with a narrow or wide canal, with a stove pipe and fluted femur. Conversely, two femurs with similar canals (width and flaring) could exhibit very different lateralizations. Lateralization does not increase with the width of the medullary canal or with the size of the prosthetic stems. This advocates for a non-homothetic neck; a prosthetic neck always identical placed on the prosthetic stem, regardless of the size of the latter. The Corail® stem has a non-homothetic neck. The prosthetic lateralization increases with the size of the stem through the increase of the medio-lateral width of the stem.

Our population exhibits a broad variability and scattering of the lateralization for a single head centre. This of course causes a practical problem when the femur anatomical parameters are to be restored – lateralization – to reproduce the ALA, and when the height of the head centre is to be respected to ensure equal lower limb length. It is possible to adjust the height of the head centre by means of the depth at which the stem is introduced. Thirty percent of the patients exhibited a lateralization well beyond what can be restored by a standard implant, even in a long neck configuration. This is why the ARTRO Group has decided to use standard and lateralized implants in order to achieve the best possible restoration of this parameter and in respecting hip biomechanics. The Corail® stem – an internationally recognized implant – had to cover all the architectural specificities of the various populations throughout the world.

A modular neck could have been used but was not selected since modular implants produce particles and debris and it could have caused incipient fractures in certain systems. Finally, this modularity offers too many surgical options – often useless, not to say dangerous – if not associated with a reliable navigation system.

Conclusions

A large variability of femoral lateralization is observed in the population. There is no correlation between the femoral lateralization and any other anatomic characteristic. Therefore, in routine hip surgery, standard and lateralized prosthetic ranges should be used and this is the option selected for the Corail® stem.

Key Learning Points

> The design geometry must respect the biomechanics.

> There is no correlation between the endomedullary and the lateralization that could justify a non-homothetic neck on a Corail® stem.

> In order to respect the architecture of the hip, the Corail® stem comes in a standard and lateralized range.

> Planning is justified and validated to select the implant offset.

> The notion of standard and lateralized range imposes the use of trial implants in order to validate the choices made preoperatively.

> A modular neck is not necessary. Considering the current status of science, it is a source of complications.

References

1. Amstutz HC, Sakai DN (1975) Total joint replacement for ankylosed hips: indications, technique and preliminary results. J Bone Joint Surg Am 57(5):619–625
2. Devane PA, Horne JC (1999) Assessment of polyethylene wear in total hip replacement. Clin Orthop Relat Res 369:59–72
3. Fessy MH (1992) L'extrémité supérieure du fémur: étude anatomique. Application aux implants. Thèse Sciences, LIPS éditions, Lyon
4. Pauwels F (1976) Biomechanics of the normal and diseased hip. Springer, Berlin
5. Rubin PJ, Leyvraz PF, Heegaard JH (1989) Variations radiologiques des paramètres anatomiques du fémur proximal en fonction de sa position de rotation. Rev Chir Orthop 75(4):209–215
6. Sakalkale DP, Sharkey PF, Eng K et al (1999) Effect of femoral component offset on polyethylene wear in total hip arthroplasty. Clin Orthop Relat Res 369:59–72
7. Steinberg B, Harris WH (1992) The “ offset &rdaquo; problem in total hip arthroplasty. Contemp Orthop 24(5):556–562

2.1.2.2 Impingement: How to Avoid the Risk

Michel-Henri Fessy and Michel Bonnin

Prosthetic femoroacetabular impingement is characterized by abnormal contact between the prosthetic neck and the rim of the acetabular cup. According to the literature, the incidence of impingement after total hip arthroplasty (THA) is high, as confirmed by implant retrieval studies. This phenomenon is an important cause of adverse outcomes. It reduces the range of motion, which in turn causes:

- Dislocation
- Wear debris and osteolysis
- Implant migration and loosening
- Damage to the components

The aetiology of hip impingement is multifactorial. The important factors include:

1. Acetabular implant parameters:
   The plane of the cup opening
   The anti-dislocation elevated rim
   Wear

2. Femoral implant parameters:
   The head–neck ratio
   The prosthetic neck design
   The Morse taper

3. Implant positioning parameters

We advocate the use of practical strategies to prevent impingement.

Introduction

Impingement is a disorder of the hip caused by abnormal contact between the neck of the femoral stem and the rim of the acetabular cup. Contact may also occur between bone and soft tissue, but this article focuses exclusively on the contact occurring between the prosthetic components. This contact is an undesirable outcome which the surgeon should endeavour to prevent during the procedure by appropriate implant selection and correct implant orientation.

Impingement: A Sad Reality

Cup retrieval analysis demonstrates that impingement causes damage to the prosthetic components both on the femoral and acetabular sides. According to the literature, cup retrieval studies have reported impingement-related damage in 30% of the cases.

Impingement and Its Consequences

Impingement may have disastrous consequences. It reduces the range of motion, thus limiting the functional benefits of arthroplasty. It causes subluxation and even dislocation. It probably constitutes the *primum movens* of prosthesis dislocation. According to the literature, impingement can lead to accelerated wear and osteolysis. This was demonstrated by Urquhart et al. [5] in 1998 by comparing skirted femoral head components with standard head implants. This was confirmed by Efthekar [3] with respect to the Charnley long posterior wall cup design. These observations confirm our opinion about the risks of using anti-dislocation elevated rim cups.

Impingement promotes implant migration and loosening. Charnley had already made the hypothesis that these repeated impacts could lead to component loosening when using the McKee Farrar prosthesis. He wrote: 'In the case of the 41 mm McKee prosthesis a common observation at secondary interventions is a bright spot on the neck corresponding with a point of impingement on the rim of the socket. McKee himself frequently attributed loosening of one or other of the components to the patient sustaining trauma as the result of a fall.' Several observations confirm that impingement may cause component damage. Since impingement has a deleterious effect on arthroplasty, it should therefore be anticipated and prevented postoperatively. Therefore one should be aware of the risk factors and mechanisms associated with the occurrence of prosthetic impingement. Impingement is influenced by:

- Acetabular implant parameters
- Femoral implant parameters
- Implant positioning parameters

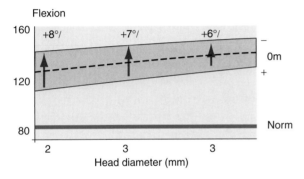

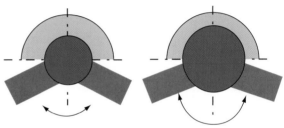

Fig. 2.13 Influence of head diameter

Fig. 2.12 Flexion and plane of the cup opening: this *graph* represents the relation between the diameter of the prosthetic head (*x-axis*) and the maximum flexion angle of the hip before impingement (*y-axis*). The *dotted line* represents the contact if the plane of the cup is equatorial. The *solid lines* represent the contact if the plane of the cup is below (−2 mm) or above (+2 mm) the equator of the prosthetic head

Table 2.2 Influence of head diameter on mobility in flexion–extension

Head	22 mm	26 mm	28 mm	32 mm	36 mm
Flexion	93°	102°	107°	112°	117°
Extension	64°	73°	78°	84°	89°

Neck: 13 mm – anteversion 15°
Cup: angle 45 – anteversion 15°

Acetabular Implant Parameters

The Plane of the Cup Opening

When the cylindrical part of the cup extends beyond the equatorial plane, it reduces the angular range of motion and promotes impingement whereas any material removal relative to the equatorial plane has the opposite effect (Fig. 2.12).

The Anti-dislocation Rim (on an Acetabular Cup)

According to the same principle, the use of an anti-dislocation rim, congruent or not, reduces the angular range of motion and promotes early contact between the neck and the cup.

Wear

Linear wear of the polyethylene (PE) decreases the angular range of motion. In the Charnley system featuring a 22.2 mm femoral head, 1 mm linear wear will reduce the angular range of motion by 6% and 5 mm wear will reduce the range of motion by 30%. As demonstrated in low-friction arthroplasty [2], the wear–loosening–dislocation triad is a well-known phenomenon. For that reason, we advocate the use of a standard cup which does not extend beyond the equatorial plane. Moreover, in young and active patients we recommend the use of a hard-on-hard, ceramic-on-ceramic bearing combination to prevent long-term wear phenomena.

Femoral Implant Parameters

Femoral Head Diameter

The femoral head diameter is a key element (Fig. 2.13). An increase of 4 mm in femoral head diameter will increase the range of motion by 5%, thereby delaying the onset of impingement. Therefore, we systematically use the maximum head diameter available and suitable with the selected bearing couple. If a hard-on-hard, ceramic-on-ceramic bearing couple is used, we advocate the use of a 36 mm femoral head whenever possible (Table 2.2).

Neck Diameter

An increased neck diameter promotes the occurrence of impingement and reduces the range of motion (Fig. 2.14). The use of a skirted implant would further reduce the range of motion in all directions and make impingement more likely.

The Femoral Head–Neck Ratio

It is widely acknowledged that the femoral head–neck ratio may be a contributing factor in the impingement process. The combination of a small head with a large neck is the worst configuration.

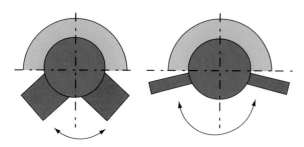

Fig. 2.14 Influence of femoral neck diameter

Table 2.3 Influence of the neck design on the range of motion (head: 28 mm, neck: 13 mm – anteversion 15°, cup inclination 45° – anteversion 15°)

Neck	Trapezoidal	Circular
Flexion	124.8°	114.6°
Extension	40.2°	22.2°
Abduction	60.4°	40.8°
Adduction	67°	27.8°
Int. rotation	48.2°	35°
Ext. rotation	37.8°	26.2°

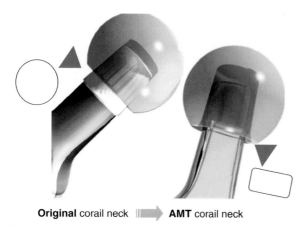

Original corail neck ▶ **AMT** corail neck

Fig. 2.15 The AMT femoral neck (circulo-trapezoidal neck and mini taper) (Copyright DePuyInternational Limited)

The Prosthetic Neck Design

As demonstrated in the literature, the prosthetic neck design is a key factor which greatly contributes to improving the joint range of motion in a specific direction. A circular and trapezoidal neck design will increase hip joint mobility in flexion and extension by 20% when compared to a circular neck of identical diameter. The Articul/eze® Mini Taper (AMT) femoral neck (Fig. 2.15) was thus selected by the ARTRO Group to be combined with the Corail® implant, in order to reduce impingement in flexion–extension (Table 2.3).

The Morse Taper

In most implants available on the market today and featuring a long neck configuration, the femoral neck overhangs underneath the head. In this case, the neck is no longer likely to be in contact with the acetabular cup, but rather the Morse taper which has a larger diameter. For this reason, the Corail® femoral stem has a 10 mm mini taper (Fig. 2.15).

Positioning Parameters

Prosthetic parameters provide a specific angular range of motion. Implant positioning within the space orientates the angular range of motion within the space, thus defining the range of motion of the joint. This range of motion should be sufficient for the range of motion needed by the patient. However, it has been demonstrated that achieving optimal implant positioning is a challenging objective [1, 4]. Fortunately, as demonstrated by Charnley, there are some adaptive processes, which help the patient achieve a wide range of activities in most cases. These processes, however, account for the high frequency of impingements reported in retrieval studies. Therefore our current objective is to optimise implant positioning through computer-assisted navigation. Figure 2.16 displays the range of motion in flexion of both prosthetic components as a function of the cup abduction and

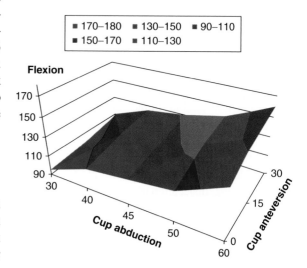

Fig. 2.16 Range of motion in flexion according to the cup abduction and opening angle for a given orientation of the Corail® stem (head: 28 mm, neck: 13 mm – femoral anteversion 15°)

opening angle for a given orientation of the Corail® stem. The Corail® stem is automatically positioned, without the ability to make any adjustment during its insertion into the femur (Fig. 2.16).

Conclusions

The use of a circular trapezoidal and mini-neck on the Corail® femoral stem (AMT neck), combined with a femoral head of maximum diameter and the selected bearing couple, greatly improves the functional outcome in terms of range of motion. Computer-assisted surgery should enhance cup positioning relative to the implanted Corail® stem.

Key Learning Points

> Impingement severely worsens the functional result (range of motion) and the long-term outcome of hip replacement.
> The AMT femoral neck of the Corail® stem, which combines a circular trapezoidal neck with a mini-neck, significantly increases joint mobility in flexion–extension.
> For a given bearing couple, the largest head diameter available should be chosen to delay the onset of impingement.
> Skirted implants and anti-dislocation rims should be avoided.
> Computer-assisted navigation remains the current research objective to ensure optimal orientation of the cup relative to a given implanted stem.

References

1. Adam P, Béguin L, Grosclaude S et al (2008) Functional range of motion of the hip joint. Rev Chir Orthop Reparatrice Appar Mot 94(4):382–391
2. Charnley J (1979) Low-friction arthroplasty of the hip. Theory and practice. Spinger, New York
3. Efthekar NS (1993) Total hip arthroplasty, 7th edn. Mosby, St. Louis
4. Herrlin K, Selvic G, Petterson H et al (1988) Position, orientation and component interaction in dislocation of the total hip prosthesis. Acta Radiol 29:441–444
5. Urquhart A, D'Lima D, Venn-Watson E et al (1998) Polyethylene wear after THA: the effect of a modular femoral head with an extended flange reinforced neck. J Bone Joint Surg Am 80:1641–1647

2.1.2.3 Collar and Collarless: Belt and Braces

Tarik Aït Si Selmi, Camdon Fary, and Guillaume Demey

When the Corail® femoral stem was designed 25 years ago there was debate among the designers about the benefits of a collared stem. Research since then has proven the benefits of a collared prosthesis. The authors believe that a collar adds extra protection by increasing the immediate stability of the construct. The collar acts as a 'safety belt'. However, it is not a substitute for incorrect technique or grossly incorrect sizing. Despite the benefits and routine use of a collar by the majority of the Corail® design team, it is not routinely used by the majority of other surgeons, perhaps because they just have not been exposed to it.

What Is a Collared Stem?

A collar on a femoral stem allows additional contact with the femoral calcar (Fig. 2.17). It is from this contact that the benefits provided by the collar occur. The collar size and contact area vary according to stem size. The collar length is from 6 to 9 mm and width is from 22 to 24 mm. The collar contact area varies from 78 to 105 mm^2.

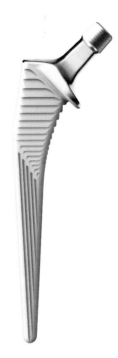

Fig. 2.17 Standard Corail® stem with collar (Copyright DePuyInternational Limited)

How Does Technique Change with the Use of a Collar?

Routine technique does not change when a collared stem is used. As described in Sect. 3.3.2, once the appropriate-sized broach has been impacted into the femur a calcar reamer is used over this broach. This gives the perfect calcar–collar contact required for a collar. This routine step is performed regardless of whether the stem is collared or collarless.

What Are the Benefits?

Improved Immediate Vertical Stability

Immediate stability forms the platform required for secondary ingrowth and bone integration. During this period the stem is at risk of subsidence both vertically and rotationally (Fig. 2.18). Secondary integration may occur in an unintended position. This can have a detrimental effect on the functional outcome. Collared stems are significantly more stable in the immediate postoperative period than collarless stems. They are able to withstand greater vertical force before they subside [1].

Improved Immediate Rotational Stability

The collar decreases the lever arm and so the moment of the torque is greater in the collared stem. The collar also impinges on the calcar, preventing rotation. Rotation of a collared prosthesis can only occur if it is withdrawn from the calcar or the calcar is fractured. The axial compression exerted upon the stem by the patient's body weight prevents the stem from withdrawing [1].

Preoperative Templating Equals Postoperative Stem Position

Templating the femur is based on using the calcar cut as the primary reference for stem placement, as described in Sect. 3.2. So if the appropriate calcar cut is replicated intra-operatively, the stem cannot be over or under impacted inadvertently (Fig. 2.19). Also, as the collar increases the immediate stability, secondary integration is more likely to occur in the intra-operatively obtained position. If the stem has undergone subsidence before secondary integration, there is the risk of leg-length inequality and impingement due to templating mismatch. If the stem has undergone a change in version before secondary integration, there is increased risk of dislocation.

Immediate Weight Bearing

Both collared and collarless stems are suitable for immediate full weight bearing. The collared stem is significantly more resistant to rotation prior to secondary integration in at-risk situations (e.g., stumbling, pathological bone or revision) than a collarless stem. It

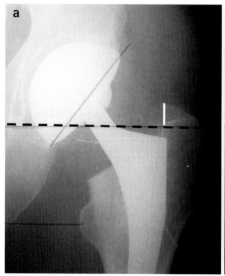
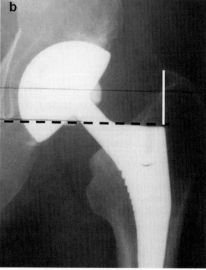

Fig. 2.18 Postoperative x-ray of collarless stem (**a**) and of same stem after 6 months implantation showing subsidence of the prosthesis within the femur (**b**)

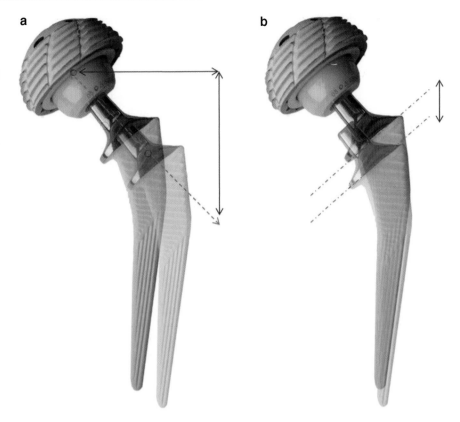

Fig. 2.19 The standard leg-length adjustment with the use of a longer neck option increases the overall offset (**a**). Length adjustment obtained by an accurate cut determined from templating will not affect the hip offset (**b**) (Copyright DePuyInternational Limited)

is not possible to rotate a collared stem in the femur without simultaneously distracting the stem, unless the cortical bone under the dorsal part of the collar is crushed or fractured. By using a collar we can utilise the vertical component of the forces to help prevent rotation prior to secondary fixation. For both collared and collarless stems vertical subsidence after stem insertion occurs at such a great force that any difference in force is clinically insignificant.

Increased Confidence with Complicated Patients

1. Neck of femur (NOF) fracture

This often occurs in osteoporotic bone in the elderly. Following NOF fracture the greater immediate stability of a collar adds a safety belt to secondary integration in the position it was implanted. In addition, were the patient to stumble, the risk of subsidence will be decreased. This is of particular importance in the immediate postoperative period.

2. Osteoporosis/Pathological bone

In these situations the benefits, as mentioned above, of greater immediate stability and the ability to withstand greater forces before both the initiation of subsidence and subsequent fracture enable the surgeon to treat the patient with greater confidence.

3. Dorr Type I femur

A collarless stem has increased distal fixation due to a narrow diaphysis and a relatively wide metaphysis. With a collared stem load sharing occurs between the collar–calcar contact and the diaphysis contact. This increases immediate stability and decreases the risk of sole distal fixation and possible thigh pain.

Decreased Risk of Femur Fracture

When the appropriate-sized broach has been inserted into the femur, as per the recommended surgical technique, a calcar reamer is used to obtain perfect calcar–collar contact. When the definitive femoral stem is inserted the collar indicates to the inexperienced surgeon when to stop, preventing stem over-impaction, which can result in fracture of the femur.

Intra-operative Calcar Fracture

Very occasionally, when broaching the femur to determine the correct stem size, a calcar fracture may occur. As this happens during the broaching stage the surgeon has the option to change to a collared stem (unless it is already their standard choice!). In our experience these fractures can be divided into two types depending on what happens when the broach is inserted. These types are stable or unstable. An unstable fracture requires a cerclage femoral wire prior to insertion of the definitive prosthesis. We pass the cerclage wire via a drilled tunnel through the lesser trochanter. The use of the tunnel creates greater stability by preventing distal migration of the wire and resulting in loss of tension.

Stress Transfer with Long Offset Stems

Recently the neck offset options have increased with the addition of varus and high offset stems to the existing range. Both designs come with a +7 mm offset as compared to the standard neck length. For such stems the varus stress is increased and there may be a risk of increased proximal micromotion or instability, especially when combined with a narrow femur and predominantly distal fixation (Dorr type I). The use of the collar may facilitate homogeneous stress transfer along the medial shaft (Fig. 2.20).

Revision

The above are also reasons for using a collared stem in revision. Often in revision the bone is of poor quality or is deficient. All methods that increase the immediate stability of a stem will improve successful secondary integration in the intended position. However, primary fixation must be achieved from the metaphysis and must not rely on the collar only!

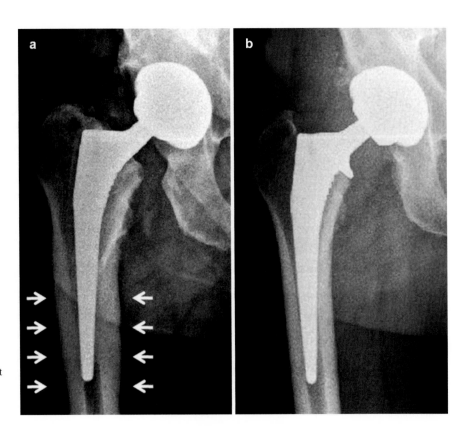

Fig. 2.20 (**a**) Fluted femur with distal fixation and 'window wiper' motion of the femoral prosthesis resulting in distal cortical hypertrophy, proximal lucency and pain (Collarless Corail® stem). (**b**) Similar situation demonstrating distal fixation and proximal calcar–collar contact without alteration of the bone (Collared varus Corail® stem)

In some revision cases there is insufficient calcar remaining for collar contact. In this situation a calcar graft may be used. It will make stem positioning and leg-length restoration easier. This graft after secondary integration may be absorbed or integrated depending on the circumstances (e.g., depending on the forces acting on the graft, see also Sect. 5.4).

Barrier

Coverage of the neck resection and 'sealing' of the medullar canal are facilitated by the collar. Theoretically there is decreased blood loss and debris migration from the shaft. These can be a cause of multiple complications such as haematoma collection or heterotropic ossification.

No Long-Term Disadvantages

In the long run there is no difference in survival rate with or without a collar. Similarly, the radiological results are the same with or without a collar. With a collar calcar resorption occurs frequently, but no more frequently than with collarless stems (see Sect. 4.2.5) (Fig. 2.21).

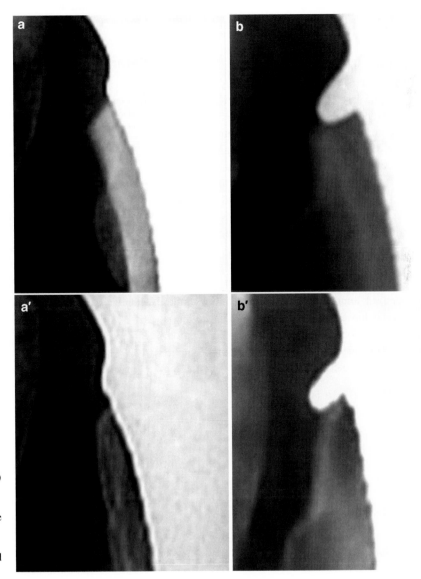

Fig. 2.21 Immediate postoperative appearance of the calcar with a collarless (**a**) and collared stem (**b**). Appearance of the calcar 10 years after implantation of the same stems. Calcar reshaping is very limited with both the collarless (**a′**) and the collared stems (**b′**)

Reasons Against Use of a Collar

No Long-Term Advantages

The use of a collar provides no long-term benefits once secondary integration has occurred. All the benefits are short term in providing improved primary stability, which is needed for successful secondary integration.

More Difficult Extraction

A well-fixed, uncemented stem is by definition difficult to remove. If routine extraction techniques as described in Sect. 5.2. are not suitable, due to poor-quality or deficient bone, a routine extended greater trochanteric osteotomy can be done, just as it is done when removing a well-cemented femoral prosthesis along with its cement.

With collarless stems there is a tendency to use bigger stems. The ease of extracting the stem can be predicted from preoperative x-rays by the amount of medullary space between the cortical bone and the stem. When a collar is used there is often a 2 mm medullary sleeve around the stem. In this situation extraction may be relatively easy, since there is sufficient room for flexible osteotomes to be inserted around the stem. Less than 2 mm space implies an overimpacted stem and results in more difficult extraction.

Risk of UnderSizing

An undersized femoral stem, despite using a collar, may become loose and may subside. The collar is not intended to be the principal means of fixation. Rather it is intended to be in addition to other means (double tapering, etc.). The importance of achieving

appropriate canal preparation and broach stability cannot be overemphasized. The calcar reamer is then used to determine the final stem position and to thereby avoid misplacement, either with the stem being proud or being overimpacted.

Conclusion

We use the collared version of the Corail® stem in our daily practice of total hip replacement and we believe that it provides useful short-term benefits. It makes the surgical technique easier, safer and more reproducible. We expect a progressive increase in the use of this option.

Reference

1. Demey G, Fary C, Lustig S, Neyret Ph, Aït Si Selmi T (2011) Does a collar improve the immediate stability of uncemented femoral hip stems in total hip arthroplasty? A bilateral comparative cadaver study", Accepted for publication in The Journal of Arthroplasty. Manuscript # 10-0205ER2. In Press

Further Reading

Berend ME, Smith A, Meding JB et al (2006) Long-term outcome and risk factors of proximal femoral fracture in uncemented and cemented total hip arthroplasty in 2551 hips. J Arthroplasty 21(6 Suppl 2):53

Froimson MI, Garino J, Machenaud A et al (2007) Minimum 10-year results of a tapered titanium, hydroxyapatite-coated hip stem: an independent review. J Arthroplasty 22(1):1

Gandhi R, Davey JR, Mahomed NN (2009) Hydroxyapatite coated femoral stems in primary total hip arthroplasty: a meta-analysis. J Arthroplasty 24(1):38

2.1.3 Bone–Implant Interface

2.1.3.1 Manufacturing Process: All White Powder Is Not HA

Carole Reignier and Valéry Barbour

During the last 25 years over 900,000 Corail® stems have been manufactured using the same manufacturing processes. These processes are forging and machining. They transform the raw material, titanium alloy, into a femoral stem of the required size and shape. These processes give the stem its final shape and its mechanical strength. Hydroxyapatite (HA) coating is then applied to the stem surface in the intramedullary region. This coating gives the stem its unique long-term fixation ability. The different manufacturing steps are described in this article.

Introduction

Over the past 25 years over 900,000 Corail® stems have been manufactured using the same manufacturing processes. These processes are forging and machining. They transform the raw material, titanium alloy, into a femoral stem of the required size and shape. HA coating is then applied onto the stem surface in the intramedullary region.

Manufacturing Process Selection

A number of material and process combinations have been used successfully in the manufacture of total hip replacements. Materials have to be biocompatible and approved by governmental agencies. There are several manufacturing strategies for producing total hip stems. The dimensions and complexity with regard to shape of the parts have a major bearing on the manufacturing process to be selected: flat parts with thin cross sections cannot be cast properly, whereas complex parts cannot be forged easily.

The Corail® stem has a trapezoidal cross section. In the frontal plane the stem has a lateral flare and a medial curve. In the lateral plane it has a progressive anterior to posterior tulip flare. These design features are such that forging could be selected as the best method for manufacturing the Corail® stem.

Moreover, the forging process can produce a part that is stronger than an equivalent cast or machined part. As the metal is shaped during the forging process, its internal grains deform to follow the general shape of the part. As a result, the grains are continuous, giving rise to a part with improved strength characteristics.

Forging technology occupies a very important place among the manufacturing processes of the Corail® stem and consists of the following steps:

1. Cutting the billet

The Corail® stem is manufactured from titanium alloy bars (Ti6Al4V). This bar is billeted to the desired length according to the size of the stem and the necessary amount of material to fill the forging die (Fig. 2.22).

2. Preforming

The billet is heated in an induction furnace to 920°C. The sample is then preformed to shape in two steps and is then air cooled (Figs. 2.23 and 2.24).

3. First forging step

The parts are heated on an induction furnace at 920°C. Then, the hot preform is forged by a press to the desired shape. These first stamp dies do not have the final shape of the stem and other forging steps are required before the final shape is reached (Fig. 2.25).

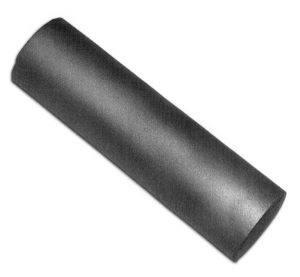

Fig. 2.22 Cutting billet to length (Copyright DePuy International Limited)

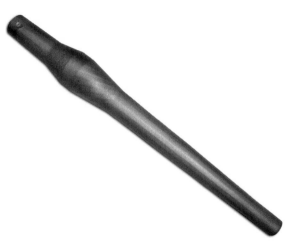

Fig. 2.23 Preforming – first step (Copyright DePuy International Limited)

4. Trimming

Once the parts have cooled down excess flash is removed using a trimming press. Grinding is also used to remove any remaining flash and surface defects (Fig. 2.26).

5. Second forging step

Stems are heated to 880°C. The hot parts are then forged using a forging press to produce the macrostructures on the anterior and posterior faces (Fig. 2.27).

6. Trimming

Excess flash produced during the second pressing is removed with this operation (Fig. 2.28).

The forging process does not produce the finished part and additional operations are necessary to reach

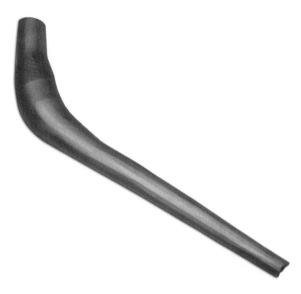

Fig. 2.24 Preforming – second step (Copyright DePuy International Limited)

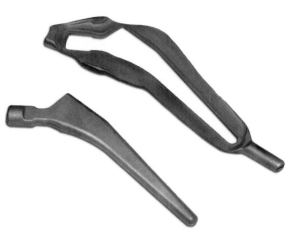

Fig. 2.26 First trimming (Copyright DePuy International Limited)

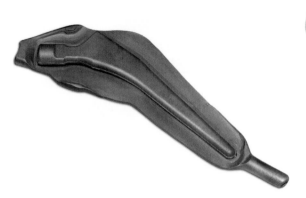

Fig. 2.25 First stamp (Copyright DePuy International Limited)

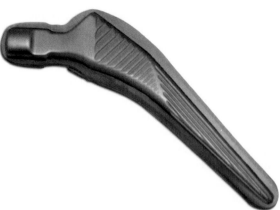

Fig. 2.27 Second stamp (Copyright DePuy International Limited)

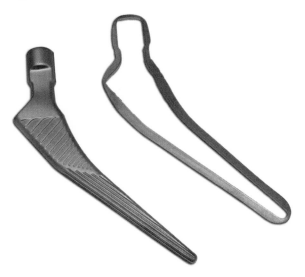

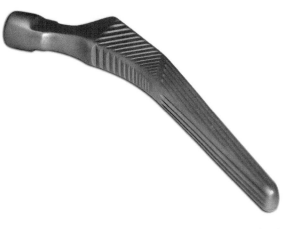

Fig. 2.29 Grooves machining (Copyright DePuyInternational Limited)

Fig. 2.28 Second trimming (Copyright DePuyInternational Limited)

the desired dimensions and surface finish. The Corail® has horizontal grooves around the circumference of the stem and vertical grooves on the distal faces. The neck is polished and a 12/14 Articul/eze® Mini Taper is machined at its end. In order to facilitate stem insertion and extraction, the stem has a threaded hole compatible with inserters.

As a result, the following operations are necessary to finalise the part:

7. Machining the grooves

Grooves are manufactured using a computer numerical control (CNC) machine, while deflashing is also performed on the neck area. After this step the shape of the stem in the intramedullary region is completed. It will become the substrate for the HA coating (Fig. 2.29).

8. Machining and polishing

The taper is machined into the proximal end of the neck and the tolerances are tight, so that the taper can be combined properly with the femoral head. The threaded hole is also machined at this stage to be compatible with the stem inserters. The neck is then polished in order to obtain a smooth surface finish and to improve fatigue strength (Fig. 2.30).

Before the stem can be implanted additional processes are performed such as coating, cleaning, packaging and sterilization.

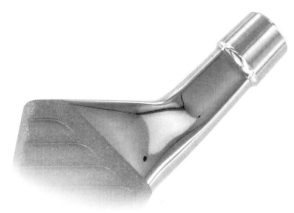

Fig. 2.30 Taper machining and neck machining and polishing (Copyright DePuyInternational Limited)

What Is a Hydroxyapatite Coating

HA is a biocompatible and bioactive material with a chemical and crystalline composition similar to that of the mineral part of bone. It has strong osteoconductive properties. It promotes bone ongrowth through the multiplication of osteoblast cells and the generation of new bone in contact with the coating. HA also prevents the formation of a fibrous membrane at the stem surface. It is composed of calcium and phosphate ions which are used by the bone to remodel. Its chemical formula is $Ca_{10}(PO_4)_6(OH)_2$.

HA coatings have been used for orthodontic implants since the mid-1980s and in 1986 the Corail® HA coating for total hip arthroplasty (THA) was introduced.

How Is Corail® Hydroxyapatite Coating Produced?

The Corail® HA coating is applied onto the surface of the implant by plasma spraying. During this process the HA powder is introduced into a plasma jet, produced by a plasma torch, as illustrated in Fig. 2.31. It is the difference of applied voltage between the cathode and the anode of the torch which creates the plasma jet. The HA powder fed into this plasma jet is melted and propelled onto the implant. There are a large number of parameters controlling the process such as powder size, plasma gas composition and flow rate, energy input, torch offset distance and substrate cooling. Throughout the process the stem is cooled by cold air jets.

The plasma gas causes the HA powder particles to become partially molten and to accelerate. Upon impact on the substrate the powder particles produce pancake-like lamellae. The thickness of a lamella is in the micrometre range and the lateral dimension of a lamella is in the hundreds of micrometre range. The core of a lamella is crystalline HA and the outer shell is a mixture of amorphous HA with traces of other calcium phosphates (tricalcium phosphate, tetracalcium phosphate, calcium oxide) as described in Fig. 2.32.

The coating consists of a multitude of lamellae stacked together resulting from several HA powder particles impacting into each other. The amorphous shell around each of the lamellae acts as glue and bonds the

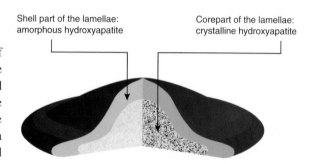

Shell part of the lamellae: amorphous hydroxyapatite

Corepart of the lamellae: crystalline hydroxyapatite

Fig. 2.32 Typical structure of flattened HA lamellae after impact on the implant (Copyright DePuyInternational Limited)

lamellae together. Figure 2.33 shows the microstructure of a typical HA coating. The small voids or pores can be seen (Fig. 2.33).

Prior to coating, the implant is prepared. The neck that is not to be coated is protected and the surface that is to be coated is roughened. This surface preparation, grit blasting, modifies the texture of the surface in order to create mechanical anchorage sites for the HA lamellae. It creates peaks and valleys, where upon impact the partially molten HA particles will lock onto the surface. This surface preparation is a key process, since it enhances the adhesion of the coating. It consists of making the surface of the implant rough by spraying the implant surfaces with hard, ceramic particles of alumina. The parameters controlling this process are the size of the ceramic particles, the pressure, the spraying duration and the spraying distance.

Hydroxyapatite Characteristics

The action of HA coating is to promote good osteointegration [6], which means uniform ongrowth of bone onto the implant surface without the formation of a fibrous membrane. The factors that influence the performance of the HA coating include its compositional and its physical and mechanical properties. Critical quality specifications for HA coatings include the purity (phase composition), crystallinity, Ca/P ratio, microstructure, porosity and thickness of the coating, the composition of the implant alloy and its surface roughness and the coating adhesion and cohesion [6].

1. Crystallinity/crystalline phase composition

The proportion of crystalline to amorphous phase in the coating influences the process of bone remodelling

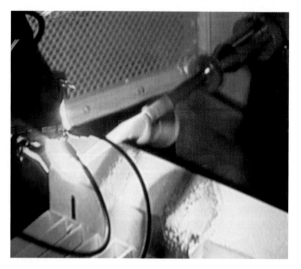

Fig. 2.31 Picture of the plasma torch used to apply the HA Coating onto the Corail® implant

Fig. 2.33 Typical micro-structure of an HA coating cross section and a picture of the HA coated surface (Copyright DePuyInternational Limited)

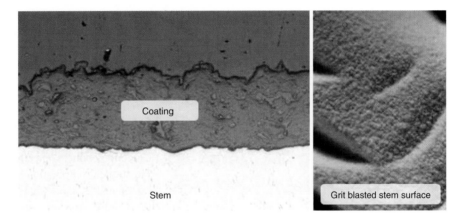

around the stem. The amorphous phase of the coating partially dissolves and promotes early bone ongrowth [1, 4]. This dissolution produces a supersaturated environment, which allows physiologically produced HA to precipitate onto the coating enhancing bone ongrowth. Bone grows towards the implant and collagen incorporates the HA crystals in the body, thereby producing a strong interface. The dissolution rate of the amorphous phase and of the other crystalline phases formed during the spraying are much higher than the dissolution rate of the HA phase [3, 5]. The Corail® coating crystallinity and phase composition have been tailored to promote early osteointegration and the coating thickness has been tailored to provide long-term effectiveness.

2. Coating thickness

The Corail® coating thickness of 155 µm is sufficient even though the coating partially dissolves over time. The coating needs to be thick enough to enhance the bone remodelling process over a long period of time. Clinical results have shown that HA coating dissolution takes place mainly in the metaphyseal region of the stem. Thanks to its thickness, the coating remains in place on the Corail® stem even after nearly 2 years of implantation [2]. The 25 years experience of Corail® has confirmed the design rationale of the coating.

3. Adhesion

Corail® coatings have been tailored for good cohesion due to the combination of crystalline and amorphous phases. As described earlier, the HA particles partially melt during the plasma process. It is the amorphous phase around the crystalline core of these particles that provides the high cohesive strength. The coatings adhesion to the stem is produced by the mechanical interlocking of the HA lamellae that cool rapidly upon impact and then shrink on the projections in the grit-blasted surface of the implant. As already stated, grit blasting is a key process in the adhesion of the coating.

The mechanical interlocking of the implant with the bone is also promoted by the Corail® grooves, which increase the contact area between the coated surface and the bone.

4. Purity

It is important that the coating is biocompatible and does not contain impurities that could compromise the safety of the implant. The Corail® coating is ISO 13779-2 (Implants for surgery – Hydroxyapatite – Coatings of hydroxyapatite) compliant in terms of its heavy metals content.

5. Porosity/density

Coating porosity has a harmful effect on the cohesion and mechanical properties of the coating. Therefore the Corail® coating is dense and has a porosity level below 10%. Admittedly, there are some small pores, but these are well distributed within the coating and do not have an adverse effect on the coating cohesion.

Conclusion

Twenty-five years ago the HA coating process was very innovative and even today it still meets modern requirements. The plasma spray process is still the most widely used industrial process to coat stems with HA. Experience has shown that the forging process was well suited to the production of Corail® stems, even though they have a complex shape, and enhances the mechanical properties of the stem. The chosen manufacturing processes have contributed to the clinical success of the Corail®.

References

1. De Bruijn JD, Bovell YP, van Blitterswijk CA (1994) Structural arrangements at the interface between plasma sprayed calcium phosphates and bone. Biomaterials 15:543–550
2. Frayssinet P, Hardy D, Hanker JS et al (1995) Natural history of bone response to HA coated prostheses implanted in humans. Cells Mater 5(2):125–138
3. LeGeros RZ (1993) Biodegradation and bioresorption of calcium phosphate ceramics. Clin Mater 14:65–68
4. Maxian SH, Zawadsky JP, Dunn MG (1993) Mechanical and histological evaluation of amorphous calcium phosphate and poorly crystallized hydroxyapatite coatings on titanium implants. J Biomed Mater Res 27:17–28
5. Radin SR, Ducheyne P (1992) Plasma spraying induced changes of calcium phosphate ceramic characteristics and the effect on in vitro stability. J Mater Sci Mater Med 3:33–42
6. Sun L, Berndt CC, Gross KA et al (2001) Material fundamentals and clinical performance of plasma-sprayed hydroxyapatite coatings: a review. J Biomed Mater Res 58(5):570–592

2.1.3.2   The Cancellous Bone Environment: A Privileged Partner

Jean-Christophe Chatelet

The design rationale for the Corail® stem is based on the fixation of the hydroxyapatite (HA)-coated stem in cancellous bone. Cancellous bone compaction during the surgical preparation of the proximal metaphyseal femur makes it possible to seat, stabilize and anchor the Corail® stem in a cancellous bone bed. Primary stability is provided by the cancellous bone sleeve and this is sufficient to achieve secondary osseointegration. This fixation, achieved over the whole stem surface is enhanced by the HA coating and evolves with time owing to the various forces and stresses imparted to the bone by the stem. These forces and stress cause stress-induced remodelling, which enables the fixation to adapt as the bone ages and the patient's activity level changes.

There are more than 500 models of total hip prostheses available today on the world market. All these models, albeit different in design, have similar shapes, materials or coatings. However, minor modifications made to an implant can potentially cause big changes in the long-term behaviour of that implant. There have been only rare new and decisive innovations in total hip arthroplasty (THA) in the last two decades. New models replace old ones as fashion evolves and according to economic constraints.

Twenty-five years ago, the Corail® stem started a new era because of its HA coating and its tapered shape, but mainly because of the unique biological fixation which uses cancellous bone to provide biomechanical support. The concept of cancellous bone compaction is the basis of this relationship, which for the last 25 years has enabled bone and prosthesis to achieve a successful union between inert and living materials.

The Implant Environment: The Cancellous Bone

The proximal metaphyseal end of the femur consists of compact cortical bone and trabecular cancellous bone. The compact cortical bone forms the hard, dense, external shell. The Haversian canals (feeders) are surrounded by concentric lamellae called osteons. These lamellae are composed of collagen fibres in which mineral crystals deposit. The assembly constitutes a compact and stiff structure. The cancellous or trabecular bone comprises the osteons with unfolded lamellar structures, which when assembled, form the bone trabeculae. At the microstructure level, this composite material is made of water, an organic phase (collagen fibres) and a mineral phase (crystals of calcium and natural hydroxyapatite). At the cellular level, there are three types of cells: the *osteoblasts*, which are mononuclear cells, and are located at the surface of the bone trabeculae. They produce the lattice that contributes to bone formation and calcification. The *osteoclasts* are polynuclear cells, which move along the surface of the bone trabeculae and control bone resorption, bone remodelling and the maintenance and repair of the bone. The *osteocytes* are differentiated osteoblasts embedded in the bone material. They are connected to the osteoblasts by means of fine tissue extensions. These are mechanical receptors (mechano-sensitive cells), which are sensitive to pressure variations. They manage the resorption and new bone apposition activity.

Architecture of the Cancellous Bone Tissue

The trabeculae, or lamella bone, form bony sheets which are oriented so as to exhibit the highest possible tensile strength. They bear on the compact bone to which they transmit forces. These trabeculae exhibit resistance to bending, tensile, compression and shearing stresses. In 1866 Culmann demonstrated that the architecture of the proximal end of the femur corresponds to the tensile lines in the femur [1]. In 1892 Wolff showed that any modification of the function or shape of a bone leads to modifications of its internal structure [5]. The bone is sensitive to static pressures generated by the weight of the body, but also to tensile stresses generated by muscle contractions. Hence the bone adapts itself to the mechanical stresses to which it is subjected. The osteocytes therefore act as internal sensors able to measure the forces and to translate this data into signals that will activate bone reconstruction (Fig. 2.34).

Bone Remodelling

Bone is under constant turnover and remodelling. The osteocytes regulate the activity of the osteoclasts and osteoblasts. Our bone mass increases until the age of 20; it then stabilizes and starts diminishing after the age of 40. With age, the destruction mechanisms outdo the construction mechanisms. This process is called osteoporosis. Bone remodelling is also subject to hormonal regulation and to mechanical regulation. The osteoblasts create bone at locations where the forces are greatest and the osteoclasts resorb the bone where there is no mechanical need. This mechanism also occurs in the natural state in the formation and evolution of micro-fracture healing, but it also occurs when bone is subject to the stresses generated by an intramedullary implant such as a femoral stem.

Corail® and Cancellous Bone

The implantation of the Corail® prosthesis completely modifies the distribution of the mechanical stresses in the proximal femur. The host bone reacts to the stresses generated by the metallic implant inside its

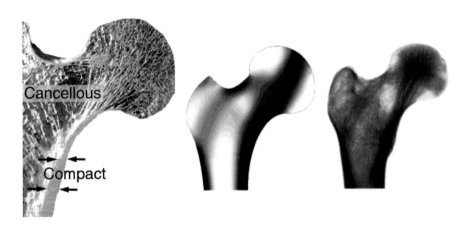

Fig. 2.34 Transmission of stresses from cancellous bone to cortical bone

medullary cavity. In the natural femur, the stresses applied to the cortical walls decrease from the proximal part to the distal part. Following the insertion of an implant, this decreasing stress gradient must be maintained. It is achieved by the shape of the Corail® stem which changes from a proximal quadrangular cross section to a distal conical section with a stiffness gradient which is gradually decreasing (Fig. 2.35). The bone will integrate with the prosthesis wherever it is in contact with the HA-coated stem and stress is applied. This fixation will depend on the shape, the design, the coating, the materials, the size of the implant and the mechanical stresses. In this equilibrium three phases will take place over the 25 years.

Phase 1: Implantation of the Corail®
Stem – Primary Stability

The bed of compacted bone prevents any direct contact between the implant and the cortical walls. Primary stability must be achieved in a *bed of cancellous bone*,

and not by means of localized cortical contact. The Corail® broaches inserted into the femoral canal break the lamellar structures of the cancellous bone and form a compacted, lamellar bone sleeve around the stem (when it is implanted). This sleeve covers the cortical bone and acts as a "biological cement" (Fig. 2.36).

At this stage of primary mechanical stability, the interface is subjected to two types of stresses: shear compression (parallel with the interface) and radial compression (perpendicular to the interface). Mechanical studies have shown that the maximum sliding is higher at the cortical contact than at the cancellous points of contact [3, 4]. The mechanical strength of the bone sleeve will depend on its volume and hence on the pre- and perioperative condition of the compacted cancellous tissue. A young patient will have very dense cancellous bone, whereas an elderly patient will suffer from bone loss due to the depletion of the bony lamellae.

Regardless of the condition of the cancellous bone – dense or osteoporotic – there will always be enough cells and collagen to activate secondary osseointegration.

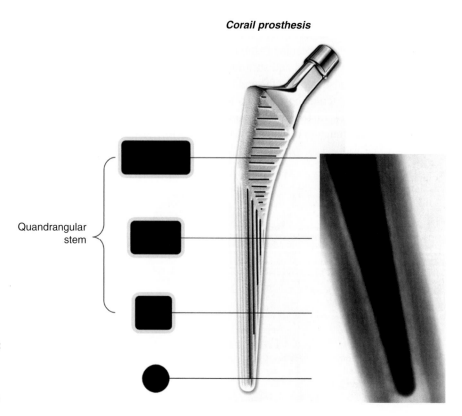

Corail prosthesis

Quandrangular stem

Fig. 2.35 Corail® prosthesis: quadrangular section with degressive stiffness gradient (Copyright DePuyInternational Limited)

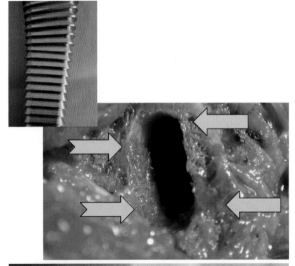

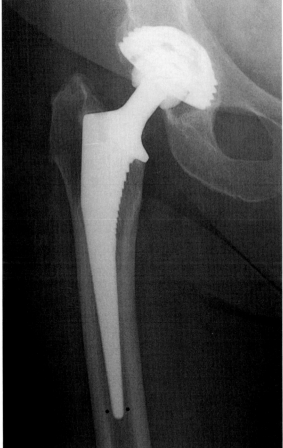

Fig. 2.36 Cancellous bone sleeve around the Corail® stem

Phase 2: Secondary Osseointegration

The HA coating of the Corail® stem encourages direct osseointegration and reduces the formation of a layer of fibrous tissue between the bone and the implant. Resorption of the HA gradually generates new bone in direct contact with the metallic surface of the implant. This phase has been studied in depth by Hardy [2], who performed histological studies on HA-coated implants and bone. Rapidly and during 6 weeks, a repair and mineralization process evolves as a fracture would owing to the local environment of the surgical hematoma and fractured cancellous bone. Just as in a fracture, the repair process is promoted by immobilisation of the bone fragments (e.g., using a plaster cast or by means of internal fixation). Hence, this second osseointegration phase, in contact with the HA, is promoted by the primary stability of the stem in the impacted cancellous bone sleeve. This osseointegration will take place along and around the whole Corail® stem, if the compaction sleeve fully covers the stem. The macrostructures of the stem surface increase the contact surface by 25% as compared with the surface area of an equivalent smooth stem. This simple healing and consolidation process is made possible by the absence of fibrous tissues in contact with the implant.

Phase 3: Stress-Induced Bone Remodelling

The first signs of remodelling appear 6–8 months postoperative. Remodelling continues for 1 or 2 years, and then stabilizes, but with the Corail® stem it has the potential to develop further over the next 25 years.

The initial bone sleeve changes as a function of the stresses imparted to the bone. Hence, all the images of bony bridges can be explained by the loading and stresses generated by the Corail® stem. The evolution of this process is influenced by numerous individual parameters and unlike the previous phase it is not uniform.

1. It depends on the mechanical stresses governed by Wolff's laws. There are four types of stress: compression, torsion, traction (tensile) and shear. Note that the patient's body weight is not the sole force responsible for mechanical stresses. Muscles and the tendons also produce forces such as the tensile force produced by the gluteal muscles at the greater trochanter.
2. It depends on the shape of the stem. Certain stems are designed to achieve a purely diaphyseal fixation. The compression loads are then transmitted

directly from the prosthesis to the diaphysis. They bypass the metaphysis and thereby create the risk of proximal osteoporosis (and thigh pain induced by stress-shielding).

Other stems are designed for a purely metaphyseal fixation. In this case the loss of diaphyseal fixation may lead to distal instability and poor osseointegration. The design of the Corail® stem with its decreasing stiffness gradient prevents stress peaks and stress-shielding, but increases stresses at the corners of the quadrangular prosthesis and in the grooves of the macrostructures. The fixation is elastic and soft and it allows the bone to grow again wherever bone growth is needed as a function of the applied loads. The development of bony bridges therefore corresponds to the new stress transfer pattern.

3. It depends on the shape of the femur. The modulus of elasticity of titanium is close to that of cortical bone, which is higher than that of cancellous bone. The stiffness of the femur is determined by the diameter of the diaphysis and the thickness of the cortical walls. There is a difference between the champagne flute femur and the cylindrical (stove pipe) femur, just as there is a difference between the femur of a young patient with thick cortical walls and narrow canal and the femur of an elderly osteoporotic patient with thin cortical walls and a large empty medullary canal. Cancellous bone compaction helps avoid high peak stresses due to localized cortical contact. In stove pipe femurs, the cancellous sleeve, although thin, means that there is no need to fill the intramedullary space with a large metallic mass in direct contact with the cortical walls. In champagne flute femurs, distal diaphyseal reaming makes it possible to transfer load proximally, thereby compressing the metaphyseal cancellous bone without the need for distal locking.

4. It depends on the stress transfer zone. X-ray images are different between the proximal and distal femur, between zone I or zone VII, where tensile or compression loads are applied

5. It depends on the quality of the secondary fixation and of the surface condition. Bone is in a state of constant renewal and the fixation develops as a function of the increase or decrease in the patient's activity level and as a function of the aging of the femoral bone that supports the Corail® stem.

Conclusion

The relationship between cancellous bone and a Corail® stem is a long cohabitation, as it may be for any couple! The first encounter (impaction of the cancellous bone) and the first many months (osseointegration) are a beautiful time. During this period the linkage between the bone and the Corail® stem takes place in a uniform and standardized way. The following years are more tumultuous (bone remodelling) determined by the influences of several external factors and agents. The relationship is different and specific for each prosthesis femur couple. Yet we can state today that in most cases it can last more than 25 years.

Key Points

> The design rationale for the Corail® stem is based on the fixation of the stem in cancellous bone.

> The compaction of the cancellous bone – a surgical technique specific to the Corail® – enables the implant to be stabilized and then fully fixed within a bed of cancellous bone. This bed of cancellous bone prevents, as much as possible, contact between the implant and the cortical walls.

> The only explanation for the excellent long-term survival and the radiological silence observed on x-rays with more than 25 years of follow-up is the gradual transfer of loads from the prosthesis to the bone. This transfer is designed to eliminate unwanted stress peaks and to protect the bone from damage, which would otherwise be caused by the implant.

References

1. Culmann C (1880) Die graphische static,Zurich,Meyer und Zeller 1866 (traduction francaise traité de statique graphique). Dunod, Paris
2. Hardy D, Frayssinet P et al (1995) Natural history of bone response to hydroxyapatite coated hip prostheses implanted in human. Cells Mater 5:2
3. Rubin PJ, Rakotomanana RL, Leyvraz et al (1993) Frictional interface micromotions and anisotropic stress distribution in a femoral total hip component. J Biomech 26(6):725–739

4. Terrier A, Rakotomanana RL, Ramanikara N et al (1997)
    Adaptation models of anisotropic bone. Comput Methods
    Biomech Biomed Engin 1:47–59
5. Wolff J (1986) The law of bone remodelling (translation of
    the German 1892 edition). Springer, Berlin/Heideleberg/
    New York

2.1.3.3 Natural History of Osteointegration: Looking Through the Microscope

Dominique C.R.J. Hardy

A unique series of 47 human femora previously implanted with a Corail® stem as a treatment for displaced femoral neck fracture has been obtained during autopsies. This material allows the whole – and successful – history of the osteointegration process from the early period (5 days postoperative) until late follow-up (10 years postoperative) to be retraced. This history includes (1) the genesis of osteointegration, (2) the remodelling period, and (3) the resorption phase of the coating, with subsequent modifications of the stem attachment. Fixation of the implant occurs in every patient, whatever the age, the sex or the filling of the femoral cavity. Remodelling is predominant after 6 months of implantation and completely transforms the bone implant interface according to Wolff's laws. Resorption is always encountered after 1 year of implantation, and does not affect the fixation, as no signs of micromotion, fibrous development or cortical hypertrophy are seen. Even where there is osteoporotic bone loss, the hydroxyapatite (HA) coating is effective in obtaining stable implantation, without any relevant adverse reactions.

Introduction: A Few Properties of Hydroxyapatite

The first use of calcium Hydroxyapatite dates back to 1981, when it was used as particulates to fill periodontal lesions [2]. Around the same period, solid HA was used to fill bony deficits [23]. These first uses demonstrated two of the main properties of HA: (a) its excellent biocompatibility (there is a total absence of local or systemic toxicity and of inflammatory or pyrogenic responses) and (b) its osteoconductive potential.

The biocompatibility of HA in bony sites when the implantation is mechanically stable has been confirmed by numerous teams. Among the numerous experimental articles on the subject, we should mention Hoogendorn et al. [20], who showed the absence of inflammatory signs around HA blocks implanted in a dog's femur with a 3.5-year follow-up. Gumaer et al. [15] came to a similar conclusion following more than 8 years of observation of HA granules implanted in a dog's femur. Klein et al. [21] implanted cylinders of porous calcium phosphate in the shin bones of rabbits and, after periods ranging from 3 weeks to 9 months, they demonstrated that all specimens were biocompatible and induced no inflammatory reactions.

According to Furukawa et al. [13], even when HA particles migrate in soft peri-prosthetic tissues, they do not cause any inflammatory response. Anderson et al. [1] demonstrated the same absence of inflammatory reactions even when the intra-osseous implantation fails mechanically.

This excellent biocompatibility takes its origin from the basic chemical nature of HA, which is composed solely of calcium and phosphates. De Groot's works [8,9] demonstrated that the dissolution of HA causes no pathological increase of the blood level and urine rate in the calcium and phosphorus concentration. The mechanisms that ensure the homeostasis of these ions are sufficient not to be overtaken by the excess of ions released during the dissolving of the ceramics.

Osteoconduction is defined as the ability of the HA implanted into a bone site to guide the osteogenesis on its surface, as opposed to *osteoinduction*, which is the ability to induce the osteogenesis directly regardless of the environment in which the implantation is made. Osteoconduction implies the presence of the whole biological mechanism (cells, substrates, various stimuli) leading to osteogenesis [27].

Several founding works, including those by de Bruijn [7], have taught us that the osteoconduction mechanism involves at least five steps:

1. Partial dissolving of the coating, mainly in its amorphous phase.
2. Creation of a solution supersaturated in calcium and phosphates in the immediate vicinity of the implant.
3. Formation of carbonated apatite microcrystals in that zone.
4. Association of these microcrystals with an organic matrix and deposit on the implant surface. This deposit, which appears dense in the electron microscope after decalcification, morphologically translates into something similar to a *lamina limitans* [22].
5. Immobilization of precursor cells on this assembly. They undergo a pre-osteoblast differentiation and initiate the process.

Under load HA exhibits poor mechanical properties in a solid or particulate form. Hence, it was decided to deposit HA on a metallic substrate as a coating. The same works as those carried out on pure HA implants have been carried out on metallic implants of different nature, with or without HA coating. The method of transfemoral pegs, used by Geesink et al. [14], has confirmed radiologically and histologically that osteointegration occurred after 6 weeks for coated implants, whereas it took more than 12 weeks for non-coated implants. The difference is not only in the timing. It is also in the volume of interfacial bone observed around the pegs, with a greater volume occurring around the coated pegs. The "push-out test" method has made it possible to quantify the pull-out strength of the pegs. Cook and his collaborators [6] were thus able to demonstrate – after 32 weeks of residence time – that the HA-coated pegs exhibited a pull-out strength of around 6–7 megapascals (MPa), whereas that of the non-coated pegs was only 1 MPa. Thomas et al. in 1989 [25] implanted hip prostheses, both HA-coated and uncoated, in dogs that were retrieved after 52 weeks. This experiment was possibly less meaningful since it concerned implantation in cancellous bone and in the cortico-diaphyseal zone (the results were difficult to interpret as the measures of skeletal attachment were derived both from intracancellous fixation and cortical fixation), yet it was still interesting for surgeons since pull-out tests were done on the prostheses. Moreover, the tests showed that the osteointegration process was slightly better and faster with the coated implants, which exhibited pull-out strength values seven times higher than for the uncoated implants. Histologically, it was also possible to demonstrate that the fracture produced during the retrieval of the peg took place at the bone–implant junction for non-coated implants, whereas it took place within the HA coating for the coated implants. This enabled a third fundamental property of HA to be discovered, i.e. the nature of the bone–HA junction.

One of the bonds that forms between bone and HA is covalent in nature. This bond forms between the hydroxyl group of the hydroxyapatite and the hydrogen radicals of the collagen molecules [5]. This bond is extremely strong and explains why all types of loads, including tensile, can be transmitted from the bone to the HA and vice versa. This enables the bone tissue to maintain its trophicity over time through mechanical stimulation.

These various properties explain the exceptional success of HA-coated implants. The Corail® stem was one of the very first implants to use this technology. In order to understand the mechanism of action of HA in the human body and to elaborate on the story of osteointegration, a study of human explants was undertaken as early as 1988 and published regularly [16–18]. This unique material serves as a basis for this chapter.

Explants

In our orthopaedics department, all patients over 65 with a displaced fracture of the femoral neck – Garden type III or IV – received a hip arthroplasty. Starting in 1988, we used the Corail® stem, which was initially reserved for patients who exhibited normal femoral morphology. Patients with bone mineralization that seemed deficient and those in whom stable implantation of the prosthesis seemed impossible due to a cylindrical femoral medullary cavity were excluded. Then, the indications were extended to all patients, regardless of their age, gender, mineralization rate or femoral morphotype. All received a Corail® femoral stem (DePuy) fitted with a bipolar head (BHP™, Zimmer, Warsaw, Indiana, USA).

The femurs of 47 of these patients were harvested during systematic autopsy. The autopsy included the whole femur and the acetabulum, which was separated from the pelvis by three saw cuts (pubis, ilium and ischium). Informed consent had been obtained antemortem from the patients or from their family or doctor. The excised femur was replaced with a telescopic rod. Each time the specimen was photographed, x-rayed and fixed in Karnovsky liquid (4% formaldehyde solution in phosphate buffer) for at least 7 days.

The 47 specimens were distributed as shown in Table 2.4. The explants thus obtained had been implanted for a period ranging from 5 days to 123 months.

Histological Processing

Following fixation, the specimens were pre-cut and then refixed in Karnovsky liquid. Then, the specimens were washed in water, in toluene and dehydrated in solutions with increasing ethanol concentration, before being placed in methylmethacrylate. Fine slides (2 mm), without preliminary decalcification, were thus produced using a low-speed cooled diamond saw. The slides were then reinserted in vinyl and were polished for examination under an optical reflection microscope. Other slides were surface-coloured with a Fucsine-Toluidine solution or with Cole Hematoxyline and 1% Eosine, after they were etched for 2 min in 2% formic acid solution and 2 h in a 20% methanol solution, and examined under a transmission light microscope (Reichert, Polyvar). Other colours were also used to carry out specific investigations under a transmission light microscope. Slides were also examined under polarized light for the detection of polyethylene (PE) particles. Some slides were coloured using silver methanamine deposits at 1% (pH 9.6) for 1 min at 2,450 MHz in a 100 W microwave oven. The colouring solution was then reduced with a thiocarbohydrazide (TCH; Sigma-Aldrich, St-Louis, MO, USA) solution for 5 min for examination under an optical microscope. These slides, after application of a carbon coating, were also studied in an electron microscope in backscattering mode, operating at an accelerating voltage of 25 kV. Energy-dispersive x-ray (EDAX) microanalysis was also performed on some slides using an EDAX-5000 (Philips, Mahwah, NJ) system equipped with an Auger element detector [10].

Some of the slides were processed for microradiography before colouring, in order to better determine the bony nature of the HA–bone interface.

Table 2.4 Length of implantation, number of retrievals, sex ratio, clinical details and ambulatory/non-ambulatory ratio for the 47 human explants

Year	1	2	3	4	5	6	7	8	9	10	total
Number	15	7	4	5	3	4	2	4	2	1	47
M/F ratio	12/3	6/1	4/0	3/2	3/0	3/1	1/1	4/0	2/0	1/0	39/8
Relevant details	1 sepsis	1 (non union of an intertrochanteric fracture)			1 (non union of a basal fracture)						
Ambulant/non ambulant ratio	9/6	4/3	2/2	4/1	2/1	2/2	1/1	4/0	2/0	1/0	31/16

Specimens that had a follow-up of at least 3 years were also treated in histomorphometry, using image analysis (AES software, AES-Image, Toulouse, France). Using this technique it was possible to measure the thickness of the residual coating, together with the exact length of the perimeter of the prosthesis and the portion of that perimeter in contact with the bony tissue. The bone affinity index (BAI) was then calculated.

$$\text{B.A.I.}\left(\text{Bone Affinity Index}\right) =$$

$$\frac{\text{Length of the interface implant } - \text{ bony tissue}}{\text{Length of the prosthetic perimeter}}$$

The thickness of the HA coating was measured on the same slides every 500 μm.

The PE inserts were sampled 16 times. Extraction of the PE inserts was performed using a rongeur to ensure that the inserts would not be touched by fingers. The inserts were then treated with NaOH at 10% for 20 days, in order to eliminate any organic material. Then their surface was examined using a scanning electron microscope, selecting the zones which seemed to be macroscopically unpolished.

Among the specimens which, when using standard x-rays, exhibited ectopic ossifications within the capsular or muscular tissues, samples were taken and examined without preliminary decalcification after Von Kossa colouring to identify the nature of the ossifying incrustations and to find possible HA particles.

Macroscopic Observations

At the macroscopic level, all specimens were identical. There was no inflammatory granuloma, no sign of metallosis and no palpable lymph nodes in the lymphatic drainage zones adhering to the anterior capsule or to the psoas tendon (Fig. 2.37).

The joint cavities were opened in the autopsy room for inspection. Each of the cavities contained a small amount of synovial fluid, albeit never an excessive quantity. Twice the liquid sampled for biochemical analysis was found to have a physiological composition without specific anomaly.

During the pre-cutting step, some of the implants were found to be poorly fixed, especially if there was massive fat involution of the bone marrow. In these cases, several secondary fixation processes were necessary in order to be able to proceed with the subsequent steps.

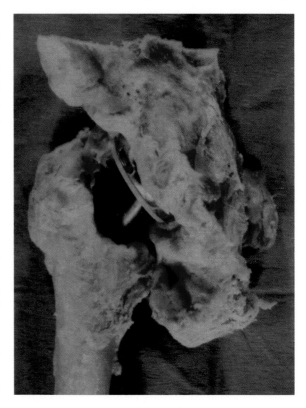

Fig. 2.37 Macroscopic view of a specimen, including the femur and the acetabular bone. Joint cavity has been opened for inspection

Microscopic Observations

Osteointegration

All the explants harvested showed various levels of obvious osteointegration coherent with their residence time.

1. In the immediate postoperative days the periprosthetic interface showed the presence of endomedullary bony trabeculae compacted around the implant as a consequence of the broaching process. These bone trabeculae ensure the primary mechanical stabilization of the implant (Fig. 2.38).
2. In the postoperative months, the organic material synthesizes at the HA surface, to form a material known as the osteoid matrix. This is a proteic material, directly synthesized by osteoprogenitor cells. This osteoid matrix exhibits a high affinity for the collagen-specific histological colourings, and is found over the whole HA surface. The importance of this osteoid neoformation varies from one specimen

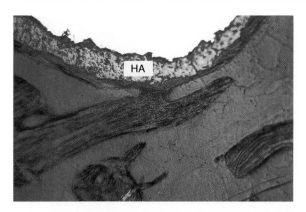

Fig. 2.38 Bone–HA interface. A sleeve of bone covers the coating and is connected to peri-prosthetic trabeculae (Specimen 24. Implantation time: 13 months. Reflected light microscopy. Bar = 150 μm)

to another and it was not possible to identify a single factor which could account for this difference. Age, gender, bone–implant proximity or the location on the implant did not appear to be able to modify the synthesis of the osteoid matrix.

3. Simultaneously, within the peri-prosthetic space, bony neoformation islands appear, composed of an ovoid assembly of osteoblastic morphology cells, surrounded by a deposit of osteoid matrix (Fig. 2.39). This reaction is morphologically comparable to that observed after medullary reaming and injury of the endomedullary cancellous bone, whether or not implantation is performed. There is also a superficial bony neoformation of compacted trabeculae, which is formed by the surgical preparation of the medullary

cavity before the stem is implanted. This illustrates the second reason that justifies the compaction of the endomedullary cancellous bone, i.e. the contribution of primary mechanical stability and the support of post-implantation repair neo-osteogenesis.

4. As of the seventh postoperative week, the first signs of osteointegration appear: creation of osteoid bridges between the osteoid matrix deposited at the HA surface and the osteoformation islands found in the peri-prosthetic space.

5. As of approximately the third postoperative month, there are signs of mineralization of the osteoid material. Thus, the bone resulting from this mineralization displays a lamellar arrangement. This process produces a lamellar bony formation that covers the whole HA surface, with the appearance of the bony sleeve surrounding more or less completely the implant. Newly formed trabeculae, in continuity with the endosteal bone of the femur, cross the peri-prosthetic space. They are largely interconnected with each other and constitute many bone bridges developed between the host bone and the peri-prosthetic sleeve (Fig. 2.40).

Bone Remodelling

Generally, the material explanted after at least 2 years exhibits similar bone neoformation phenomena. Osteointegration is most obvious in Gruen zones I and VII, on the internal and external surfaces in zones II, III, V and VI, and zone IV, at the tip of the implant.

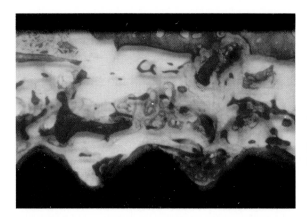

Fig. 2.39 Bone–HA interface. The implant is covered with a discontinuous sleeve of bone. At the top, the host bone, of Haversian type. In between, multiple areas of new bone formation, filling progressively the peri-prosthetic space (Specimen 6. Implantation time: 8 weeks, Fuchsin-Toluidine blue staining. Bar = 200 μm)

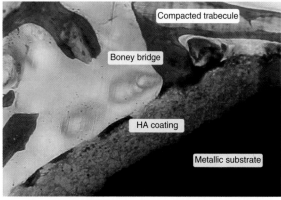

Fig. 2.40 Bony bridge and osteogenesis on the periphery of one compacted trabecule surrounding the prosthesis. Newly formed bone is darker because of its higher proteic contents. (Specimen 19. Implantation time: 23 months. Fuchsine-Toluidine blue staining. Bar = 150 μm)

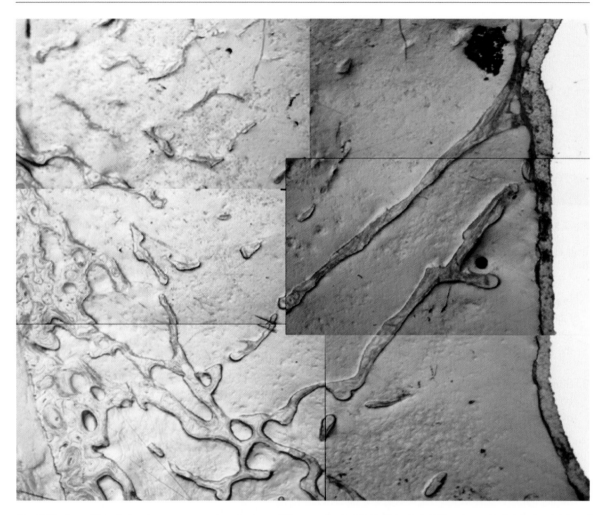

Fig. 2.41 Assembly of six views reconstructing the bone–HA interface in the vicinity of the greater trochanter. Note the long, thin trabeculae running parallel from the HA coating (onto which they are firmly attached) to the largely osteopenic area in the vicinity of the greater trochanter (Specimen 16. Implantation time: 24 months. Toluidine blue staining. Reflected light microscopy. Bar = 300 μm)

This similarity within the specimens makes it possible to accept the hypothesis that the neoformed bone is distributed in agreement with Wolff's laws that govern the intensity of bone remodelling as a function of the nature and intensity of the mechanical loads.

1. Zone I. The trochanteric zone is biomechanically critical. Most uncemented prostheses fail because of the lack of bone fixation in this zone. This proximal fixation failure almost inevitably causes a deviation of the stresses towards the distal part of the implant, leading to disuse osteopenia. This set of signs is usually referred to as 'proximal stress-shielding'. Unlike with the other zones, zone I exhibits systematically and by the end of the first year, thin, parallel bone trabeculae which stretch between the lateral edge of the implant and the greater trochanter (Fig. 2.41). These trabeculae are continuous and display the histological signs of an intense bone remodelling. Indeed, they exhibit constantly and simultaneously numerous active osteoblasts, osteoclasts and even, in five prostheses examined, Haversian remodelling within the trabeculae.

2. Zones II, III, V and VI. In these zones, the implant is often seated in the endosteal bone (Fig. 2.42). Infrequently, the implant is in contact with the cortical bone itself. The presence of trabeculae that join the HA surface with the endosteum is most often limited to the internal and external surfaces of the implant as well as to its corners. If the implant is not centred within the medullary cavity, it can be observed that the zone most remote from the

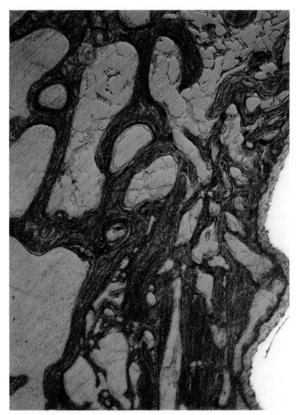

Fig. 2.42 Bone–HA interface. Typical trabecular morphotype (see text) (Specimen 12. Implantation time: 24 months. Reflected light microscopy. Bar = 500 μm)

endosteum has the lowest number of bone trabeculae. In these regions, the only visible ossification results from a more or less continuous bone sleeve that coats the HA, but without any connection to the host femur. None of the specimens examined – even those coming from bedridden and non-ambulatory osteoporotic patients – exhibited fibrotic tissues at the bone–implant interface.

3. Zone IV. The tip of the implant is always rich in peri-prosthetic osteogenesis. The trabeculae that form are dense, compact and oblique between the surface of the implant and the closest endosteum. None of the specimens examined exhibited any ossification at the extreme tip of the implant, thus making it possible to exclude the formation of a pedestal. The rule concerning the off-centring of the tip within the medullary cavity also applies here, with connecting trabeculae more developed at the location where the implant is closer to the endosteum.

Peri-prosthetic Bony Morphotypes

An examination of hundreds of the available slides revealed that the neoformed bone may take three morphological arrangements (in order of decreasing frequency): trabecular, digitiform or Haversian [10, 18].

1. *The trabecular morphotype* – the most frequent one – is composed of a thin peri-prosthetic bone sleeve, connected with a lattice of short trabeculae bridging the endosteum to the prosthesis coating with numerous cross-linking trabeculae (Fig. 2.42). For this morphotype to be present, the implant must be fairly close to the endosteum (1–2 mm).

2. *The digitiform morphotype* is found essentially in the metaphyseal zone. It is made of long trabeculae, roughly perpendicular to the coating, bridging the endosteum to the prosthesis coating with no cross links between the different trabeculae (Fig. 2.43).

3. *The Haversian morphotype* – very rare in our experience – results from the implantation in contact with the cortical bone. The neoformed bone exhibits a Haversian arrangement, but its protein content is higher than that of the host bone and so it has a higher tinctorial affinity to toluidine.

Bone Affinity Index (BAI)

On seven specimens with more than 3 years of residence time (specimens *n°* 12, 17, 18, 19, 24, 31 and 39), at least three slides were made in the metaphyseal zone, six in the diaphyseal zone and three near the tip of the implant. The mean BAI measured on each of these slides is 39%

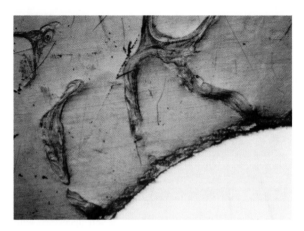

Fig. 2.43 Bone–HA interface at the calcar area. Typical digitiform morphotype (see text). (Specimen 12. Implantation time: 24 months. Reflected light microscopy. Bar = 500 μm)

in the metaphyseal zone, 51% in the diaphyseal zone and 66% near the tip of the implant. Globally, if we work out the mean BAI on all the observed sections, the value is 48%.

HA Coating Resorption

All the explants obtained after 1 year of residence time exhibited signs of HA resorption. This resorption is most often partial (Fig. 2.44) and shows a reduction of the nominal thickness of the coating. Sometimes it is complete, with the metallic substrate being exposed. The resorption zones comprise:

(a) Multinucleic cells, about 100 µ in diameter or larger, provided with a brush-like edge and set closely to the outer surface of the coating and/or the lamellar bone layer which envelops the HA coating. This morphology is similar to that of the osteoclast. These cells, sometimes called ceramoclasts, contain carbonic anhydrase and acid phosphatase, which resist sodium tartrate (=TRAP+ cells).

(b) Mononucleic cells, which are grouped near the resorption zones. The cytoplasmic compartments of these cells contain phagocytosis vacuoles, which in turn contain HA debris, sometimes in large quantities.

HA resorption is therefore a cellular mechanism. The cell elements present remind us of the physiological resorption of the bony tissue, and animal experiments confirm that there is a net parallel between the two

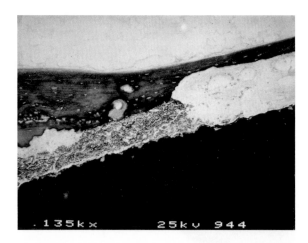

Fig. 2.44 Resorption of HA in the zone left uncovered with bone (*B*). Partial resorption leaving an irregular remnant or coating (*P*). Complete resorption leaving the metallic substrate in contact with bone marrow (*C*) (Specimen 34. SEM + silver methenamine. Bar = 200 µm)

resorption mechanisms – bone and HA – such as described by Frost in 1969 [12].

As shown in Fig. 2.45 HA resorption is initiated by the activation of osteoclastic cells, which degrade the coating, leaving numerous fragments on site. The osteoclastic cells migrate, leaving the degraded zone to the macrophages, which phagocytose most of the fragments which are thus degraded in terms of calcium ions and phosphate. Like the bone resorption–reconstruction process, and whenever the biomechanical context justifies it, osteoprogenitor cells are activated. These cells set in the resorption zone and synthesize an osteoid matrix, which will undergo a secondary mineralization.

The presence of this resorption–reconstruction mechanism leads to the simultaneous presence of several types of interfaces:

1. The succession of these resorption–reconstruction cycles explain the images very frequently observed where a thin layer of coating remains under a bone that exhibits signs of intense remodelling, as demonstrated by the presence of cementing lines within the neoformed bone. These cementing lines, the composition of which is similar to that of the *lamina limitans* mentioned above, are composed of bone proteins which are above the neoformed bone at the end of the neo-osteogenesis process. The presence of several cementing lines probably means that several cycles have taken place successively (Fig. 2.46).

2. Sometimes, this succession of cycles leads to the full resorption of the HA coating, with the formation of a direct interface between the metallic substrate and the bone. Even then, there is no fibrotic interface between the bone and the metal. This type of interface is found in most cases in zones with a high remodelling potential, such as the Gruen zone VII, or the internal face in zone VI or the external face in zone III of the implant (Fig. 2.47).

3. Certain zones show no bone reconstruction. The HA coating disappears leaving the metallic substrate in direct contact with the bone marrow. This is the interface usually visible on the anterior and posterior surfaces of the implant in Gruen zones II, III, V and VI.

Peri-Articular Soft Tissues

The joint capsules, the psoas tendon or the gluteus medius tendon have been submitted to histological investigation when heterotopic ossification was visible

Fig. 2.45 Turnover of interfacial bone. (1) During the rest phase, bone and HA are preserved from resorption. (2) Activation, by retraction of the resting cells, providing access to the underlying bone for the osteoclasts. (3) Osteoclast-mediated resorption of bone, and of HA. (4) Removal of the remaining fragments by macrophages. (5) If no bone reconstruction, back to the resting phase. (6) If bone reconstruction on the degraded coating, then back to the resting phase

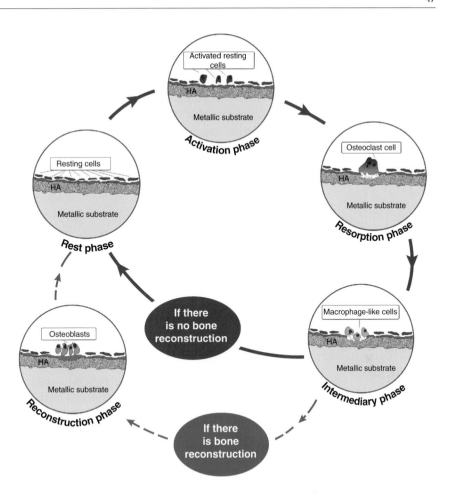

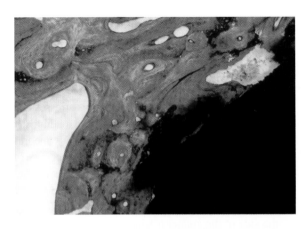

Fig. 2.46 Intense Haversian remodelling of the interfacial bone, with multiple cementing lines, large resorption of the coating with a remaining flake of HA (Specimen 22. Implantation time: 49 months. Cole hematoxylin staining. Bar = 150 μm)

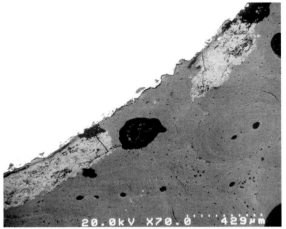

Fig. 2.47 Bone reconstruction on a previously highly degraded coating (Specimen 31. Implantation time: 56 months. SEM + Back Scattering. Bar = 429 μm)

in these tissues on the post-mortem x-ray, i.e. in 21 patients. Using the Brooker classification there were type I ossifications in 7 cases and type II in 14 cases. No type III or IV ossification has been submitted to histological investigation. Each time, it was a differentiated bone tissue, morphologically comparable in all aspects to the ossifications reported with other types of prostheses. The calcification is obvious, as demonstrated by the Von Kossa colouring. No HA particles were found in the specimens.

Polyethylene Insert

It has been possible to identify 51 particles in the 16 inserts available. These particles were embedded in the PE, in most cases at the end of a scratch caused by the particle itself. Using x-ray spectrometry, it has been possible to determine that all these particles were metallic and that they came from the femoral head (steel). No calcium or phosphorus-containing particles were identified.

Synthesis and Discussion

Osteointegration

The biocompatibility and osteoconductive properties of the phosphocalcic coatings have been properly established. The bone-bonding ability (osteointegration) is specific to so-called bioactive materials [19]. A definition of the term 'bone bonding = osteointegration' has been defined during successive consensus conferences [27]. It is defined as *the creation by means of physicochemical processes of continuity between the implant and the bone matrix.* For HA, osteointegration can only occur after implantation in a bone environment. This limitation defines the osteoconductive property of HA.

The definition of these properties is essential for the surgeon. Indeed, to achieve high-quality osteointegration the Corail® implant must be located within a bone environment that is both alive – hence reactive – and mechanically stable. Thus the preparation must be stringent, with the cancellous bone compacted inside the medullary cavity to create a congruent bony bed. This is why the broaches have been designed so as not to remove the cancellous bone but rather to compact it progressively. The ideal implantation must take place in the endosteal envelope, the space that corresponds to the interface between the bone marrow, the surface of the cancellous trabeculae and the internal cortical walls. Within this endosteal envelope, a so-called 'junction zone' seems to be the seat of a very intense bone remodelling potential. In the same line of thinking, in order to preserve the bone marrow it is preferable to avoid undue lavages of the medullary cavity or the introduction of solutions potentially cytotoxic for the medullary cells. The future osteoprogenitor cells are located in the bone marrow, and more specifically in the junction zone; hence they should be preserved.

At the experimental level, the importance of the stability of the HA-coated implant has been underlined several times [24]. The creation of a bony bed made of compacted cancellous bone serves that purpose. It is worth noting, however, that even in conditions where mechanical stability was not optimal (see photos), there have always been clear signs of osteointegration, no matter how small, without fibrotic interposition. This success is attributed to the HA, since with other types of surface treatment, it is probable that some of these patients would not have been able to achieve such a reliable fixation.

Bone remodelling is crucial. It depends on the prosthetic design, the intensity and kinetics of the host bone and also of the neoformed bone. It is indeed determined by the shape of the implant, the position of the contact points and the nature of the load transfer. Three design parameters of the Corail® stem seem to have a very specific influence on the remodelling: (1) the proximal flaring, (2) the presence of grooves and (3) the quadrangular section.

1. *The proximal flaring* increases the transfer of stresses in zone VII and especially in zone I. The radiological aspect of this zone which exhibits long radial bone trabeculae and the histological correspondence calls for some comments. We know from biomechanics that this zone is submitted to numerous stresses and loads. The bending forces applied during loading and the tensile forces generated by the gluteus medius explain why a large proportion of these forces are of the traction type. For a tensile stress to be able to cross a bone trabecula, the two ends must be solidly attached to the zones where the stress is applied. On the side of the greater trochanter, this is an anatomical continuity between the bone and the trabeculae, but on the prosthesis side, there must be a powerful fixation between the bone and the HA, and between

the HA and the metal. The pull-out resistance of the metal coating interface is higher than 35 MPa, a value much higher than the tensile forces which are applied in that region.

2. *The presence of grooves* in the prosthetic design actively influences bone remodelling, since each of these grooves generates a stress peak which increases bone trophicity. The horizontal grooves in the proximal and medial aspect of the stem act as superimposed microflanges, generating each time a compression stress peak.

3. *The quadrangular section* makes it possible to define the corners, which also generate stress peaks. These stress peaks are mainly rotation stresses when torque is applied to the implant, when the patient sits down, gets up from a chair or climbs stairs. This feature is essential for stability, especially in osteopenic patients (Fig. 2.48) in whom implant–bone contact is difficult to obtain. Stability results from the development of bone bridges at each corner. It is probably because of the rotary nature of these stresses that the trabeculae which react to them are often stocky, wide and round.

Coating resorption can, in theory, be linked to three main mechanisms: (1) osteoclastic resorption, (2) delamination and (3) dissolution at neutral pH.

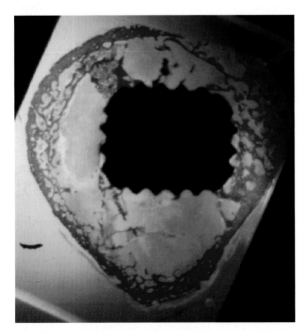

Fig. 2.48 Macroscopic view. Section obtained 3 cm over the tip of the stem (Specimen 36. Implantation time: 4 years. Cole hematoxyline staining. Bar = 1 cm)

1. *Osteoclastic resorption* seems to be the main mechanism as confirmed by most of the authors. Therefore, this mechanism is part of the bone turnover physiological process, and is even one of its first steps. The physico-chemical properties of the HA make it a natural substrate for these osteoclastic morphological cells.

2. *Delamination*, i.e. the loss of adhesion of the HA coating, has only been observed in two specimens: and specimen 31 after 7 years of implantation also in zone II. Wherever delamination takes place, it is much localized and covers a very small area (only a few square millimetres). The coating detached from its substrate is surrounded by bone not only on its external surface but also on the surface that is opposite the metallic substrate, without gigantocytes, without histiocytic proliferation, without fibrosis and without loosening. These detached fragments are nearly always engulfed into newly formed bone and do not seem to cause any form of secondary effect, such as loosening.

3. *Dissolution in neutral pH* exists, albeit it is as a marginal phenomenon. Experimentally de Groot [9] tried to measure it and came to the conclusion that a layer of 15 μm is lost each year, which is negligible for a 155 μ ± 35 μ coating. This dissolution, at least in the first months after implantation, is necessary to initiate osteointegration [7]. The bioactivity of a phosphocalcic compound is indeed proportional to its solubility.

In theory, there are three side effects of coating resorption:

1. *Progressive loosening* may be reasonably expected to occur as the coating resorbs. However, this is not the case as evident from the examination of all specimens implanted for more than 1 year which exhibit more or less obvious signs of HA coating resorption. Loosening did not occur in any of these specimens. There seems to be no problems as long as the loss of HA stock is associated with bone reconstructed on the HA residues: a bone tissue capable of stabilizing the prosthesis and of transmitting stresses to the host femur. Our data at 10 years, confirmed by others, make it possible to exclude any form of prosthetic loosening. The degree of bone fixation of the implant is independent of the amount of HA residue. Yet, our material comes from poorly mobile patients, most often victims of severe osteoporosis in whom the osteoclasts

are known to be activated. It should also be noted that signs of active bone remodelling, such as the presence of osteoclasts, macrophages or osteoblasts in the immediate vicinity of the implant, are rare after 4 years of implantation.

2. *The initiation of inflammatory reactions* around released HA particles has always been feared. However, the literature shows that even as particulates, the HA remains biocompatible. Wang et al. [26] have demonstrated that HA particles of a diameter less than 5 μm implanted in harvested bone chambers do not disturb the bone formation process.

3. *Intra-articular migration of HA particles* can ensue, with a subsequent damage to the prosthetic joint surfaces, by a third body wear mechanism. Numerous different types of particles can migrate within the joint, especially cement particles, barium sulphate, bone fragments and metallic particles. Hence, specific attention must be paid to possible HA debris migration. Bloebaum and co-workers [3, 4] have mentioned this possibility, with the formation of an acetabular cystic granuloma that contains HA debris as well as cement particles (their observations were made from hybrid implants). Despite repeated and detailed investigations, our studies could hardly show any loose hydroxyapatite granules away from the coating, and the presence of HA fragments in the joint has never been noted in our material. Moreover, certain studies on polyethylene inserts retrieved from revised cemented prostheses have demonstrated that calcium phosphate particles could form and become embedded by precipitation in the prosthetic joint surface [11]. This finding indicates that any calcium phosphate body found in the prosthetic joint is not necessarily the result of a particulate migration.

Acknowledgement I wish to thank the members of the ARTRO Group for their unfailing friendship during these 25 years and their encouragement in continuing my work. Special thanks to Dr. Frayssinet who introduced me to bone biology and who has provided me with significant material to better understand and illustrate the mode of operation of bioactive coatings.

References

1. Anderson GI, Orlando K, Waddell JP (2001) Synovitis subsequent to total-hip arthroplasty with and without hydroxyapatite coatings: a study in dogs. Vet Surg 30:311–318
2. Block MS, Kent JN (1984) Long term radiographic evaluation of hydroxyapatite augmented mandibular alveolar ridges. J Oral Maxillofac Surg 42:793–796
3. Bloebaum R, Dupont J (1993) Osteolysis from a press fit hydroxyapatite-coated implant. A case study. J Arthroplasty 8:195–202
4. Bloebaum R, Beeks D, Dorr LD et al (1994) Complications with hydroxyapatite particulate separation in total hip arthroplasty. Clin Orthop 298:19–26
5. Bonel G, Heughebaert JC, Heughebaert M et al (1988) Apatitic calcium orthophosphates and related compounds for biomaterial preparation. Ann N Y Acad Sci 523:115–130
6. Cook SD, Thomas KA, Dalton JE et al (1992) HA coating of porous implants improves bone ingrowth and interface attachment strength. J Biomed Mater Res 26:989–1001
7. de Bruijn JD, Klein CPAT, de Groot K et al (1992) The ultrastructure of the bone hydroxylapatite interface in vitro. J Biomed Mater Res 26:1365–1382
8. de Groot K (1983) Bioceramics of calcium phosphates. CRC, Boca Raton
9. de Groot K (1988) Effect of porosity and physicochemical properties on the stability, resorption, and strength of calcium phosphate ceramics. Ann N Y Acad Sci 523:227–233
10. Frayssinet P, Hardy D, Hanker JS et al (1995) Natural history of bone response to hydroxyapatite-coated hip prostheses implanted in humans. Cells Mater 5:125–138
11. Frayssinet P, Vidalain JP, Ranz X et al (1999) Hydroxyapatite particle migration. Eur J Orthop Surg Traumatol 9:95–98
12. Frost HM (1969) Tetracycline based histological analysis of bone remodeling. Calcif Tissue Res 3:211–237
13. Furukawa T, Matsusue Y, Yasunaga T et al (2000) Biodegradation behavior of ultra-high strength hydroxylapatite/poly (L-lactide) composite rods for internal fixation of bone fractures. Biomaterials 14:403–406
14. Geesink R, de Groot K, Klein C (1987) Chemical implant fixation using hydroxyapatite. Clin Orthop 225:147–170
15. Gumaer KI, Salsbury RL, Sauerschell RJ et al (1985) Evaluation of hydroxylapatite root implants in baboons. J Oral Maxillofac Surg 44:73–79
16. Hardy DCR, Frayssinet P, Guilhem et al (1991) Bonding of hydroxyapatite-coated prostheses. Histopathology of specimens from four cases. J Bone Joint Surg Br 73:732–740
17. Hardy DCR, Frayssinet P, Bonel G et al (1994) Two-years outcome of hydroxyapatite-coated prostheses. Two femoral prostheses retrieved at autopsy. Acta Orthop Scand 63:253–257
18. Hardy DCR, Frayssinet P, Delincé P (1999) Osteointegration of hydroxyapatite-coated stems of femoral prostheses. Eur J Orthop Surg Traumatol 9:75–81
19. Hench LL, Wilson J (1984) Surface-active biomaterials. Science 226:630–636
20. Hoogendorn HA, Ronooij W, Akkermans LMA et al (1984) Long term study of large ceramic implants (porous hydroxyapatite) in dog femora. Clin Orthop 187:281–288
21. Klein CPAT, Driessen AA, de Groot K et al (1983) Biodegradation behaviour of various calcium phosphate materials in bone tissue. J Biomed Mater Res 17:769–784

22. Orr RD, de Bruijn JD, Davies JE (1992) Scanning electron microscopy of the interface with titanium, titanium alloy and hydroxyapatite. Cells Mater 2:241–251

23. Osborne JF, Weiss T (1978) Hydroxylapatite-ein knochenahnlicher Blowerkstoff. Schw Mechr Zahnheik 88:118–124

24. Søballe K, Hansen ES, Rasmussen HB et al (1992) Tissue ingrowth into titanium and hydroxyapatite-coated implants during stable and unstable mechanical conditions. J Orthop Res 10:285–299

25. Thomas KA, Cook SD, Haddad RJ et al (1989) Biologic response to hydroxylapatite-coated titanium hips. A preliminary study in dogs. J Arthroplasty 4:43–53

26. Wang JS, Goodman S, Aspenberg P (1994) Bone formation in the presence of phagocytosable hydroxyapatite particles. Clin Orthop 304:272–278

27. Williams DF, Black J, Doherty PJ (1992) Second consensus conference on definitions in biomaterials. In: Doherty et al (eds) Biomaterial-tissue interfaces: advances in biomaterials, vol 10. Elsevier Science Publishers, London, pp 525–533

Contents

J.-P. Vidalain et al. (eds.), *The CORAIL® Hip System*,
DOI: 10.1007/978-3-642-18396-6_3, © Springer-Verlag Berlin Heidelberg 2011

3.1 Selection Criteria: *Prêt-à-Porter*

Markus C. Michel

Corail® implants suit most femoral anatomies (Dorr-types A, B and C). Nevertheless, in all cases the indications need to be planned carefully taking account of the specific demands of the individual patient. It is important for the surgeon to understand the principle of 'compaction broaching' and the mechanism of fixation using a fully hydroxyapatite-coated (HAC) stem as well as the correct implantation technique in order to achieve the best possible result for all patients. Even then, the surgeon needs to be aware that there might be some rare situations in which a different surgical technique is needed.

So, is this already the end of the chapter? Are there really no selection criteria? Is it really possible that one stem is suitable for all indications?

Yes, after having used the stem for many years and having implanted more than 2,000, I have the personal experience to say that the stem, the Corail® implant, really fits most femora. It certainly fits all Dorr-type femora, including type C.

There are special types of Corail® stem designed to cope with different neck lengths and offset, to take into account the wide variety of human femora. For very thin femora, I use special dysplastic stems and for very big femora, I may use a Corail® Revision stem.

So the answer to the initial question should rather be that the Corail® implant family is able to cope with nearly all anatomical variations. It is pivotal to use the optimal Corail® implant to restore leg length and offset in order to achieve the optimal functional outcome. Most experienced surgeons use a standard stem in about 75% of cases and a high offset or varus stem in about 25% of cases. These percentages are quite uniform in Europe, but different percentages would apply for different patient populations. For example, the percentages among an Asian population would be different.

In my opinion it is vitally important to use the correct implant templating to match the patient's anatomy.

It is essential to restore size, offset and caput–collum–diaphyseal (CCD) angle. There are, however, more factors to be considered. Age, which may affect bone density, is important and there are specific considerations for young and active patients and, at the other end of the age spectrum, for elderly patients with lower bone density. These considerations are of great importance and there are two specific chapters on these subjects (Sects. 4.4.1 and 4.4.2).

Another criterion for an implant might be the approach to the hip. In our hospital we use a direct anterior approach (DAA) (Sect. 6.1.3). This procedure was optimized to minimize soft tissue damage. Special care is taken in this procedure not to damage the hip deltoid or the abductor tendons. The Corail® stem with its low shoulder profile and the biological fixation is entirely compatible with this approach.

Figure 3.1 shows the Corail® stem compared to a complete straight stem. This image illustrates how the Corail® stem easily bypasses the greater trochanter and therefore also the abductor tendons, whereas a complete straight stem passes through the tendons of gluteus medius or minimus. This is one reason why the Corail® stem not only suits most anatomical situations, but can also be used with tissue-sparing approaches such as the DAA.

The Corail® stem is certainly a forgiving implant, but the surgical technique needs to be followed carefully and in a few situations the technique needs to be adapted to patient-specific circumstances. One of the anatomical variations that needs specific consideration is the severe champagne flute femur (Fig. 3.2). If a small Corail® is implanted into a fluted femur, fixation will occur in the diaphysis only. Diaphyseal fixation on its own is contrary to the principles of Corail® fixation, as there will be no proximal fixation. Absence of proximal fixation may lead to early loosening, particularly in high-demand patients. Therefore in this situation it is better to over-ream the medullary cavity with a canal reamer to accommodate a bigger implant allowing better compaction of the proximal metaphyseal bone. It has to be emphasized that this is an unusual step in the technical procedure, but one which is necessary to allow the principle of bone compaction to be respected (Fig. 3.3).

3.2 The Art of Planning and Restoration of Biomechanics: A Good Plan for a Good Construct

Tarik Aït Si Selmi and Camdon Fary

Restoration of hip anatomy is the key to successful total hip arthroplasty (THA). Planning the procedure is the only way to reliably achieve a good construct.

Fig. 3.1 The Corail® stem compared to a complete straight stem (Copyright DePuyInternational Limited)

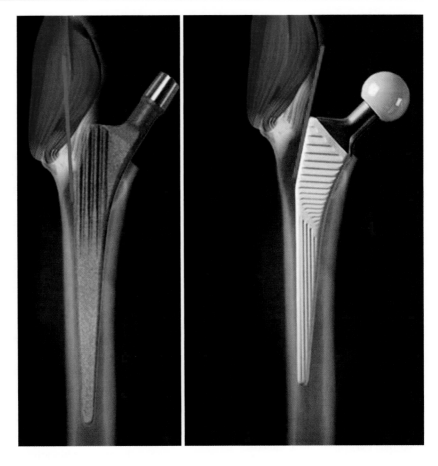

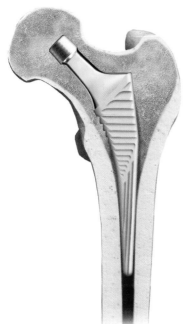

Fig. 3.2 Severe champagne flute femur (Courtesy of David Beverland) (Copyright DePuyInternational Limited)

Despite variations related to local anatomy, bone quality and radiological magnification mismatch, planning provides the surgeon with a guideline for reproducible results. A record of the templating also illustrates the surgeon's effort to address unique patient anatomy and pathology. This is important if any complication, such as leg length discrepancy or dislocation, occurs.

Clinical Evaluation

Planning is more than just templating. Planning involves clinical and radiological assessment.

Checking for a leg-length discrepancy (LLD) is the first priority. When observed it must be discussed with the patient and the clinical and functional relevance of the LLD must be determined. The origin of the LLD must be determined. The first step is to distinguish between intra-articular and extra-articular causes; the latter, usually, cannot be addressed by a total hip arthroplasty (THA). The patient's history will reflect the effect of the LLD on their gait, including whether a shoe raise is required. Examination will recognize false LLD due

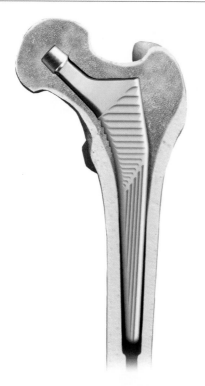

Fig. 3.3 The medular cavity over-reamed with a canal reamer to accommodate a bigger implant and compacting the proximal metaphyseal bone much better. This is rarely indicated especially in Dorr type A femurs (Courtesy of David Beverland) (Copyright DePuyInternational Limited)

to flexion deformities. In chronic LLD some patients develop responsive changes that are sometimes irreversible such as a fixed foot equinus deformity or a fixed pelvic tilt. Realignment may be compromised by the limb or spinal adaptations. In fixed spinal deformities the clinical examination and associated radiographs assess the reducibility of any adaptation deformity. On the anteroposterior (AP) pelvic radiograph pelvic tilt is easily recognized. It must be measured and the effect on the hip position, which itself may be affected by bone wear, protrusion, subluxation, etc., recognized. Long leg radiographs can be useful to identify the origin of the LLD, when this is unclear on standard radiographs. Most cases of LLD are found to be from an intra-articular origin and will be addressed by the THA, if the anatomy of the contralateral hip is reproduced. In the case of chronic diseases which occurred during childhood, the hip and surrounding soft tissues may display some degree of atrophy. This is typically observed in paediatric arthritis and developmental dysplasia of the hip (DDH). In this

particular situation it is often impossible or undesirable to reproduce the 'ideal' anatomy. In such situations it is important to discuss with the patient the resulting true or observed LLD and the options for its management.

Secondly, the range of motion of the arthritic hip must be determined during the examination. Special attention should be paid to a fixed external rotation deformity. When the hip is externally rotated, the neck-shaft angle appears greater on the AP radiograph, and subsequent templating may underestimate the true offset of the hip.

Finally, sagittal spinal and pelvic balance must be assessed in each case as adjustment of the cup positioning may be required to decrease the risk of dislocation or impingement. Special attention must be paid to patients with ankylosing spondylitis.

Templating with Standard Radiographs

Templating requires a standardized step-by-step procedure. Having good-quality radiographs is crucial. Also, it is essential to know the radiographic magnification. The standard way to determine the magnification is to use a spherical marker on the x-ray at the level of the hip joint. Once the magnification is known, the appropriate templates must be used. An AP pelvis in the standing position is the minimum requirement. The knees must be internally rotated to reveal true offset to compensate for the femoral neck anteversion. In arthritic hips, fixed external rotation tends to minimize the neck-shaft angle, and the contralateral hip, if normal, can be used for reference. AP-centred and lateral hip radiographs must show the proximal third of the femur to assess the shaft.

There are five consecutive formal steps to templating.

Step 1: Acetabular Cup Placement and Selection

The ideal cup position is usually clear and determines the *prosthetic* hip centre as opposed to the *native* hip centre. The template is placed over the radiograph to ensure the cup is covered, 45° abducted and against the medial wall of the acetabulum. With this technique there is a tendency to slightly over-medialise the prosthetic hip centre. In some instances, one may consider a shallower cup position if sufficient coverage is provided. The sizing of the cup is difficult on the AP film, but can be approximated by matching the cup with the acetabular contour on the lateral view. More often the cup centre that is templated is slightly medial compared to the pathological or contralateral normal native hip centres (Fig. 3.4).

with the tip of the greater trochanter overhanging the metaphysis. As a result, it is common to insert the stem in a varus position. If varus placement is combined with the use of a coxa vara stem, the correction of the offset may be too great. In the situation in which a varus placement of the stem is predicted, it is recommended to use a standard stem.

Step 2: Femoral Stem Selection

Stem selection is less critical, since several head, neck and stem combinations may result in the same overall restoration of anatomy. The initial reference point for Corail® templating is the metaphyseal placement of the stem. A template that matches the metaphyseal anatomy of the femur is placed over the femoral radiograph with the stem centred along the shaft. The template is then moved proximally or distally along the femoral axis in order to determine the best match of the femoral neck axis with the prosthetic stem neck. The standard, high offset and coxa vara options can be tried against the femoral radiograph to determine the best match for the neck-shaft angle and offset (Fig. 3.5). In the coxa vara femur the neck-shaft angle is 125°. In this particular femoral configuration, not just the neck, but often the proximal femur tends to be in varus

Step 3: Neck Length Selection

After the templates that best match the anatomy are selected as described in step 2, it is recommended to position the template so that it coincides with a +5 (medium) neck (Fig. 3.6). This allows the benefit of fine-tuning intra-operatively, although one must keep in mind that changing the pre-selected neck length will also change the offset. Implanting a stem that differs in size by a factor of 1 from the stem size which was templated is common, but the Corail® hip system is designed so that neck size does not change significantly between stem sizes. Thus, the neck length selection does not have to be modified if the stem finally inserted is not the templated size. It must be remembered that templating is only a guide and, ultimately, it is the operative findings that will take precedence.

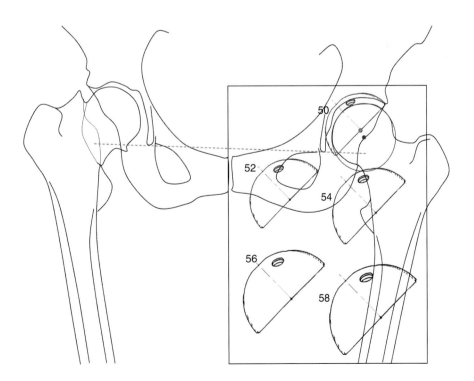

Fig. 3.4 Cup placement (Copyright DePuyInternational Limited)

Fig. 3.5 Offset selection
(Copyright DePuyInternational
Limited)

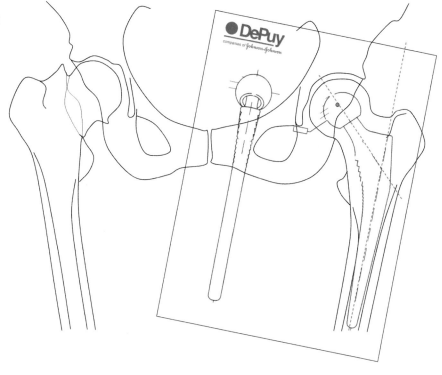

Fig. 3.6 Neck length
determination. A medium
neck (+5 mm) was selected
here (Copyright
DePuyInternational Limited)

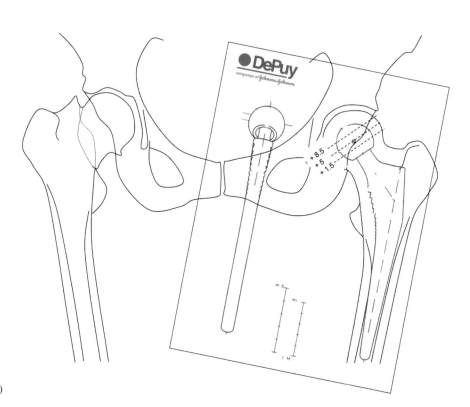

Step 4: Neck Resection Level

The Corail® stem is designed to be placed accurately within the stem.

Templating for the Corail® stem allows the calcar cut to be determined providing a precise preoperative reference (Fig. 3.7). The Corail® template is placed on the x-ray and the level of the cut determined. The calcar length is measured relative to the lesser or greater trochanter (piriformis fossa) bony landmarks. At surgery the level determined by the templating is measured with reference to the surgeon's preferred intra-operative landmark. The proximal aspect of the lesser trochanter is the most commonly accepted and reliable bony reference. The use of a collared stem guarantees the correct stem positioning. If the calcar is cut at the templated level, the collared stem cannot pass beyond the level of that cut.

Step 5: Stem Sizing

Stem sizing is the last, but not least, important step. The correct stem size (8–20) is selected using the template. The correct size is the size that fills the femoral cavity to within 1–2 mm distance from the cortices (bone compacted sleeve). This will vary according to the magnification and, importantly, with the bone quality. In a type C osteoporotic femur, the stem will fill the canal nearly reaching the cortices before good initial fixation is achieved. In a younger patient, or in a type B femur with a narrow canal, a smaller stem than anticipated will achieve good initial fixation (Fig. 3.8). In some instances, where the isthmus is excessively narrow, the need to ream the femur can be predicted. This avoids distal locking and the possible risk of proximal instability. The lateral view should be assessed for marked bowing of the sagittal femoral shaft, as such bowing will result in the use of a smaller stem than the one selected using the AP radiograph.

After a short period of practice the surgeon is able to select the stem 'at a glance'.

Digital Templating

Digital templating is becoming the standard x-ray format in hospitals. It offers faster availability and greater accuracy. The principles are similar. The first step is to determine the image magnification by measuring the

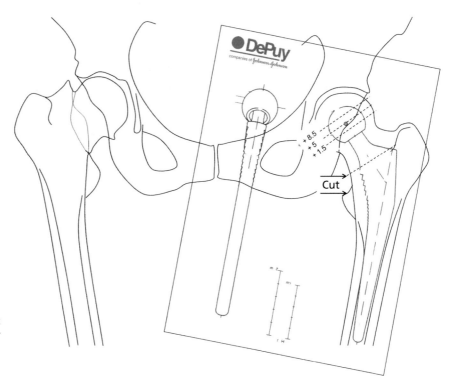

Fig. 3.7 Cut level assessment as the distance from the lesser trochanter to the neck osteotomy (Copyright DePuyInternational Limited)

Fig. 3.8 Stem sizing. *Left*: Osteoporotic bone with a narrow cancellous sleeve surrounding a relatively large stem. *Right*: Large shaft of a young male where the compacted bone mantle is greater than 2 mm in thickness

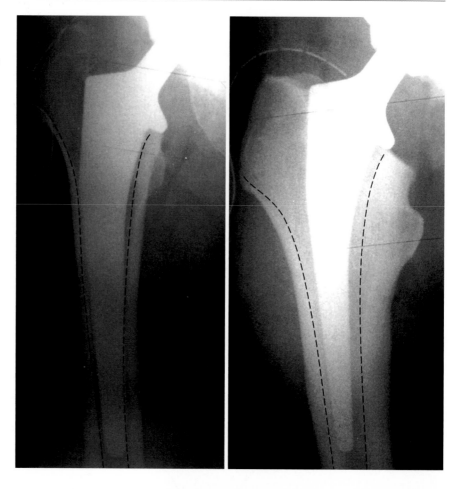

size of a marker of known length. The digital templates are then changed to the appropriate magnification. The digital software templating package will also contain different tools. Tools are available to assess and measure pelvic tilt and limb length discrepancy. Other applications allow the image of the femur with the template superimposed to be moved into its final position (Fig. 3.9). Finally, digital templating may be semi-automated and will detect the hip contours on x-ray and then offer the surgeon selected templates. The final construct can be recorded in the patients' notes or on a dedicated database.

Navigation Systems

Navigation systems are not designed as substitutes for templating. They are used to achieve a more accurate intra-operative execution of the preoperative templating. Navigation relies upon the data that is fed into it

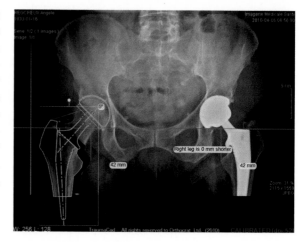

Fig. 3.9 Digital templating

and appears to be most useful in cup placement. Digital templating can be connected to the navigation tools. CT scan reconstruction may provide more accurate placement of the prosthetic components, as it allows orientation in three dimensions and, therefore, provides a greater understanding of cup and stem placement interdependent of each other.

Further Reading

Bayne CO, Krosin M, Barber TC (2009) Evaluation of the accuracy and use of x-ray markers in digital templating for total hip arthroplasty. J Arthroplasty 24(3):407–413

The B, Verdonschot N, van Horn JR et al (2007) Digital versus analogue preoperative planning of total hip arthroplasties. J Arthroplasty 22 (6):866–870

Debarge R, Lustig S, Neyret P et al (2008) Confrontation of the radiographic preoperative planning with the postoperative data for uncemented total hip arthroplasty. Rev Chir Orthop Reparatrice Appar Mot. 94(4):368–375

3.3 Surgical Technique

3.3.1 How to Implant the Stem: Respect the Advice of Your Elders

Jean-Charles Rollier and Jean-Claude Cartillier

When implanting a Corail® stem the surgeon must implement a specific technique that meets the mechanical and biological requirements of the stem. The aim of the procedure is to preserve the bone stock, and the compaction of the metaphyseal cancellous bone is the essential step since it provides the primary mechanical stability for the implant. The adequacy of the stability is checked after the trial reduction has been carried out using the final broach fitted with the selected neck segment and trial femoral head. The femoral neck resection level is another important factor. This level is determined preoperatively during the templating. A preliminary cut is made and the final cutting adjustment is carried out at a later stage during the procedure using a calcar reamer. The Corail® stem is introduced by hand into the femoral canal until about 1 cm of the stem protrudes above the femur cut. The stem insertion is then completed by careful impaction. The success of the stem implantation also relies upon accurate acetabular component positioning. The selected component must ensure adequate stability of the bearing surfaces and must provide an optimal range of motion without the risk of impingement.

Introduction

When implanting a cementless total hip prosthesis [1], the surgeon must create close contact between the host bone and the implant. In fact, the surgical technique serves two essential requirements: providing the best mechanical fit (this is what creates primary stability) and promoting secondary biological osseointegration. Each implant has distinctive features, which must be factored into the standard technique. The specific requirements for the Corail® system should be known and respected.

Surgical Technique

Preoperatively, the surgeon determines the most suitable bearing surface and the appropriate size, position and fit of the stem and acetabular component based on the patient's characteristics.

The patient is positioned appropriately depending upon the surgical approach used. This stage should be standardized, safe and comfortable for both the patient and the surgical team.

The selected approach must minimize surgical trauma. It should provide sufficient exposure to visualize the exposed femoral neck and the anatomical landmarks previously determined during the preoperative planning (greater and lesser trochanter, digital fossa, etc.).

The resection of the femoral head may be performed before or after the hip dislocation. The initial femoral neck cut should be positioned just above the preplanned final neck resection level. A resection guide can be used to make the cut at the appropriate angle on the neck. The initial femoral neck cut should be approximately 5 mm above the required level (assessed using a small ruler) and later converted to a final resection level using the calcar reamer.

The resected femoral head is stored for use as autologous grafting material at a later stage, if necessary.

The Preparation

The preparation of the acetabulum is carried out first in order to position the selected trial cup and its liner. The soft tissue capsular releases performed at that stage of the procedure facilitate subsequent exposure of the femur.

The preparation of the femoral canal begins with an adequate exposure of the neck. Following resection of the femoral head a rongeur forceps or specific chisel may be used to excise the residual proximal femoral neck (Fig. 3.10).

The next step in preparation of the stem is to check the axis of the femoral shaft. A blunt 8 mm reamer can be used as a canal or pathfinder. This blunt instrument preserves the cancellous bone but still demonstrates the axis of the canal to be followed by the broaches. This assists in accurate alignment of the component, particularly avoiding varus.

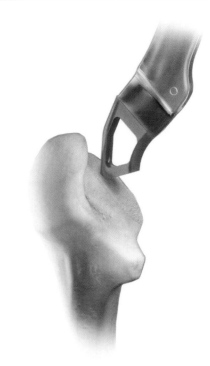

Fig. 3.10 Rongeur forceps or a specific chisel is used to excise the residual proximal femoral neck (Copyright DePuyInternational Limited)

The preparation of the metaphyseal cancellous bone can then be carried out and is the crucial stage in Corail® stem implantation. The technique is called compaction broaching.

Firstly, the bone impactor is used to compress a wedge of cancellous bone to create a cavity through which the insertion of the broaches can begin (Fig. 3.11).

Secondly, the metaphyseal cancellous bone is compacted by means of specific bone-sparing broaches. This stage begins with the smallest broach.

Broaches of increasing sizes are introduced (Fig. 3.12). The patient's own anteversion must be respected; this is facilitated by the shape of the broaches which will naturally follow the patient's own version. The broach handle should be tapped with the hammer to prevent any varus tilt during impaction into the femoral canal. The compaction broaching technique should enable a cancellous bone envelope to be achieved without cortical contact of the stem inside the femoral canal.

Femoral broaching is completed once adequate stability of the broach has been achieved. Initially axial stability is felt with the broach. Once this has been

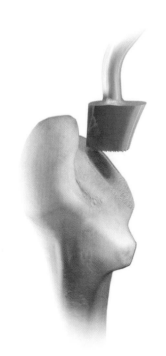

Fig. 3.11 The bone impactor is used to compress a wedge of cancellous bone to create a cavity

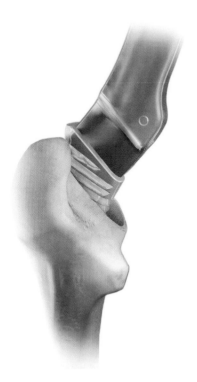

Fig. 3.12 Broaches of increasing sizes are introduced (Copyright DePuyInternational Limited)

achieved the rotational stability of the final broach is assessed. These stages should be performed in the right sequence. Rotational stability should not be repeatedly checked for during the broaching process as this could cause the cancellous bone cavity to be enlarged.

The size of the final broach should match the size of the stem templated using the preoperative radiographs. It is not unusual for there to be a difference in one size between the templated stem and the actual stem implanted. However, if this does occur it is important to consider the possible causes. If the stem implanted is smaller than that templated, the early locking of the broach during femoral preparation could be attributable to (1) incorrect insertion axis, either in a varus/valgus or rotational direction, (2) a tulip-shaped femur, which may require distal diaphyseal reaming, or (3) high-density cancellous bone commonly found in young patients. A size larger than that templated could be due to (1) the cancellous bone being of poor mechanical quality, (2) fracture, or (3) misalignment. The intra-operative results should be compared with the preoperative planning data.

Check that the final broach, once fully inserted, is recessed 2–3 mm below the planned level. The calcar mill is placed onto the stud of the broach to make height and orientation adjustments. The calcar reaming is mandatory whether a collared Corail® stem is used or not (Fig. 3.13).

Caution must be exercised during the calcar reaming step. Ream first at a low speed to prevent the risk of a calcar crack and to preserve soft tissue integrity. Then ream at a higher speed to achieve a flat surface on the medial cortex upon which the Corail® collar will seat.

At this stage, using a ruler the level of the femoral neck cut is measured relative to the selected landmark (inferior aspect of the lesser trochanter, tip of the greater trochanter or digital fossa). If the neck cut is too high, it may be necessary to insert the broach a few millimetres and then to ream down to the required level.

The appropriate trial neck segment is then fitted to the final broach in situ (Fig. 3.14). It should correspond to the selected femoral stem (STD, KLA and KHO). At this stage, the level of the final broach may also be checked by placing a horizontal wire into the trial neck (Fig. 3.15), so that it seats flush with the tip of the greater trochanter. The level of this wire can then be

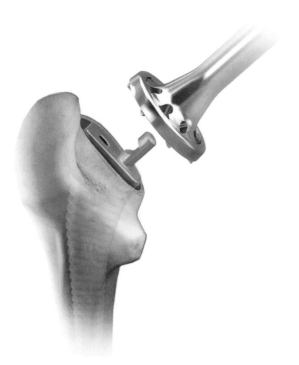

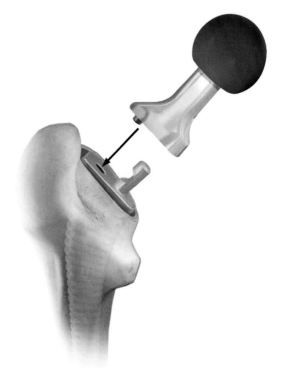

Fig. 3.13 The femoral cut level is perfected by the calcar reamer when using a collared stem (Copyright DePuyInternational Limited)

Fig. 3.14 The appropriate trial neck segment is then fitted to the final broach in situ for reduction and hip testing (Copyright DePuyInternational Limited)

compared with the pre-planned level. The trial head, of a predetermined diameter (28 mm, 32 mm or 36 mm) and length (+3.5, +5.0 or +8.5), is then placed onto the selected trial neck segment (Fig. 3.16).

With the trial acetabular and femoral components in situ, the hip is then reduced to assess the soft tissue tension, the stability of the bearing couple and the risk of impingement throughout the full range of motion. Should one of these parameters need adjustment, this can be done by repositioning the cup or by changing the femoral neck segment or the length of the trial head. The various components of the prosthetic hip should fit together well before final implant insertion. Once satisfactory results have been achieved, the hip is dislocated once more and the trial components are removed.

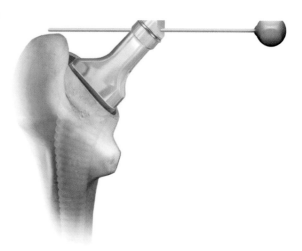

Fig. 3.15 The level of the final broach may also be checked by placing a horizontal wire into the trial neck (Copyright DePuyInternational Limited)

The Definitive Stem

The definitive acetabular cup is impacted with the same orientation as the trial component. Through the apex hole, assess the implant–bone contact and ensure a congruent fit. There should be no anterior overhang to avoid the risk of contact with the psoas tendon. The cup orientation should be 40–45° of abduction. The

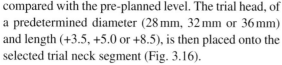

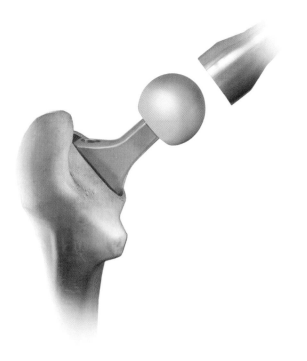

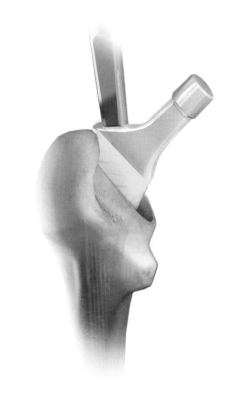

Fig. 3.16 The trial head, of a predetermined diameter and length, is then placed onto the selected trial neck segment (Copyright DePuyInternational Limited)

Fig. 3.17 The Corail® stem introduction should be easy until the stem stands proud 2 or 3 cm above the neck cut (Copyright DePuyInternational Limited)

anteversion is determined by the transverse acetabular ligament (TAL). The selected liner (polyethylene [PE], alumina or metal) is then placed into the metal shell, which must be clean and dry. Note that ceramic liners should be positioned with the greatest care and must be coaxial with the shell. The dedicated inserter can be used for this purpose. The liner/cup interface should be inspected for proper seating prior to final impaction.

The final Corail® stem can then be inserted into the femoral canal. Prior to the removal of the broach, rotational and axial stability should be reassessed. This is done by reattaching the broach handle and trying to rotate the broach within the stem. If there is any movement, the next size of broach must be used.

Upon completion of the trial stage, suction may be used in the canal but the femoral canal should not be cleaned or irrigated with antiseptic or antibiotic solutions. The definitive Corail® implant (of same size and type as the trial stem) is inserted into the femoral canal. The stem should be introduced by hand into the prepared compacted cancellous bone envelope while ensuring that the correct anteversion is maintained.

The introduction should be easy until the stem stands proud 2 or 3 cm above the neck cut (Fig. 3.17). At this stage only, impaction may be completed using a hammer – regular tapping being applied on the stem impactor – until the collar seats flush against the calcar or up to the level of the hydroxyapatite (HA) coating in collarless implants.

Once the femoral stem is implanted, check for calcar cracks. Any defects between the cortices and the implant are filled with cancellous bone from the resected femoral head. After removal of its protective cover, the taper should be cleaned and dried to ensure it is free of debris. The prosthetic head of the selected diameter, length and type is then placed onto the taper by applying torsional/axial pressure followed by light impaction. The hip is then reduced and the stability checked. The joint capsule is repaired and the wound closed.

Key Learning Points

> Preoperative planning helps determine the neck resection level and the exact Corail® stem positioning. It also helps select the implant lateralization and size.

> The Corail® stem is designed to seat in metaphyso-diaphyseal compacted cancellous bone and 'fit and fill' cortical contact should be avoided. Trial components are useful in assessing stability and range of motion and in avoiding impingement. All necessary adjustments should be made prior to definitive implantation.

Reference

1. Nourissat C, Cartillier JC (2007) Technique de mise en place des prothèses totale de hanche sans ciment. EMC (Elsevier Masson SAS, PARIS) techniques chirurgicales. OrthopédieTraumatologie 44:667

3.3.2 The Art of Compaction: Make Your Bed and Lie in It

James T. Caillouette

Femoral canal preparation is a critical step in total hip arthroplasty (THA). The Corail® system uses a compaction broach method that enhances initial implant stability, maximizes bone/implant contact and creates a more biologic environment than the diamond tooth broaches common in North American systems. This chapter will briefly review the various methods of femoral canal preparation with emphasis on the advantages of compaction broaching.

Introduction

'First do no harm' was the principle of Hippocrates that has been adopted by modern medicine. As surgeons, our goal in the preparation of the endosteal canal of the femur for total hip arthroplasty (THA) is to be as biologic as possible to enhance the long-term fixation of the prosthesis that is implanted. Femoral canal preparation and prosthetic implantation took two distinct paths during the evolution of THA. Beginning in the 1960s, Sir John Charnley promoted the concept of cementation of the femoral component. This technique allowed for rapid fixation of the implant and immediate weight-bearing. However, as we now know, there are potential pitfalls with cement pressurization.

Complications

Cement pressurization is known to increase the risk for intra-operative and post-operative fat embolism as well as post-operative deep vein thrombosis. The interaction of cement has been known to cause irreversible hypotension intra-operatively. In fact, a study by the Mayo Clinic of 7,316 patients demonstrated '30-day mortality with significantly higher, at 4.7% where patients receiving a cemented implant, compared to a 1% mortality rate observed for those receiving an uncemented implant ($p < 0.0001$)' [5].

In addition to these complications, there was an increased risk of cardiac failure following over-hydration during cementation by anaesthesiologists and, as life expectancy increases, there is concern about skeletal fixation of cemented devices in osteoporotic patients when the diameter of the medullary canal increases over time. If we acknowledge these risks and then compare this technique to cementless canal preparation and insertion, the differences are significant. Not only is there a lower risk of morbidity and mortality with cementless preparation, but it is a more rapid and reproducible procedure for surgeons in general.

Techniques

Cementless femoral canal preparation followed two separate courses between Europe and North America. In Europe, the broach-only technique was favoured as early as the 1970s. In North America, cementless THA began to become popularized in the 1980s, with a combination of reaming and broaching or reaming and milling of the femoral canal. The earliest proponent in North America of the ream and broach technique was Dr Charles Engh, with the AML® prosthesis (DePuy). The goal of this technique was to machine a cylindrical diaphyseal 'line-to-line fit' followed by broaching of the metaphyseal region (Fig. 3.18). This was a

common technique, simple and reproducible and has an excellent long-term track record.

The ream and mill technique was most commonly associated with the S-ROM® prosthesis (DePuy). Again, using a reamer, the diaphyseal canal was machined for a cylindrical 'line-to-line fit'. Proximally, the femoral metaphysis was milled and this was followed by positional calcar milling (Fig. 3.19). This technique in combination with the modular S-ROM® implant allows for infinite version options and excellent torsional stability.

Preparation of the femoral canal for the Corail® implant involves a 'broach-only' technique. There is no reaming of the femoral canal and the broach design differs from the typical diamond tooth broach pattern used following diaphyseal reaming. Where reaming the diaphyseal canal followed by broaching of the metaphysis with a diamond tooth broach typically crushes and extracts bone, a 'broach-only' technique with a chipped tooth or ribbed broach will radially compact and preserve bone (Fig. 3.20). Figure 3.21 shows a photomicrograph of an animal tibia demonstrating the difference between canal preparation with a diamond tooth and that with a chipped tooth broach. The larger teeth of the diamond tooth broach crush and remove cancellous bone whereas the smaller teeth of the chipped tooth broach actually compact the cancellous bone.

Evolution of cementless canal preparation

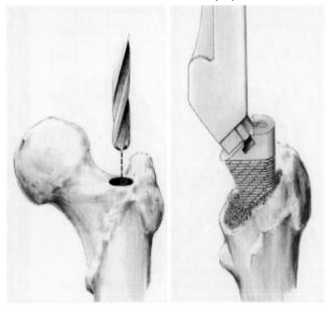

■ Ream and broach
  — Machine a cylindrical diaphyseal <u>line to line fit</u> with Prosthesis - AML

  — Broach the metaphyseal region

Fig. 3.18 Diagram of the reaming and broaching technique (Copyright DePuyInternational Limited)

Fig. 3.19 Diagram of the reaming and milling technique

Evolution of cementless canal preparation

- Ream and mill
  - Metaphyseal milling
  - Calcar milling

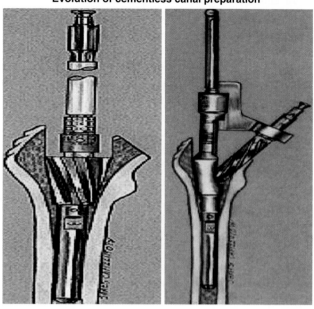

Evolution of cementless canal preparation

- Compaction broaching

- No reaming
- Different broach tooth design

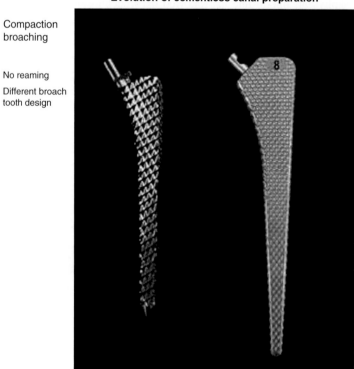

Fig. 3.20 Photograph of the diamond tooth and compaction broaches – note the difference in tooth design

Fig. 3.21 Photomicrograph demonstrating the difference in canal preparation when using diamond tooth versus compaction broaching

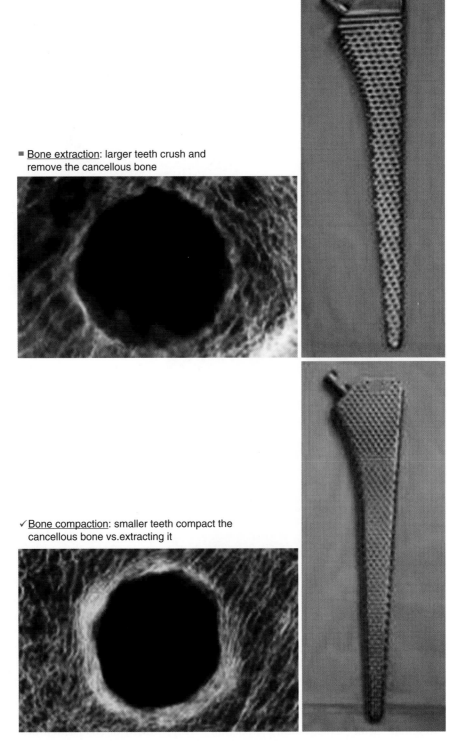

■ <u>Bone extraction</u>: larger teeth crush and remove the cancellous bone

✓<u>Bone compaction</u>: smaller teeth compact the cancellous bone vs.extracting it

Fig. 3.22 Close-up of the diamond tooth broach filled with extracted cancellous bone

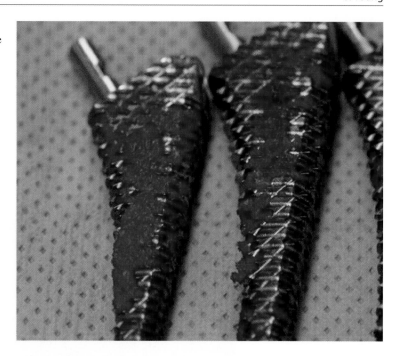

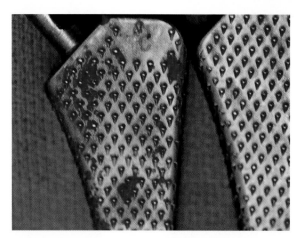

Fig. 3.23 Compaction broach (chipped tooth pattern) showing minimal bone extraction after use

In addition to the photomicrographs shown are intra-operative photographs of diamond tooth, chipped tooth and ribbed broaches demonstrating the marked difference in bone extraction seen with diamond tooth broaches and the minimal bone extraction with compaction broaching (Fig. 3.22–3.24).

The Advantages of Compaction Broaching

Compaction broaching has significant advantages beyond bone preservation. As discussed in detail in other chapters of this book (Sects. 2.1.3.2 and 2.1.3.3), preservation of the unique biochemical inductive compounds that reside within the host marrow is best achieved by the relatively atraumatic effect of compaction broaching of the femoral canal. Early in the evolution of cementless THA, David Hungerford and Peter Walker noted that 'In order to establish initial torsional stability, both clinical and laboratory studies have shown that a close geometric fit between the implant and the supporting bone is critical' [3, 6]. Bench-top laboratory studies have demonstrated that torsional stability is actually greater with compaction broaching than with reaming and broaching. In fact, torsional stability is improved with cemented femoral components in conjunction with compaction broaching as well [2]. Studies by Vail at Duke University compared reaming and broaching, reaming and milling, and compaction broaching for bone implant contact and demonstrated that bone implant contact was greatest with compaction broaching (Fig. 3.25) [1] (Vail TP, personal communication). Beyond this, prosthetic

Fig. 3.24 Corail® compaction broaches showing minimal bone extraction after use

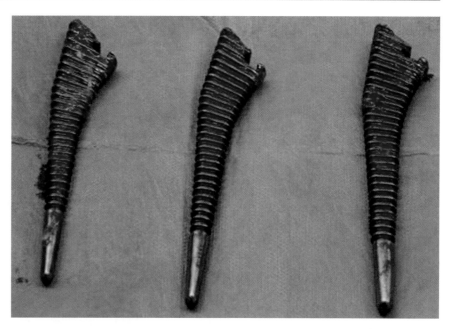

Benchtop analysis: improved bone implant contact with bone compaction

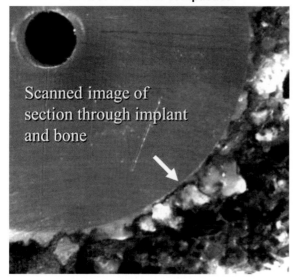

Scanned image of section through implant and bone

Fig. 3.25 Photomicrograph showing bone–implant contact with compaction broaching

fixation was greater in vivo using compaction broaching and this was demonstrated by bench-top analysis through pull-out testing.

Conclusion

In summary, femoral canal preparation through compaction broaching has biologic advantages in bone preparation; in addition, it has a biomechanical advantage of improved fixation and immediate torsional stability, and avoids the risks of morbidity and mortality associated with cement. The broach-only femoral canal preparation technique, specifically compaction broaching, is rapid and reproducible. It is clear why this is now the preferred technique of the majority of hip surgeons worldwide.

With compaction broaching, we are able to prepare the endosteal canal of the femur optimally to enhance the long-term fixation of the prosthesis implanted. In addition, through this technique we follow the dictum 'first do no harm'.

References

1. Channer MA, Glisson RR, Vail TP (1996) The use of bone compaction in total knee arthroplasty. J Arthroplasty 11(6):743–749
2. Chareancholvanich K et al (1997) Stability of primary cemented femoral implants with compaction of existing cancellous bone. In: 43rd annual meeting, Orthopaedic Research Society, Hilton Head Island, 1997, p 316

3. Coombs R, Gristina A, Hungerford D (eds) (1990) Joint replacement – state of the art. Orthotext, London
4. Cusmariu J, Glisson R, Seaber T et al (1998) Cortical strain associated with press-fit stems in revision total knee arthroplasty. J Bone Joint Surg Br 80(Suppl I):35
5. Lewallen D (2001) Current concepts in joint replacement (Lecture)
6. Walker PS, Schneeweis D, Murphy S et al (1987) Strains and micromotions of press-fit femoral stem prostheses. J Biomech 20:693–702. doi: 10.1016/0021-9290(87)90035-2

3.3.3 Restoring Femoral Anteversion: Let It Be

Sébastien Lustig and Tarik Aït Si Selmi

Restoring the anatomy in the horizontal plane is one of the keys to a successful arthroplasty. However, planning to restore the anteversion of a hip on an anteroposterior (AP) x-ray of the pelvis is not easy and there are only a few reports on this subject in the literature. In this chapter we report the results of a dedicated computed tomography (CT) study, the purpose of which was to determine to what extent the patient's original anteversion was restored using the Corail® stem. The horizontal positioning of the hip implant relies primarily on the stem design and to a lesser extent on the surgical technique.

Clinical Implications of the Femoral Stem Anteversion

When planning the implantation of a femoral stem, the surgeon's main concern is to restore the proximal anatomy of the femur. While the offset, the cutting angle and the varus or varus angle can easily be assessed using 'standard' x-rays, the position in the horizontal plane (the anteversion) is much more difficult to determine. There are mathematical formulae for the acetabulum, yet the only way to measure precisely the femoral anteversion is to use a CT scanner, which is never done in routine practice. Indeed, measuring the anteversion of the femur is not necessary when a Corail® stem is used (except in the case of major dysplasia), since the anteversion of the stem is imposed by its design.

Several authors (users of computer-assisted surgery [CAS]) have recently studied femoral anteversion and recognize the significant patient-to-patient variability of this parameter. Thus, the use of a stem with automatic positioning would make it possible to respect the patient's anteversion without formal measurement. The surgeon could then adjust the acetabular anteversion to achieve the required 'combined anteversion' (femur + acetabulum) [2].

Any modification of the femoral anteversion has clinical consequences. Firstly, incorrect anteversion can affect the *step angle*. This produces a tendency for the patient to walk with the foot in internal rotation if the femoral anteversion is too excessive and, conversely, with the foot externally rotated if the anteversion is less than normal.

Secondly, incorrect anteversion can affect the stability of the prosthesis, which will increase the likelihood of anterior dislocation, especially if the surgeon uses a postero-lateral approach. A large error also causes a reduction of the femoral *offset*, which in turn contributes to a reduction of the lever arm of the gluteus medius and an increase in prosthetic instability.

Thirdly, excessive anteversion can cause a *risk of impingement* (cam effect) between the posterior portion of the neck and the acetabulum. This in turn can cause metal–metal contact and potential anterior instability. Even without unwanted contact, a poor orientation of the femoral neck could create a zone of hyperpressure (anterior in the case of excessive anteversion). This may cause premature wear when a metal polyethylene (PE) bearing is used, or squeaking when a ceramic–ceramic bearing is used.

Analysis of 100 Patients Using Scanning Computer Tomography

Our intention was to investigate whether the use of the Corail® stem could reproduce the correct femoral anteversion. We therefore carried out a prospective study of 100 consecutive patients having primary total hip replacement for unilateral osteoarthritis. All patients were operated by the same surgeon, with the same surgical technique in the same institution. The surgeon (who was right-handed) used a mini-invasive postero-lateral approach with the patient in lateral decubitus. Each patient had a preoperative and post-operative CT scan to measure the femoral anteversion before and after implantation of the Corail® stem. The preoperative values of the femoral anteversion were only known to the surgeon after the procedure, so the surgeon was not aware of or influenced by these values during the implantation of the prosthesis.

The method used was validated using the contralateral side as the reference. The validation consisted of measuring the anteversion of the contralateral side both pre- and post-operatively in order to determine the difference (which should have been zero). The mean difference in these measurements was $0.05° ± 3.9°$.

This confirmed the reproducibility of the measurement to plus or minus a few degrees.

In our series 97 patients were analysed. For these 97 patients the mean increase in anteversion was $+3.5° ± 8.6°$. A significant difference ($p = 0.02$) was observed between the right hips ($n = 54$) and the left hips ($n = 43$). For the right hips the femoral anteversion had increased on average by $5.2° ± 8.9°$ (from $-10.1°$ to $15.3°$) and this increase was significant ($p = 0.002$) (Fig. 3.26). For the left hips the anteversion had increase on average by $1.3° ± 4.2°$ (from $-12.9°$ to $14.2°$), but this increase was not significant ($p = 0.23$) (Fig. 3.27).

The results of this study are given in Table 3.1. In this study the original anteversion was reproduced to within $5°$ in 45.3% of the cases, to within $10°$ in 82.5% of the cases and to within $15°$ in 90.7% of the cases.

Discussion

The stem anteversion is established by the first femoral broach, which reproduces the patient's femoral anteversion as it is hammered into the femoral canal. The calcar of the cut neck provides a guide to the anteversion necessary although the final version is dictated by the implant design itself. The initial broach should be implanted parallel to the posterior calcar of the neck (posterior approach) or slightly more anteverted than the anterior calcar (anterior or antero-lateral approach). The axis of the lower limb can also be used as a reference to the stem anteversion but is again only a guide. Then the broaches are driven in successively – with the same anteversion – until the required size is reached. As the definitive-sized broach is reached the anteversion will be 'fine-tuned' automatically by the broach. Broaching stops at the first size that is stable in rotation and in the longitudinal axis. Stability is achieved due to the compaction of the cancellous bone by the successive broaches. Cortical contact is not the intended end point. If the stem is inserted correctly, anteversion is quasi-automatic, ensured by the 'flaring' of the broach (which is the same as that of the prosthesis). Our scanner study has shown that in this way the femoral anteversion was reproduced satisfactorily.

With respect to positioning of the femoral stem in the horizontal plane, we consider that Computer Assisted Surgery (CAS) offers no significant advantage. The shape of the prosthesis imposes the correct

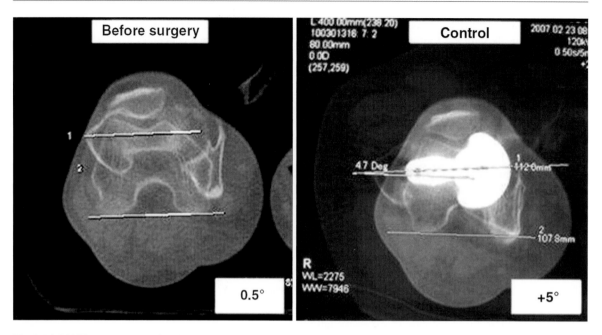

Fig. 3.26 RH Hip, 5° increase of the femoral anteversion

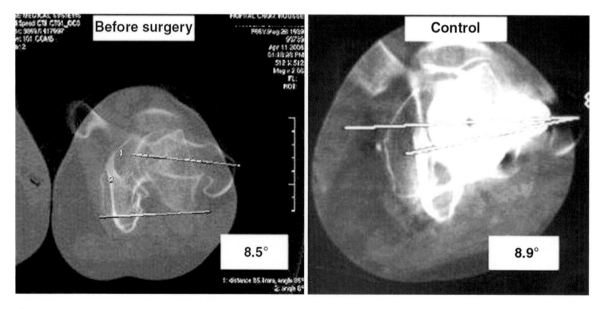

Fig. 3.27 LH Hip restoration of the femoral anteversion to the nearest 1°

anteversion, to within a few degrees, assuming that we use good surgical technique. The offset of the hip operated on, the handedness of the surgeon (right-handed or left-handed) and the surgical approach can affect this anteversion, but only to a limited extent. The anteversion of the stem is automatic to plus or minus a few degrees.

The results of this study confirm that the use of a *modular neck* is not necessary with the Corail® stem, since the correct anteversion is 'automatically' obtained to plus or minus 10° in 82.5% of cases. Moreover, the use of *large diameter heads* (36 mm in most cases) allows the 5–10° anteversion variation not to significantly affect stability, angle of motion and possible

Table 3.1 Results of the computer tomography study on 97 patients

	Anteversion		Anteversion modification	
	Preop	Postop	(Pre-op–post-op)	
Non-operated hip	13.2° ± 8.6°	13.2° ± 8.7°	0.05° ± 3.9°	NS
Global series	11.3° ± 9.2°	14.9° ± 9.7°	3.5° ± 8.6°	NS
RH hip (n = 54)	10.1° ± 8.7°	15.3° ± 10.4°	5.2° ± 8.9°*	P = 0.02
LH hip (n = 43)	12.9° ± 9.6°	14.2° ± 8.6°	1.3° ± 4.2°*	NS
	NS	NS	*P = 0.01	

neck–acetabulum impingement [1]. We also consider that the hip articulation has a certain amount of *adaptability* (a few degrees) to reproduce the step angle and demonstrates that an alteration of between 5° and 10° in anteversion with our current prostheses has no clinical consequences. Hence, we consider that restoring anteversion to within 15° in 91% of cases is satisfactory, particularly with the use of large diameter heads.

Conclusion

The Corail® stem enables the 'anatomical' femoral anteversion to be restored satisfactorily. There is no need for external landmarks, CAS or implant modularity. The surgeon simply needs to follow the anatomy of the femoral cut to reproduce the required anteversion.

References

1. Bargar W, Jamali A, Nejad A (2010) Femoral anteversion in THA and its lack of correlation with native acetabular anteversion. Clin Orthop 468:527–532
2. Dorr L, Malik A, Dastane M et al (2009) Combined anteversion technique for total hip arthroplasty. Clin Orthop 467:119–127

3.3.4 Specific Techniques for Specific Femurs: Variations on a Theme

Jean-Charles Rollier and Jean-Claude Cartillier

The Corail® stem implantation technique has already been described in Sect. 3.3.1. In this chapter, we describe the technical options available for implantation of this stem in some special cases. Abnormal bone shape or abnormal bone quality requires different techniques. In addition, various conditions such as Paget's disease or developmental dysplasia of the hip (DDH) may increase the complexity of the surgical procedure. Accurate preoperative planning and case-specific technical solutions can help the surgeon when these conditions occur. We believe that the Corail® stem is a suitable option in the management of most primary hip replacements.

Introduction

The main principles of conventional hip implantation with the Corail® stem have been described in Sect. 3.3.1. In exceptional cases, special surgical techniques may be needed to facilitate the reliable implantation of the Corail® stem. These techniques may be needed in cases where the shape of the femur is irregular, the bone quality is poor or a particular pathological process has

Surgical Technique According to the Femoral Morphology

The anatomical features of the proximal femur vary from individual to individual. These variations are dependent upon ethnicity or family characteristics. Intramedullary changes should be preoperatively identified during templating to decide the most appropriate surgical technique.

Three types of proximal femur are described in the Dorr classification (Fig. 3.28). Dorr type I and III femurs require specific techniques for correct implantation.

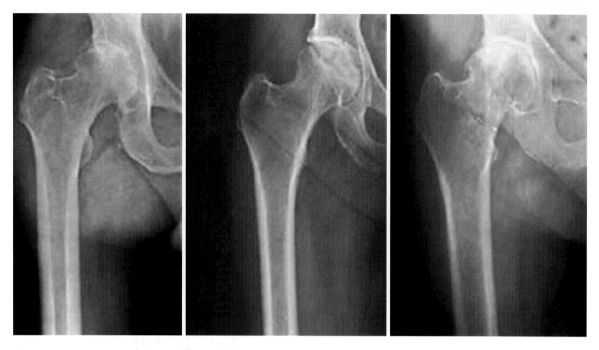

Fig. 3.28 Types of proximal femur using the Dorr classification: Dorr type I, left; Dorr type II, centre; Dorr Type III, right

Dorr Type I: The Champagne Flute Femur

The champagne flute femur has a wide metaphyseal region but a narrow diaphyseal segment usually surrounded by thick cortices. These femurs are at a greater risk for early diaphyseal blocking of the broach during femoral preparation. The application of excessive force while broaching increases the risk of femur fracture at the tip of the broach. Therefore, diaphyseal reaming is recommended to facilitate distal femoral broaching and to allow metaphyseal bone compaction. Rigid reamers of progressively increasing diameter must be used. These reamers will progressively enlarge the diaphysis. If templating and initial 'pathfinding' at surgery suggest the diaphysis is under 8 mm in diameter, rigid reamers should be used up to 11 mm. This will allow the insertion of a prosthesis with a better metaphyseal/diaphyseal match.

Dorr Type III: Stovepipe Femurs

Stovepipe femurs have a wide diaphyseal section with thin cortices. The cancellous bone required for the cancellous bone envelope of compaction broaching is

poor. It is still possible to use the Corail® in this situation. In such cases the size of the femoral broaches should be increased to fill the femoral canal with the implant, even if some cortical contact occurs. Such cortical contact is acceptable in these cases as a means of reducing the risk of femoral fracture. Broaching should be performed progressively by repeated broach insertion and progressive impaction up to the desired level at which good stability is achieved. This must be done cautiously and checks for rotational stability must only be done after axial stability has been achieved. The use of a collared stem is recommended in this case. If the obtained stability is not sufficient, a long revision Corail® stem (KAR™) should be used.

Dorr Type II Regular Femurs

This should be managed using the standard Corail® surgical technique.

Surgical Technique According to Bone Quality

Bone density decreases with age, but total hip arthroplasty (THA) is indicated even at the extreme of life regardless of age. Therefore, the femoral preparation must be adapted to take this variable into account. Two technically demanding situations may occur depending on bone quality at various stages of life such as when the bone is dense and compact, or when the bone is osteoporotic.

Dense and Compact Bone

The situation here is similar to the Dorr type I bone, but if the bone is particularly dense in the neck the entry point of the femoral component may be difficult to identify. The piriformis fossa acts as a valuable anatomical landmark. The canal explorer can be very useful in this situation in determining the alignment of the femoral canal. Cancellous bone compaction with the punch should be avoided due to the already high density of the bone. Broaching is initiated beginning with the smallest size (size 7 or 8). Rigid reamers of progressively increasing size may be used to prepare the diaphyseal region, if necessary. Care should be taken to maintain the correct orientation during broaching in order to avoid early cortical contact. Sequential broaching should be performed with great caution to reduce the risk of metaphyseal cracking.

Osteoporotic Bone

The osteoporotic femur is typically a Dorr type III femur. Preservation of metaphyseal cancellous bone is essential due to its low density. It is important to emphasize two points. Firstly, broaching is a very delicate procedure. Small taps on the broach should be used rather than heavy blows. Secondly, rotational stability should be assessed once axial stability has been achieved. This is important to maintain a bone envelope around the broach. When the bone is osteoporotic, a larger implant than that used in younger patients is commonly selected. Careful sizing of the stem is crucial to not undersize and subside, or oversize and risk fracture. The use of a collared stem in this situation is mandatory.

Surgical Technique After Fracture or Osteotomy

These two conditions require specific surgical techniques.

After Osteosynthesis

Insertion of a femoral stem at this time may be challenging. Residual evidence of pre-existing devices or fractures should be taken into account. There is a risk of stem deviation at the level of residual screw and nail holes. The presence of callus bone may also compromise the femoral preparation. It is important to check the broach orientation on a regular basis.

Osteotomy or Malunion

In these cases thorough preoperative planning is essential and a computed tomography (CT) examination may be needed to check for the existence of a rotational malunion. If a malunion is evident, a derotation osteotomy may be needed. The use of a longer Corail® Revision Stem (KAR™) might then be necessary. If varus malunion is observed, a trench may be created in the greater trochanter to ensure that the broaches and stem can be inserted. If there are changes in bone density, the greatest care must be taken and reaming must be done cautiously.

Surgical Technique According to the Aetiology

Femoral preparation may be more technically demanding in certain conditions.

Developmental Dysplasia of the Hip (Dislocation)

Excess femoral anteversion and a small upper metaphyseal region are commonly seen in patients with developmental dysplasia of the hip (DDH). The use of a Corail® stem (KA6 – collared, size 6, dysplasia stem) specifically designed for hip dysplasia is a valuable option. It is a shorter, straight, quadrangular stem featuring a horizontal neck component, which requires a horizontal neck cut.

In the case of a high hip dislocation prosthetic repositioning in the true hip centre may lead to limb length discrepancy and sciatica. A subtrochanteric femoral shortening osteotomy (± derotation) would then be advisable to avoid these complications. Femoral shortening osteotomies must be accurately planned.

Paget's Disease

Paget's bone may be highly vascular, fragile and sclerotic. Intra-operative blood loss may be reduced with administration of diphosphonates preoperatively. Thorough preoperative planning should be performed to help determine the intramedullary entry point and the axis of broach insertion. The intramedullary canal may be non-existent, which means the entry point for broaching, and broaching itself, must be carried out with care. In some cases intra-operative radiographic assessment might be helpful to determine stem position.

Rheumatoid Arthritis

This situation leads to poor bone quality, particularly after long-term steroid. The precautionary measures are similar to those taken in osteoporotic patients.

When arthroplasty is associated with *lytic lesions of the proximal femur*, bridging the defect is essential. Therefore, a longer Corail® Revision Stem (KAR™) is frequently used to provide enhanced stability over a greater distance. The defect can be filled with autograft bone from the patient's femoral head. Delayed full weight-bearing may be necessary.

Bone Islands

In some cases, *dense benign tumors (bone island)* may cause the broach to deviate as it is being inserted and may lead to mal-orientation. To avoid this problem, inter-operative radiographs should be taken.

Conclusion

In some femurs the standard surgical technique may need to be modified and a case-specific procedure used. The Corail® stem can be used in the majority of these specific cases. However, these situations can be successfully anticipated with meticulous preoperative planning combined with simple technical tricks. In this way it is possible to obtain a hip replacement stem that fits perfectly.

3.3.5 Intra-Operative Complications: How to Get Out of the Hole

Sam Sydney

Intra-operative complications while preparing the femur to accept the Corail® stem will be examined in this chapter. This is not an exhaustive examination of all complications, but will focus on those complications which occur with some frequency with the Corail® hip system. Oversizing and fracture; component malposition, varus/valgus or rotational malposition; leg length discrepancy; and avoidance of nerve damage and vascular injury will be considered. Oversizing and fracture is a complication that occurs because of the unique bone impaction technique employed with the Corail® system. The broaching technique involves bone impaction as opposed to bone extraction. Hence, careful evaluation is needed before going from one broach size to the next.

Introduction

> If you ever find yourself in a hole, stop digging.
>
> — Will Rogers

> Our greatest glory is not in never falling, but in getting up every time we do.
>
> — Confucius

Hip replacement is arguably one of the most successful surgical procedures, adding to patients' quality of life. This chapter will deal with intra-operative complications. The best way to avoid them is to anticipate and avoid the problem.

Preoperative Planning and Templating

Preoperative planning and templating is the best way to anticipate any unusual intra-operative findings such as increased anteversion and femoral deformity – either developmental, post-traumatic or post-surgical. Preoperative templating identifies the ideal level of neck resection. With the Corail® system, preoperative templating serves only as a guide to the final size of the stem, as often bone quality and the ability to compress cancellous bone will result in a size smaller than pre-operative templating would suggest.

Overstuffing, Fracture

Preparation of the canal to accept the Corail® stem is dependent on the philosophy of optimal fill rather than fit and fill. As opposed to removing cancellous bone and filling the void created with an implant, the Corail® system preserves cancellous bone and compresses the bone creating a uniform biologic bone bed. Templating serves only as a guide for the femoral size used. Corail® broaches are bone compaction broaches as opposed to bone extraction broaches, as seen in Fig. 3.29a and b. Corail® broaches, after having been used in preparing the canal, will be removed relatively clean and devoid of cancellous bone.

Once the appropriate lateral starting point is identified, axial impaction of the broach is performed. Broaches of increasing size are used until axial stability is achieved, that is until the broach will not progress or

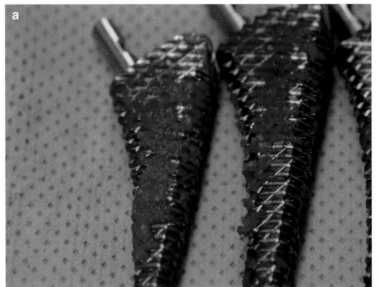

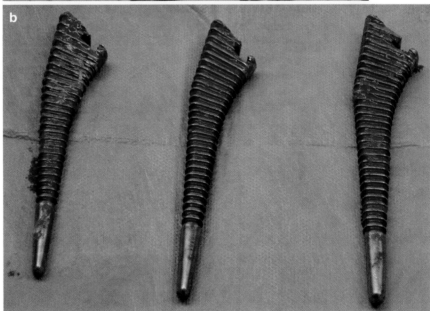

Fig. 3.29 (**a**) Summit broaches (sizes 1, 2, 3,) showing cancellous bone being removed with each broach (**b**) Corail® broaches (sizes 8, 9, 10) minimal bone removed with each broach

subside into the femoral canal. At that point, rotational stability is checked. Checking for rotational stability before axial stability is achieved results in a malformed cancellous bone bed in the proximal femur, forcing larger-sized implants to be used and risking fracture.

Note: often a change in pitch is heard during impaction when the cancellous bone is adequately compressed.

When to Progress to the Next Size?

During preparation of the femoral canal sometimes the decision as to when to proceed to the next size of broach can be difficult. Countersinking the broach about a quarter of an inch (6 mm) will often allow the surgeon to safely proceed to the next size. If the next size of broach does not adequately go down the canal, then the previous size should be used. This implant will seat further down the canal, but will have excellent stability: a longer neck may need to be used.

Fracture

When a fracture of the femur is identified, most commonly the fracture will be located in the medial calcar region. The extent of the fracture needs to be identified. The incidence of intra-operative femoral fracture for all systems is reported to be between 1% and 5 % [1–4]. Should a fracture be identified, the implant or broach needs to be removed and the fracture needs to be stabilized with a cerclage wire. In this circumstance it is recommended to use a collared version of the stem to further protect from subsidence, but this is not essential. It is very unusual for other types of femoral fractures to occur, but should they occur, standard fixation techniques should be employed (Fig. 3.30).

Mal-Position

Varus/valgus – often this is identified in a post-operative x-ray. Determination must be made as to whether this is true varus/valgus as opposed to apparent varus/valgus. The x-ray should be evaluated for lateral stem parallelism. With the Corail® system, varus/valgus position of the stem appears to be very well tolerated and can result in an excellent clinical outcome.

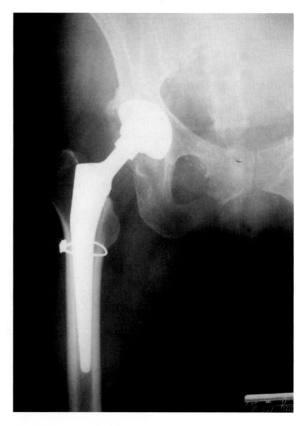

Fig. 3.30 AP radiograph showing proximal femoral fracture treated with a cerclage wire, stable fixation

Rotational Mal-Position

The best way to avoid rotational mal-position complications is to have good information preoperatively as to the relative version of the femoral neck and to have adequate visualization of the proximal femur intra-operatively. In the majority of cases, a femoral anteversion of between 15° and 20° should be aimed for. The broaches with the Corail® system tend to follow and seat in the natural host anteversion. The surgeon should always employ landmarks, local or distal, to ensure the desired version is achieved. Local landmarks include rotation of the stem relative to the neck osteotomy angle. Distal landmarks include rotation of the stem relative to the flexed knee or the axis of the distal femur. If gross mal-rotation is identified, the broach or stem needs to be removed and reinserted in the desired rotation. Proximal femoral cancellous autograft may be required to fill the bony voids created. Computer navigation may also help avoid this complication.

Stem Does Not Fully Seat

If the trial broaches sit fully, the stem will sit fully, provided it is inserted in the same direction. If the stem gets hung up, it should be removed and put in the correct position. The stem should initially be inserted by hand. It should seat to about a finger's breadth from its final position before impaction with a mallet begins. This guide should be followed in all cases. Removal of a mal-positioned stem can be very difficult. A stem that is inserted down the canal in a position that is not correctly prepared by broaching can result in fracture.

Leg Length Discrepancy

The goal of hip replacement arthroplasty is to achieve a stable hip that reconstitutes normal soft tissue tension. The surgeon should rely on adequate preoperative templating and planning to determine acetabular position and femoral neck resection level. The surgeon should also employ a method of measuring leg length that he/she is most comfortable with – either intra-operative landmarks, pin measurement guides, clinical measurement of leg length, x-ray calibration or computer navigation. Preoperative assessment and discussion with the patient about their perception of their leg length and the potential for leg length discrepancy needs to be carried out in all cases.

Nerve Damage

This complication is often related to preoperative variation in anatomy, scarring and tension of the soft tissues. Nerves commonly affected are the sciatic, obturator, femoral and lateral femoral cutaneous nerves. Careful handling of soft tissue and careful placement of retractors can largely eliminate this complication. Damage to the lateral femoral cutaneous nerve is most commonly seen with the anterior hip approach (modified Smith-Peterson). This complication can be largely eliminated by making an incision lateral to the path of the lateral femoral cutaneous nerve and dissecting the interval between the tensor fascia lata muscle and sartorius. This can be achieved by staying within the facial envelope of the tensor fascia lata muscle. Should this complication occur, it often resolves over time.

Vascular Injury

This is a known, but exceedingly rare, complication of hip replacement arthroplasty and is not dealt with in this chapter.

Conclusion

The Corail® femoral stem has been inserted for the last 25 years with no change in its intra-osseous design. It has proved to be a very reliable stem. Once the art of preparation by compaction of the cancellous bone bed is learned, it is a very reproducible and rewarding stem to use. Pitfalls that accompany all cementless stems can occur with the Corail® hip system, but with careful preoperative planning, templating and careful preparation of the femoral canal, these complications can be avoided.

References

1. Berry D (2002) Management of periprosthetic fractures; the hip. J Arthroplasty 17:11–13
2. Duncan CP, Masri BA (1996) Fractures of the femur after hip replacement. Instr Course Lect 44:293–304
3. Reis MD (1997) Hip arthroplasty: management problems; periprosthetic fractures; early and late. Orthopedics 20: 789–800
4. Taylor MM, Meyers MH, Harvey JP Jr (1978) Intraoperative femur fractures during total hip replacement. Clin Orthop Relat Res 137:96–103

3.4 Post-operative Management and Complications: All's Well That Ends Well

Bruno Balaÿ and Claude Charlet

The overall performance of hydroxyapatite-coated (HAC) implants compares well with that of both cemented and cementless implants. We report a study of 2,577 patients operated on between 1986 and 2007. All patients operated on in a single centre are reported as all had a Corail® prosthesis implanted on the femoral side. The results are reported and then recommendations made about routine post-operative management protocol, and the treatment for the complications reported.

Standard Post-Operative Management

In our study the mean hospital stay was 10 days. The patient was allowed to walk using crutches. The patient was allowed to fully weight-bear on the day after surgery. The crutches were normally discarded between 7 and 21 days.

- Physiotherapy was provided to assist the patient in walking. Standard precautions to prevent hip dislocation were given to the patient according to the approach made to the hip. No massage was given.
- Antibiotics were used prophylactically for a period of 24–48 h.
- Anticoagulant treatment consisted of low molecular–weight heparin (LMWH) followed by anti–vitamin K drugs, up to the 21st postoperative day. Support stockings were prescribed until the patient's return to normal activity.
- No treatment was given to prevent heterotopic ossification routinely. However, in ten patients Indometacin was given to prevent any ossification occurring.

Our protocol has remained unchanged except that the hospital stay has been reduced. The average stay in hospital is now 1 week.

Complications

Medical Complications

In our study 3.7% of cases had thromboembolic problems:

1. There were 80 cases of deep vein thrombosis. These patients were investigated with Doppler studies to confirm a thromboembolism and were treated with a curative regime of anti-coagulants.
2. Thirteen patients suffered pulmonary embolism. They were treated with a curative regime of anti-coagulants.
3. Four patients had a heparin allergy and were treated with Orgaran.
4. Three patients died within the first post-operative week (one patient had a myocardial infarction, one patient had a pulmonary embolism and one died from unknown causes).

We recommend anti-coagulant prophylaxis be used in all patients coming for hip surgery.

Early Surgical Complications

In our study we had the following early surgical complications.

1. Haematomas

Significant haematomata were observed in 1.33% of cases, and this is comparable with the incidence reported in the literature which ranges from 0.09% to 3.07% [3]. In 20 cases we observed superficial haematomas and in 16 cases there were deep-seated haematomas.

Ultrasonography was usually used to diagnose the condition. Surgical revision was performed in three cases urgently when there was evidence of vascular and nerve compression.

2. Infections

Seventeen cases of infection were reported within the first 90 days, which is a rate of 0.66%. We note that the incidence of infections reported in the literature varies from 0.5% to 2% [2, 9, 10]. We treated the infections as outlined in our recommendations below and we had no recurrence of infections.

We recommend antibiotic prophylaxis be used in all cases. Infection is a serious complication [8] which can be challenging to treat. We suggest a graded response strategy should be implemented as treatment for infections. In early diagnosed cases antibiotics can be administered. The choice of antibiotics should target known sensitivities of the organisms involved. This treatment protocol can only be used infrequently. In the majority of early infections occurring within the first 3–4 post-operative weeks we recommend surgical debridement and washout of the joint. At the time of this washout the revisable parts of the prosthesis, that is the acetabular liner and the femoral head, should be changed and the patient should be followed up with a prolonged course of antibiotics which may last from 3 to 12 months depending on the bacterial sensitivities. If the infection is of longer duration, we recommend surgical treatment with both stem and cup removal and subsequent re-implantation. One- or two-stage exchanges have been used in our series depending on the clinical situation. A two-stage replacement was used in clinically deeper infections if, for example a fistula was present or there were multi-resistant bacteria.

We recommend the use or re-implanting of an HAC stem. Our results have shown equally good results with cementation techniques.

3. Dislocations

In our study this was the most common complication after total hip arthroplasty (THA) [1, 2].

The incidence in our series was very low (1%). This compares with reports in the literature which range from 2.9% to 3.9% [6]. Our last 1,000 patients were operated on through a minimally invasive approach and our rate of dislocation reduced to 0.35%. In our study the surgery was carried out through an antero-lateral surgical approach, which we recognize does have a dislocation rate two or three times lower than a posterior approach [4]. The femoral head dislocated posteriorly in 85% of our cases.

We could not establish a correlation between dislocation and aetiology as, by far, the majority of our patients had osteoarthritis, and while we recognize that patients with avascular necrosis or hip replacements following a femoral neck fracture are at a higher risk for hip dislocation, this was not seen in our series. It was evident that the size of the femoral head was a contributing factor as 90% of the dislocated heads had a small diameter (28 mm).

Femoral implant mal-positioning was observed in those patients that had a dislocation. The Corail® insertion technique means that the implant follows the normal femoral anteversion and therefore this was not a

problem. However, leg length and offset problems explained why the dislocation had occurred in some instances.

On the acetabular side, the mal-positioning happened more frequently. This was apparent as excessive cup inclination or incorrect version.

We recommend that dislocation can be minimized by the following:

(a) The use of an anterior or antero-lateral surgical approach.
(b) If a posterior approach is used a meticulous repair of the posterior capsule and muscle reinsertion must be made.
(c) Femoral head diameters of 32 or 36 mm should be used.
(d) Care should be taken to ensure the cup is orientated correctly. We recommend the use of the transverse acetabular ligament (TAL) to dictate the version of the cup and we recommend that inclination of the cup should be less than 45°.

If a dislocation does occur, we recommend the following treatment plan:

(a) For a primary hip dislocation, we recommend a reduction of the joint under a general anaesthetic.
(b) Surgical revision should not be considered after just a single episode of dislocation unless there is major acetabular or femoral mal-positioning.
(c) Surgical revision is recommended after the third episode of dislocation. Usually there is a technical problem and correction of this problem will ensure a normal recovery. However, investigation, identification and correction of any other risk factors should be carried out prior to the revision surgery.
(d) If there is a problem that cannot be corrected, for example with a muscular weakness, or if the cause of the dislocation is unidentified, a bipolar cup should be used.
(e) The use of elevated rims or anti-dislocation acetabular cups is not ideal as these are associated with a higher risk of impingement and loosening, and, paradoxically, of dislocations.

4. Periprosthetic fractures

In our series we had a 0.38% rate of periprosthetic fracture. This compares with the literature in which the rate varies from 0.1% to 2.3% [7]. Our results suggest that cementless fixation was not a contributory factor. Early periprosthetic fractures in our series were clearly post-traumatic causes. When they occurred late, they were usually associated with more minor trauma reflecting that with increasing age osteoporosis increases the bone fragility and the risk of fracture.

Collared stems help prevent the risk of periprosthetic fracture occurring during the first post-operative months. The use of collared stems did not correlate with late-stage fractures associated with loosening.

We recommend treatment based on the Vancouver classification (Fig. 3.31).

Type A fractures can be managed conservatively unless there is significant displacement of the lesser or greater trochanters. In these cases osteosynthesis is necessary. A calcar fracture may require wiring (Fig. 3.32a–c).

In type B1 fractures, osteosynthesis by means of a cerclage wire is the appropriate treatment.

In type B2 and B3 fractures, the Corail® prosthesis should be converted to a long-stem Corail® (KAR™ prosthesis) or an extra-long-stem Corail® (Reef® prosthesis). We suggest that using cement is not appropriate and HAC implants appear to offer the best treatment option.

Type C fractures can be managed with open reduction and internal fixation with a plate or with an extra long stem to provide an intramedullary nailing of the fracture. We favour this method even if this means having to change a stable primary implant.

5. Heterotopic ossifications

In our study we had 4.5% of our cases with evidence of heterotopic ossification. This compares favourably with that reported in the literature, which is from 5–10% [11]. Our low rate suggests that HAC is not a contributing factor. We reported the cases in our series according to the Brooker classification:

Stage I – 72% of cases.
Stage II – 15% of cases.
Stage III – 12% of cases (no patient in this category required re-operation).
Stage IV was not observed.

We do not recommend the routine use of any specific treatment for the risk of heterotopic ossification. We do note that the pathological process starts early and

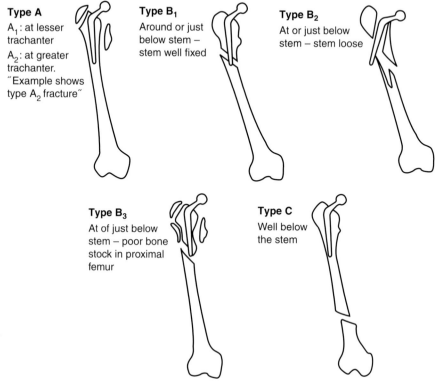

Type A
A₁: at lesser trachanter
A₂: at greater trachanter.
"Example shows type A₂ fracture"

Type B₁
Around or just below stem – stem well fixed

Type B₂
At or just below stem – stem loose

Type B₃
At of just below stem – poor bone stock in proximal femur

Type C
Well below the stem

Fig. 3.31 Vancouver classification (VanFlandern [12]. With permission from SLACK Incorporated)

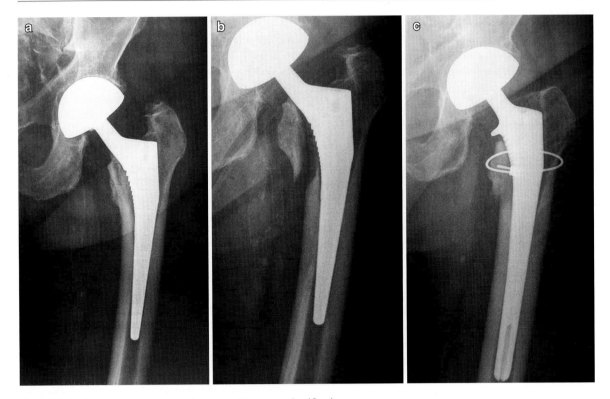

Fig. 3.32 (a–c) Type A fracture according to the Vancouver classification

therefore if prevention is to be initiated treatment should be started on the day of surgery. Medical treatment, if it is given for a patient who has had previous heterotopic ossification elsewhere or has visible ossification occurring, should consist of either Indocid or radiotherapy.

Surgical treatment should only be considered in the latter cases. It may take 2 years for the process to stop. Radiographic and scintigraphic scans must be carried out to ensure the process has stopped and surgical treatment should be preceded by and combined with medical and radiotherapy treatments for better effectiveness.

6. Limb lengthening

We stress the use of preoperative templating to prevent leg lengthening. Effective preoperative planning should allow the surgeon to accurately restore leg length and offset. At the time of surgery using the appropriately sized femoral component and introducing it with the recommended technique should prevent the stem not seating and therefore causing leg length discrepancy. If, however, the femoral stem cannot be seated to within a few millimetres of the required position, the implant can be downsized and seated properly with the use of a collar. If the limb lengthening is recognized post-operatively and is greater than 15 mm it may require re-operation. This can be achieved by converting the standard Corail® stem to a Coxa Vara stem (Corail® type KLA).

7. Stem subsidence without fracture

In our series stem subsidence was observed within the first 3 post-operative months in 0.19% of patients. The subsidence varied from 1.5 to 3 mm. We did not need to perform any revision because of stem subsidence. The stem subsided in the early post-operative period and then stabilized, achieving good secondary stability.

We recommend that if the subsidence is just a few millimetres, the implant will stabilize and will need no further treatment. If the subsidence does continue and the implant has been undersized, surgery may be necessary to prevent limping or instability from the shortened leg. If subsidence has occurred early and x-ray examination shows a fracture, we recommend surgery be performed to correct the stem subsidence and treat the calcar crack with cerclage wiring.

The use of a collar will reduce the risk of subsidence.

8. Unexplained hip pain

In our series unexplained hip pain was rare. Thigh pain was rarely reported, which may be attributable to the full length of HAC stem.

We recommend that in cases of unexplained hip pain a full history and clinical examination be carried out, and also a standard radiograph be performed. If no cause is found from this baseline assessment, further investigations should be carried out. A computed tomography (CT) scan may reveal a calcar crack or stress fracture in the pelvis. A bone scan may suggest loosening or sepsis. A hip aspiration may confirm the presence of sepsis.

If these investigations are negative, one should consider the following possibilities:

Pain in the greater trochanter region may be caused by excessive offset, leading to tendonitis of the gluteus medius or trochanteric bursitis.

Pain in the inguinal region may be caused by psoas tendinitis.

Late Surgical Complications

Specific long-term complications were observed.

1. Radiolucent lines

In our series radiolucent lines were a very rare occurrence. The precise aetiology of the lines was not fully understood. It was felt that they were most frequently seen in the metaphyseal region and were thought to represent the fact that the highest bone implant elasticity gradient occurred there. They remained static and asymptomatic.

We recommend that radiolucent lines do need to be assessed and followed. If they are present, they tend to occur in GRUEN zones 1 and 7 or 8 and 14. They fall into two categories:

(a) A radiolucent line which is a dense line 1 or 2 mm from the implant surface and outlines a clear area between the cancellous bone and the implant.

(b) A reactive line which is a dense linear image, running parallel to the implant surface and situated 2 mm from it. The area between it and the implant is of equal bone density and a match to the bone on the other side of the reactive line.

2. Osteolysis images

In our series, osteolysis occurred in post-operative radiographs infrequently. It was most often seen as a small calcar scalloping or a small lytic lesion in the greater trochanter. No osteolytic lesions were seen beyond this.

We recommend that should any lytic lesions be seen, they should be followed radiographically.

3. Loosening

In our series we did not have any cases of aseptic loosening.

We are, however, aware that loosening has occurred in some centres and we make the following recommendations:

(a) *Technical mistakes*:
  (i) Undersizing: Undersizing may lead to failure of the osseointegration process and subsidence. If this complication is detected, revision surgery should be performed and a larger prosthesis implanted.
  (ii) Inappropriate management of type A femurs: It is important to understand the basic philosophy of the Corail® implant, which must gain both metaphyseal and diaphyseal support to achieve its mechanical and then biological fixation. In type A femurs the exceptional thickness of the cortices in the diaphysis means that a small stem is inserted but becomes tight in the diaphysis

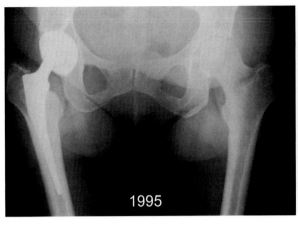
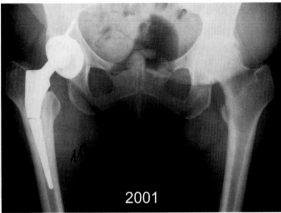

Fig. 3.33 Type A femur – distally blocked prosthesis 'Windscreen effect'

and is not supported in the larger metaphysis. This gives a combination of distal locking but inadequate proximal support and fixation. This leads to thigh pain, cortical thickening in the midsection of the stem on x-ray, proximal radiolucent lines suggesting proximal instability and in extreme situations implant fracture above the locked area (Fig. 3.33). It is preferable to recognize this particular pattern of femur prior to surgery and if necessary distally ream the cortical bone to allow a better match of proximal and distal fixation. If this complication is only recognized following implant insertion, surgical revision sometimes becomes necessary.

(iii) Varus or valgus positioning of the stem: Although seen radiographically in certain cases and may be considered a technical mistake, long-term follow-up of these patients has shown this is a radiographic issue and not a clinic issue. There are no long-term problems with this positioning of the stem.

(b) *Secondary complications to loosening*:
   (i)   Sepsis
   (ii) Cyst formation

4. Stress shielding

In our series stress shielding was uncommon and only seen in osteoporotic patients with large-diameter femoral canals. Osteopaenia of the proximal femur during prosthesis implantation has been frequently found by Vidalain. This phenomenon is less frequent with a Corail® stem compared to other implants [5].

Conclusion

Our series suggests that insertion of the Corail® prosthesis is reliable, offering a rapid post-operative rehabilitation and a small complication rate. The learning curve is short. There appear to be no specific HAC-related complications. The Corail® prosthesis has been described as a 'forgiving' implant by users and our large study supports this.

Key Points

> Hydroxyapatite (HA) is not responsible for any specific complications.
> The full coating of the stem with HA has no damaging effects and may even contribute to the good quality of long-term clinical and radiographic results.
> The very low complication rate explains why there has been no change required to the design of the Corail® prosthesis over the past 25 years.
> Revision of the well-fixed stem is exceptional, but can be done safely using a standard implant. This helps provide good preservation of the existing bone stock.

References

1. Blom AW, Rogers M, Taylor AH (2008) Dislocation following total hip replacement: the Avon Orthopaedic Centre experience. Ann R Coll Surg Engl 90(8):658–662
2. Bozic KJ, Kurtz SM (2009) The epidemiology of revision total hip arthroplasty in the United States. J Bone Joint Surg Am 91:128–133
3. Brown GD, Swanson EA, Nercessian OA (2008) Neurologic injuries after hip arthroplasty. Am J Ortho (Belle Mead NJ) 37(4):191
4. Busch JR, Wilson M (2007) Dislocation after hip hemiarthroplasty: anterior versus posterior capsular approach. Orthopedics 30(2):138–144
5. Karachalios T, Tsatsaronis C, Efraimis G et al (2004) The long-term clinical relevance of calcar atrophy caused by stress shielding in total hip arthroplasty: A 10-year, prospective, randomized study. J Arthroplasty 19(4):469–475
6. Kwon MS, Kuskowwski M, Mulhall KJ (2006) Does surgical approach affect total hip arthroplasty dislocation rates? Clin Orthop Relat Res 447:34–38
7. Lewallen DG, Berry DJ (1997) Periprosthetic fracture of the femur after total hip arthroplasty. J Bone Joint Surg Am 79:1181–1190
8. Mamoudy P (2009) Traitement des prothèses totales de hanches infectées. Conférences d'enseignement SOFCOT, 74–93
9. Moyad TF, Thornhill T, Estok D (2008) Evaluation and management of the infected total hip and knee. Orthopedics 31(6):581–588
10. Urquhart DM, Hanna FS, Brennan SL, Wluka AE (2010) Incidence and risk factors for deep surgical site infection after primary total hip arthroplasty: a systematic review. J Arthroplasty 25(8): 1216-22.e3
11. Vastel L, Kerboul L, Antrac T (1998) Ossification hétérotopique après arthroplastie totale de hanche. Rev Rhum Engl Ed 65:238–244
12. VanFlandern GJ (2005) Periprosthetic fractures in total hip arthroplasty. Orthopedics 28(9 Suppl):s1089–s1095

Corail® Outcomes

4

Scott Brumby

Contents

J.-P. Vidalain et al. (eds.), *The CORAIL® Hip System*,
DOI: 10.1007/978-3-642-18396-6_4, © Springer-Verlag Berlin Heidelberg 2011

4.1 Critical Appraisal of the Published Literature: Evidence-Based Medicine

Emilio Romanini and Attilio Santucci

The critical appraisal of the available literature together with clinical expertise is essential for the practice of evidence-based orthopaedic surgery. Good-quality clinical research provides the basis for a rational approach to evaluating and allowing the sensible and skilled application of best evidence to individual patients. This is particularly important in the adult joint replacement specialty which presents increasing volumes, the continual introduction of high-cost and relatively unproven devices into the marketplace and wide regional variations in practice patterns. Orthopaedic surgeons should gain knowledge of the most relevant issues in clinical epidemiology to be able to search and evaluate the best evidence, both in terms of type (levels of evidence) and quality of the study (outcome measures). A wide variety of scores, based on radiographs, physician assessment and patient reported outcomes are currently used to evaluate total hip arthroplasty (THA) results. The aim of this chapter is to provide a guide to the interpretation of clinical research data, in order to examine the effectiveness and safety of hip arthroplasty in general and of the Corail® stem in particular within the following chapters of this book.

Total Hip Arthroplasty: The Operation of the Century

Total hip arthroplasty (THA) has been described as the operation of the century by Learmonth et al. [6]. Only few medical treatments are able to provide such an impressive benefit to a large population of patients affected by a disabling group of conditions. THA has been adopted worldwide for the treatment of degenerative and traumatic hip problems and the worldwide number of operations is projected to continue to increase, especially in the younger population. In Italy, the total number of THAs in 2007 was close to 80,000 cases, with an almost 5% yearly increase in the last 7 years.

However, many issues are still under debate: including the role of new devices and materials in extending the long-term success of an already highly successful procedure. Unfortunately, not all attempts to improve outcomes have been successful and in some instances the early introduction of new technology has resulted in poor patient outcome.

The aim of this chapter is to provide a guide to the interpretation of clinical research data in order to examine the effectiveness and safety of hip arthroplasty in general and of Corail® in particular. It will aid the orthopaedic surgeon in making choices on the basis of the best available evidence.

Clinical Research and Hip Arthroplasty: Study Design Issues

Good-quality clinical research can provide answers to relevant questions. It is mandatory for the orthopaedic surgeon to become skilled at researching the best available published evidence to evaluate the effectiveness of the available devices and make the right choices for their patients [12, 13].

The National Institute for Clinical Excellence (NICE) in the UK published in 2000 (and reviewed in 2003) a guide for the selection of hip prostheses by arthroplasty surgeons and healthcare providers [9]. The panel assessed and graded the published literature in a structured manner. They have specified an acceptable revision rate, which is 10% or less at 10 years following implantation. Based on the NICE guidelines, the Corail® stem has a 10A rating, which is the best available rating.

Randomised controlled trials (RCTs) are generally agreed to be the most powerful methods to evaluate a medical procedure, providing robust estimates of treatment effects and therefore they are regarded as being in the highest-quality level of evidence. However, in some cases observational studies (of a lower-quality level) may present advantages over RCTs, as the design of the latter may be affected by feasibility concerns, such as the length of follow-up required to define the long-term performance of a THA. Moreover, in order to establish causality, a well-designed RCT must show high internal validity, which is gained at the expense of external validity. An RCT may answer a specific question, but as a consequence of limited surgeon involvement and restricted patient population, there may be difficulty in extrapolating these findings to community practice in order to achieve a beneficial outcome. Examples of this are when specific expertise and infrastructure used within the trial are not available in 'the real world' or when a technology has been outdated during the time of publication of the results.

This is why observational studies still play a key role in understanding the clinical outcome of THA. Most of the so-called level IV studies are single surgeon or institution case series, as are some of the studies provided in the following chapters of this book.

A more powerful example of observational studies are the arthroplasty registries, pioneered in Scandinavia in the late 1970s and now active in a growing number of nations, including Italy. Available data on Corail® stem from three major registries (Norway, Australia and UK) are presented in Sect. 4.3, depicting excellent long-term survivorship of the Corail® stem in 'the real world'.

Whilst the main outcome of joint registries is to provide survivorship outcome for implant type, patient demographics and reasons for revision, registries offer unique community-based comparative data on large patient numbers that could never be obtained through a clinical trial. The analysis of registry data provides insight into broad-based issues such as the impact of clinical experience or surgical skill and the comparison between different types of healthcare delivery systems (academic versus rural hospitals, low- versus high-volume hospitals) [4].

Statistical analysis of THA failure is generally performed using techniques such as Kaplan–Meier analysis and Cox regression; however, some methodological problems have been highlighted and discussed, including long follow-up times and low failure rates, unfulfilled assumptions of the methods, and business interests and political ambitions in comparing the results of analyses. Not surprisingly a comparison using published data from more than one register to define the performance of different hip implants could only be performed incompletely [8]. The development of common guidelines for joint registries could play an important role in enabling harmonisation of the choice of statistical methods, end points and reporting [11]. Notwithstanding all the potential benefits arising from national registries, one clear limitation of the registries is that failure is a hard end point, since revision rates do not include poorly performing patients who are unable to undergo revision surgery for various reasons. This is why more analytical outcome measures are also needed as primary or secondary end points and this is discussed in further detail below.

Clinical Research and Hip Arthroplasty: Outcome Measures

Outcome after surgery can be measured in terms of mortality, hospital stay and readmissions, morbidity, clinical and/or radiographic findings, complications, pain and health-related quality of life (HRQoL). The choice of which end point and measure to use depends on several factors (aims, funding, context). Selecting the appropriate measure is essential for the researcher when designing a study, but it is crucial also for the orthopaedic surgeon adopting an evidence-based approach when critically appraising the literature. We will briefly describe the outcome assessment tools that are used in the following chapters.

Imaging (X-Ray, CT)

The most widely used and cost-effective imaging tool is standard radiography (usually anteroposterior [AP] pelvis and hip lateral views). Radiographs, however, lack accuracy, especially if detailed analysis is needed to evaluate osteolysis over time or when the researcher needs to evaluate spatial positioning of the implant [7]. Moreover, traditional and largely adopted x-ray systems of classification (both for pre- and post-operative evaluation) are often not validated and tested for reliability. It is then mandatory to perform x-ray evaluation with validated methods and to classify findings according to well-established and comparable scientific methods, and finally to correlate these data with patient-reported outcomes (PROs). Computerised tomography (CT) is more accurate than traditional x-ray and allows three-dimensional (3D) reconstruction, but it is more expensive and not always available. This led to the development of digital measuring methods based on x-rays to improve precision and accuracy, including radio-stereometric analysis (RSA) and Einzel–Bild–Roentgen analysis (EBRA), more often used within clinical trials than for routine monitoring.

A recent RSA study analysed migration in a series of 30 Corail® stems, showing a mean subsidence of 0.73 mm at 6 months, 0.62 mm at 1 year and 0.58 mm at 2 years and a mean retroversion of 1.82° at 6 months, 1.90° at 1 year and 1.59° at 2 years [3]. This data suggests that subsidence was confined to the first 6 months, after which there was no further subsidence. This low level of stem subsidence has been shown to be a strong predictor of long-term stability.

Dual-Energy X-Ray Absorptiometry

Since the early 1990s dual-energy x-ray absorptiometry (DEXA) has been used to accurately and reliably measure changes in bone mineral density (BMD) around THA. DEXA was used in a 10-year follow-up RCT comparing 80 patients randomised to receive four different cementless stems (Corail®, Autophor 900S, Zweymuller®, Opti-Fix) [5]. At 2 years significantly less proximal bone remodelling was observed for Corail®, while a slow but progressive BMD recovery was recorded in the long term.

Physician-Derived Assessment

Commonly utilised in clinical research are mixed physician-based and functional outcome instruments, providing composite scores from questions answered by patients and physical examination performed by the outcome assessor, usually the surgeon himself or herself. Many of these instruments were conceived and used by pioneer surgeons to evaluate their own series and were not scientifically validated. For an outcome measure to be meaningful, it must be psychometrically evaluated and shown to be reliable, valid and responsive (sensitive to changes). Not only do physical examination and clinical tests have a high risk of inter-observer variability, but also the weight applied to items in mixed scales may be arbitrary, especially if scores such as pain and range of motion are combined into one single numerical measure. Among these traditional tools only the Harris hip score, originally described over 40 years ago, was recently validated and can be used by a physician or a physiotherapist to study the clinical outcome of THA in research as well as clinical settings.

Patient-Reported Outcomes

In an editorial on the *Journal of Bone and Joint Surgery* in 1993, Peter C. Amadio (at that time President of the Outcomes Committee of the American Academy of Orthopaedic Surgeons) asked 'How well do orthopaedists know what their patients really want?' and cited a study in which patients who had hip disease were asked to list and rank the disabilities that bothered them most [1]. Three items that scored high on the patients' lists were not listed in a consensus document published by the American Academy of Orthopaedic Surgeons (AAOS), the Hip Society and the International Society of Orthopaedic Surgery and Traumatology (SICOT). Such observations raised an important point; if orthopaedic surgeons do not know all that is important to their patients and if they do not measure those factors, they should not be surprised if their assessment of results and that of their patients are discordant. The following 15 years in orthopaedic clinical research have shown an increasing knowledge and awareness of the need for measurement of health-related quality of life (HRQoL) and such tools are currently largely adopted worldwide [2, 10, 14, 15]. HRQoL is a multifactorial concept comprising physical, mental and social factors which describes how a person's health affects his or her ability to carry out normal social and physical activities.

Multiple outcome scales are currently used to evaluate HRQoL of patients who have undergone THA, and they can be classified into three main categories as follows:

Generic outcome measures aim to assess all dimensions of health related quality of life. The World Health Organization Quality of Life Group has recommended that five dimensions be assessed in any generic quality of life survey: physical health, psychological health, social relationship perceptions, function and well-being. Generic outcome measures are used across a wide range of medical and surgical specialties. Commonly used measures are the medical outcomes study 36-item short-form health survey (SF-36), its 12-item reduced version (SF-12) and the European QoL 5-dimension (EuroQol) questionnaire. EuroQol was introduced in the Swedish Hip Register data collection in 2002, together with pain and overall satisfaction indicated on a visual analogue scale (VAS) scale.

Disease-specific outcome measures provide patient-centred information about a particular disease. This allows comparison of different surgical and medical treatment options for that disease. Most commonly used measures for the hip are the Western Ontario and McMaster Universities (WOMAC) osteoarthritis index and the arthritis impact measurement scales (AIMS).

Procedure-specific measures were developed to elicit the patient's perception of the outcome of THA, like the Oxford hip score (OHS). The use of universal, previously validated, patient-related outcome instruments will facilitate a comparison of results of different studies and will also facilitate subsequent meta-analysis.

Conclusions

Good-quality research can provide the clinician the basis for a rational approach to evaluating and selecting procedures and devices. Orthopaedic surgeons should gain knowledge of the most relevant issues in clinical epidemiology to be able to search and evaluate the best evidence, both in terms of study type (levels of evidence) and quality of the study, including outcome measures. A wide variety of scores, based on radiographs, physician assessment and patient-reported outcomes are currently used to evaluate THA results. However, the outcomes assessment should rely on standardised and validated tools, which provide scientifically sound and reliable data with the minimum burden possible for both the patient and the surgeon and at low cost. The critical appraisal of the available evidence together with the clinical expertise is essential to the practice of evidence-based orthopaedic surgery, the more scientific way to provide the best available care to our patients.

References

1. Amadio PC (1993) Outcomes measurements. J Bone Joint Surg Am 75(11):1583–1584
2. Ashby E, Grocott MP, Haddad FS (2008) Outcome measures for orthopaedic interventions on the hip. J Bone Joint Surg Br 90(5):545–549
3. Campbell D, Mercer G, Nilsson KG et al (2011) Early migration characteristics of a hydroxyapatite-coated femoral stem: an RSA study. Int Orthop (SICOT) 35:483–488
4. Graves SE (2010) The value of arthroplasty registry data. Acta Orthop 81(1):8–9
5. Karachalios T, Tsatsaronis C, Efraimis G et al (2004) The long-term clinical relevance of calcar atrophy caused by stress shielding in total hip arthroplasty: a 10-year, prospective, randomized study. J Arthroplasty 19(4): 469–475
6. Learmonth ID, Young C, Rorabeck C (2007) The operation of the century: total hip replacement. Lancet 370(9597): 1508–1519
7. McCalden RW, Naudie DD, Yuan X et al (2005) Radiographic methods for the assessment of polyethylene wear after total hip arthroplasty. J Bone Joint Surg Am 87(10):2323–2334
8. Migliore A, Perrini MR, Romanini E et al (2009) Comparison of the performance of hip implants with data from different arthroplasty registers. J Bone Joint Surg Br 91(12): 1545–1549
9. National Institute for Clinical Excellence. Guidance for the selection of prosthesis for primary total hip replacement. www.nice.org.uk. Accessed 05 Jan 2010
10. Poolman RW, Swiontkowski MF, Fairbank JC et al (2009) Outcome instruments: rationale for their use. J Bone Joint Surg Am 91(suppl 3):41–49
11. Ranstam J, Robertsson O (2010) Statistical analysis of arthroplasty register data. Acta Orthop 81(1):10–14
12. Sackett DL, Rosenberg WM, Gray JA et al (1996) Evidence based medicine: what it is and what it isn't. BMJ 312:71–72
13. Schemitsch EH, Bhandari M, Boden SD et al (2010) The evidence-based approach in bringing new orthopaedic devices to market. J Bone Joint Surg Am 92(4):1030–1037
14. Söderman P, Malchau H (2001) Is the Harris hip score system useful to study the outcome of total hip replacement? Clin Orthop Relat Res Mar(384):189–197
15. Wylde V, Blom AW (2009) Assessment of outcomes after hip arthroplasty. Hip Int 19(1):1–7

4.2 Clinical and Radiographic Outcome

4.2.1 25-Year ARTRO Results: *A Special Vintage from the Old World*

Jean-Pierre Vidalain

Twenty-five years ago the Corail® stem was introduced. The stem was intended to be inserted using a fixation concept, which was unique. The stem was fully hydroxyapatite (HA)-coated and had a gradually decreasing stiffness gradient due to its design. Whilst the benefits of uncemented fixation using HA-coated implants is now widely acknowledged and established, at the time of the original design it was experimental. This prospective study conducted over a 25-year period has greatly contributed to demonstrating the unmatched reliability of the Corail® stem, in terms of its functional and radiographic outcome, both of which are exceptionally good. The Corail® stem, which is a straight, proximally flared, fully HA-coated stem, offers substantial short-, mid- and long-term benefits without any harmful effects.

Introduction

Twenty-five years is a symbolic time in orthopaedic surgery and an important landmark in the life of a joint prosthesis. There are two reasons for this: firstly, because not many hip replacement implants reach this privileged age, and secondly because long-term results can undoubtedly be evoked from that date. Although more than 20,000 Corail® prostheses have been implanted by the whole group of designers during the past 25 years, we decided it would be most interesting on the occasion of this book, which is dedicated to the teachings clearly established from this quarter-century experience, to report on the original series of consecutive patients. This series of patients was operated on in the first 5 years between July 1986 and December 1990. This is a cohort of 347 Corail® stems in 320 patients with 20–25-year follow-up.

Material and Methods

This prospective and consecutive series of Corail® stems was performed in the Clinique d'Argonay (Annecy Orthopaedic Centre) by a single surgeon who is a member of the designer group but not the author. All primary total hip replacements were included, whereas all bipolar arthroplasties were excluded. This study included 347 Corail® stems in 320 patients (27 bilateral THA); 8 Corail® stems were implanted in 1986, 54 in 1987, 82 in 1988, 85 in 1989 and 118 in 1990. Therefore, the mean follow-up was 20.9 years (range 20–25). The cohort included 154 females and 166 males. The mean age at surgery was 63.3 (range 33–88 years) and greater than 40% had a high level of preoperative activity according to Devane et al. [12]: Grade 1 (sedentary, dependent, wheelchair) = 7%, 2 (semi sedentary, household works) = 20%, 3 (leisure activities, gardening, swimming) = 32%, 4 (light work, sports recreational) = 24% and 5 (power worker, sports high level) = 17%.

The aetiology was osteoarthritis of the hip (76%), necrosis (6%), neck fractures in the elderly (5%), dysplasia (5%), post-traumatic osteoarthritis (2%), inflammatory arthritis (1%) and other more unusual causes (5%).

Surgery was performed through the antero-lateral Watson–Jones approach on a traction table. As explained in Table 4.1 the Corail® stem with standard offset was used in every case, since this was the only offset option available at that time. The stem was collared in 24% and collarless in 76% of cases. Various acetabular components were implanted. These were mainly first-generation cementless cups without HA coating, since HA-coated acetabular components were introduced much later. The femoral head diameter was 32 mm in 47.4% and 28 mm in 52.6% of the procedures, and Biolox® delta ceramic femoral heads were most commonly used (318/347 cases). Metal heads were used in eight procedures. Note that information was missing in 21 files. All these cups had polyethylene (PE) liners.

In Annecy, we have prospectively reviewed all patients since the early stages of the Corail® prosthesis implantation. Despite regular patient notifications, it is reported that 9% of patients were lost to follow-up, which can be attributed to population mobility and patient ageing for whom regular clinical and radiographic examinations are unnecessary and impractical. Moreover, in the context of a Private Surgical

Table 4.1 Femoral and acetabular components implanted in this series

Femur	Standard Corail® stem:	**347**
	Collared:	83
	Collarless:	263
Acetabulum (uncemented)	HA-coated:	**268**
	Press-fit:	30
	Screwed:	238
	Non HA-coated:	**72**
Acetabulum (cemented)	Plain PE or metal-backed cups	**7**
Head	Ceramic:	**318**
	32 mm:	148
	28 mm:	170
	Metal:	**8**
	32 mm	6
	28 mm	2
	Missing:	**21**

Institution, patients own their radiographic records. All these factors explain our difficulty in obtaining a complete and exhaustive record.

The collected data were recorded in paper-based medical records and then entered into a computer-based database, whose software has been in constant evolution during the period of time. This work was done by an independent medical statistician. All traditional statistical tests were conducted using the Statview software package. Survival curves were produced according to the Kaplan–Meier method with a 1-year interval.

Results

Part 1: Previously Published Radiographic Findings

The present series of patients has already been, in the past, the subjects of independent studies with, of course, a shorter follow-up. In these works, the main features of osseointegration and peri-prosthetic bone remodelling have been described in detail. Jonathan Garino and Mark Froimson have presented the findings of their work with a follow-up of more than 10 years [17] (Sect. 4.2.2), while Jens Bolt has presented the current series analysis with more than a 15-year

follow-up, during the 2009 EFORT Congress [6]. All the findings of this present 20–25-year follow-up analysis are in total accordance with the data presented by these authors.

We will only repeat some general notions from these early series reports. On the immediate post-operative radiographic view, the stem is usually centred or in slight varus. Correction of limb length discrepancies has been performed. Unfortunately, at that time, there was no sufficient data to provide adequate analysis of joint geometry reconstruction, in particular regarding the femoral offset and abductor muscle lever arm.

Radiographic evidence of osseointegration is present in 82% of the records since the end of the first post-operative year of implantation, particularly in the more distal part of the stem, and there is no evidence of pedestal formation or radiolucent lines. These signs are still evident at the last control. On rare occasions reactive lines (0.6%) were observed in zone 1 and potential granulomas (8%) related with PE wear were observed, mostly in the trochanteric region. Implant stability is excellent and only a single case of stem subsidence of more than 3 mm was reported. Evidence of bone remodelling in the calcar region was observed in 15% of cases and only two cases of grade 3 stress-shielding were noted. Multivariate analyses confirmed that femoral remodelling was not influenced to any significant extent by either patient-related or prosthesis-related factors (such as collar, positioning and size).

Regarding polyethylene (PE) wear, there is no significant predisposing factor apart from the patient's age at the time of surgery. Younger patients commonly demonstrated earlier occurrence of PE wear. On the other hand, the femoral head diameter and the femoral head material did not appear to be significant factors.

Part 2: 20–25-Year Clinical Outcome and Survivorship

Twenty to twenty-five years after implantation, 125 patients were available for review, which represented 39% of the initial number of patients. One hundred and sixty-five patients (52%) died during the 25-year period, but for each of these patients the clinical outcome was known. Only 30 (9%) are considered as being definitely lost to follow-up. The original cohort is therefore significantly reduced due to the mortality inherent to this age bracket.

The functional results (Table 4.2) were spectacular particularly regarding the absence of pain. Eighty-three percent of the patients were pain-free at last follow-up. However, the overall score decreased slightly due to an age-related alteration of the functional score (the mean age of patients was now 80). Even so, 61% of the patients still reported a Postel-Merle d'Aubigné (PMA) score of 18 or better.

The Sedel score (Table 4.3) provides accurate information about the clinical and radiographic outcomes. There are four possible groups:

Group A: patients with no adverse functional or radiographic signs.
Group B: patients with stable clinical result, but demonstrating progressive radiographic changes.
Group C: patients with deteriorating functional score, but with a lack of any radiographic explanation.
Group D: patients with bad clinical score associated with progressive radiographic deterioration.

In our series, 83% of the patients had a totally normal hip at last follow-up and were classified in Group A. Only 15% had progressive, adverse radiographic signs. These were typically at the calcar level (scalloping or osteolysis) and more rarely proximal granulomas or lucencies. Since these patients had a normal clinical result, these cases were classified in Group B. One percent of the cohort had reduced functional scores with normal radiographic appearance. These patients were classified in Group C. Finally, 1% of the patients had poor function associated with deterioration of the femoral bone pattern and were classified in Group D. Considering the two subgroups, collared and collarless, there was less bone resorption with the collared stem (Group B: 10% vs. 16%).

Intra-operative complications (Table 4.4), in particular calcar cracks, were not attributed to the learning phase, but to the fact that when these implants were inserted it was considered good practice to have closer cortical contact than it is today.

There were 62 revisions. Most were for acetabular complications. Only two cases of unexplained thigh pain were observed. Only 12 stems (3%) were removed during the 25-year period. Four were removed for loosening, probably aseptic. Three stable stems were removed during acetabular revision due to the presence of extensive granulomas. One stem was removed for treatment of a peri-prosthetic fracture. One well-fixed stem was removed to restore leg length and offset. Finally three stable implants were removed to facilitate cup revision.

When all causes of stem removal were considered, the Corail® stem survival in this series was 97.7% at 15

Table 4.2 Functional results (PMA/HHS score)

	PMA	HHS	Pre-op		Last control	
			PMA (%)	HHS (%)	PMA (%)	HHS (%)
Excellent	18	≥98	0	0	61	0
Good	≥15	≥80	2	1	32	80
Fair	≥12	≥60	39	6	6	15
Poor	<12	<60	59	93	1	6
Mean			**10.1**	**41.3**	**17.1**	**85.1**

Table 4.3 Sedel score (function and radiographic evaluation)

	Corail® (collared) (%)	Corail® (collarless) (%)	Global (%)
A	89	81	83
B	10	16	15
C	0	1	1
D	1	1	1

Table 4.4 Distribution of the different complications

Intra-operative complications	N: 38 = 10.9%
Cracks	33
Fractures	3
Perforations	2
Early complications	**N: 65 = 18.7%**
DVT	27
PE	2
Hematoma	11
Sepsis	2
Dislocations	8
Other	15
Late complications	**N: 90 = 25.9%**
Ectopic bone	9
Pain (unexplained)	2
Recurrent dislocations	13
Revisions:	62
Cup	48
Stem	12
Liner and head	2
Other	4

years, 96.8% at 20 years and 96.3% in the 25th year (Table 4.5). On the other hand, the survivorship of the acetabular cup was 88.9% at 15 years, 84.4% at 20 years and 83.9% in the 25th year. The overall survivorship of the whole arthroplasty, stem and cup, was 87.3% at 15 years, 83.0% at 20 years and 82.5% in the 25th year (Table 4.6).

Discussion

More than a quarter of a century after the first human implantations of HA-coated implants and based on our personal experience [35], it is now possible to answer some questions and to address the concerns and doubts which were the subject of debate between the supporters and opponents of the use of HA-coated stems. The clinical and radiographic results reported in the literature at more than 20-year follow-up, in most cases reported by groups who were not inventor surgeons,

provide sufficient evidence of the long-term effectiveness of this method of bioactive fixation. The publications demonstrate that the calcium-phosphate layer prevents adverse events and represents a decisive and unequalled advance in comparison with other non-cemented techniques [2, 8, 13, 28].

The fundamental question 'Is HA just the starter in the osseointegration process or is it an essential and determining partner in the durability of arthroplasty' can now be answered. The answer, as has often been said, is that HA is not a magic powder, since an optimal coating applied to a bad prosthesis or a good prosthesis improperly implanted may predispose the stem to failure. Nevertheless, among the three important elements (the interface, the prosthetic design and the implantation technique) hydroxyapatite has proven highly effective in promoting bone ongrowth and bioactivity. Evaluation of the respective part played by each component in the quality of the final result is difficult, since it is the combination of these three

Table 4.5 Survival probability of the Corail® stem. Stem revision for any reason was the end point

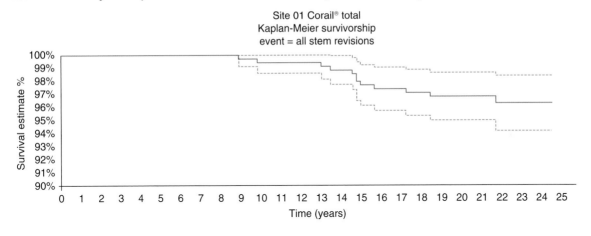

Table 4.6 Survival probability of the whole arthroplasty (stem and cup). Removal of any component as end point

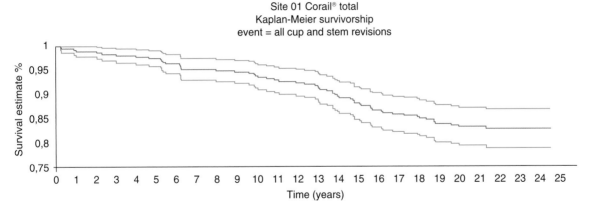

elements which ensures fixation durability and long-term quality of the functional outcome. However, gradually consensus has been reached and the benefits of full HA coating can now be classified into five categories. We will discuss them quickly as they are no longer the focus of controversy.

Osseointegration is the key element. For the first time, it is possible to create a real osseo-coalescence between the living and reactive host bone and the prosthetic implant made from inert, synthetic material. This is a continuous, reproducible and reliable integration process. It can occur at any age and in any case, whatever the bone quality of the patient. This phenomenon is not simply a transitory stage in the life of a prosthesis. Rather it is a long-term process, as demonstrated in long-term radiographs by the absence of any radiolucent lines (in other words, by the absence of any interposition of fibrous tissue). This fundamental property means that there are no restrictions with regard to clinical indications. Young and very active patients [24, 29, 30, 31, 37], older patients [15] and osteoporotic patients with poor bone stock [23] all achieved similar results. Similarly, sclerotic bone observed in revision surgeries [9, 11, 25, 26, 28] or in septic situations [36] does not constitute a contraindication.

The *stability* of the fixation is also proven. Since the experimental work of Söballe using RSA in 1995, it has now been established that HA-coated implants demonstrate early and definitive stability, significantly improved in comparison with porous metal-coated implants of similar geometry [22, 32, 33]. The various studies conducted by the ARTRO Group confirm this longitudinal stability, and a recent RSA analysis performed on the Corail® stem in Australia [7] reported good stability. In this study there was a mean vertical migration of 1 mm and a mean anteversion of 1°. These displacements occurred within the first post-operative weeks.

The *absence of unexplained pain* is also a determining factor as emphasised by all authors. Whatever the chosen method for functional evaluation, the usual absence of pain, particularly in the thigh and inguinal regions, with the Corail®, strongly contrasts with complaints reported by patients with conventional cementless implants [2].

It is known that *bone remodelling* occurs after any prosthetic implantation. The quality of bone remodelling perfectly reveals the fact that the load transfer to the bone is homogeneous [1, 10, 13]. The quality of the bone remodelling has been the subject of several independent studies. The neoformed bone trabeculae are long lasting and reflect the tensile, compressive and rotational forces which maintain bone trophicity. The calcar region is subjected to changes in 34% of cases with thinning of Merckel's femoral thigh spur and rounding of cortical ridges, but no diaphyseal anomalies (such as cortical inflation, hypertrophy or atrophy) are usually observed and the rate of grade 3 stress-shielding is lower than 1%, which may be considered insignificant. Numerous densitometry studies have also confirmed this benefit with regard to bone sparing [21].

The excellent quality of the bone implant interface causes the stem to be *embedded* and this embedding slows down wear particle migration responsible for granulomas and bone resorption. This specific point has been accepted for a long time. Granulomas may appear proximally, particularly in the calcar region (Fig. 4.1), but they are slowly progressing and never observed in the diaphyseal region. Thus, complete osseointegration around the stem provides more secure fixation.

These advantages explain why, in the majority of the cases, no radiographic changes of the implantation site are reported even after many years of implantation (Fig. 4.2). This clinical result confirms the principle of a 'silent hip' or a totally forgotten surgery.

In the 1990s, the potentially harmful effects of HA were described in a few articles [4, 5]. During the past few years, an extensive literary output has reduced these doubts [7, 8, 14, 20, 27, 34].

The more or less complete *resorption of the coating* is now a well-accepted phenomenon [3, 17, 18]. However, in mechanically loaded areas, this phenomenon is always followed by the formation of lamellar bone attached to the residual coating and this provides long-term fixation. The metallic surface may be exposed at the level of the medullary cavities, but fibrous tissue never develops. This key point has been emphasised by Dominique Hardy based on his retrieval studies [19].

The risk of *delamination* is now perfectly documented. With the current coating technologies described in a previous chapter, this theoretical risk can be considered negligible up to a ceramic thickness of 150 μ. In histological studies, notably those of Dominique Hardy et al. [19], HA fragments have never been seen in soft tissues and the rate of ectopic bone formation is not significantly increased in comparison with procedures using non-HA-coated implants.

The phenomenon of *osteolysis* has only been described in some articles and remains a marginal event. Hydroxyapatite does not cause osteolysis. Rather osteolysis is caused by the migration of other particles, which

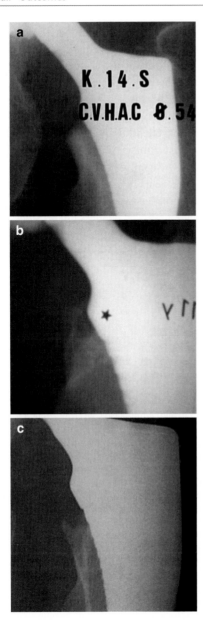

Fig. 4.1 Slow progression of granuloma at the calcar level. Scalloping process 5 years after implantation (**a**). Cortical resorption is evident at 11-year follow-up (**b**) and at 15-year follow-up (**c**). There is no evidence of radiolucencies at the interface. Excellent stability of the stem

are either the main predisposing factors or are the consequences of loosening. It is an established fact that hydroxyapatite has no inflammatory or allergising effects; nor does it have any toxic or carcinogenic potential.

Excessive *wear* might occur as a result of third-body abrasive wear, if coating fragments were present within the joint space [30]. However, this theoretical risk has never been proven. Fragments released after coating degradation

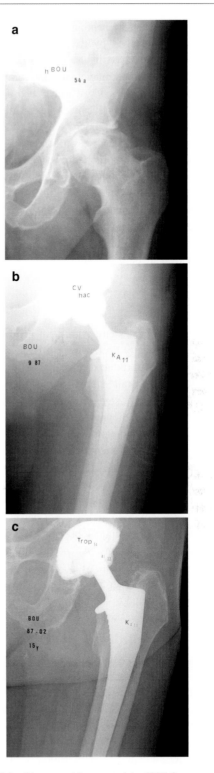

Fig. 4.2 Male, 54 years old, operated in 1987 for avascular necrosis (**a**). Immediate post-operative image (**b**). The Corail® KA11 stem had a ceramic on PE bearing. Nice reconstruction of the hip geometry. Image 20 years later: note the radiological silence with no significant modification of the peri-prosthetic bone pattern (**c**)

remain in the immediate environment of the intramedullary stem and are resorbed by the cells (osteoclasts, macrophages, etc.) involved in the local bone metabolism. These fragments do not migrate into the surrounding soft tissues or into the joint cavity. Calcium phosphates sometimes observed over the polyethylene liner surface are from natural origins and commonly appear with cemented implants. In fact, the wear rates in long-term series using HA-coated implants are reported to be not significantly different from those using other types of arthroplasties.

Lastly, the *extraction* of a well-osseointegrated implant has long been considered a challenging procedure. However, if the technique described elsewhere in this book is used, the risks and complications associated with stem removal are considerably reduced.

> › The quality of the overall outcome results from the combination of three key elements: (1) a completely bioactive interface, (2) a suitable prosthetic design and (3) a bone-sparing surgical technique.
> › All national joint replacement registers confirm the excellent survival of the Corail® stem. The oldest clinical series reports a survival rate at 20 years of more than 95%.
> › After 25 years of clinical experience, the Corail® prosthesis can be considered a Gold Standard among cementless hip prostheses.

Conclusions

A fully HA-coated stem, with stem geometry which provides a gradually decreasing stiffness gradient, is a concept that was introduced 25 years ago by the ARTRO Group with the Corail® stem. This long-term prospective and consecutive study confirmed the durability of the functional and radiographic results. Osseointegration was a continuous phenomenon, which occurred on a regular basis in all patients. Good stem stability was responsible for the absence of any unexplained pain. Early return to normal activity was allowed. The absence of adverse radiographic evidence ('radiographic silence') was common and was not dependent on the implant position. Aseptic loosening was rare despite acetabular complications. All acetabular components had a polyethylene liner, which demonstrated significant wear in more than 50% of the cases. Granulomas were always limited to the metaphyseal region and the Corail® stem survival was 96.3% in the 25th year.

Key Learning Points

> › It has now been clearly established that HA coating of hip prostheses offers a reliable osseointegration process, does not induce any adverse effects, promotes bone ingrowth and provides unequalled stabilisation.
> › The international literature confirms that the Corail® prosthesis is a well-documented and reliable implant.

References

1. Al Hertani W, Waddell JP, Anderson GI (2000) The effect of partial vs. full hydroxyapatite coating on periprosthetic bone quality around the canine madreporic femoral stem. J Biomed Mater Res 53:518–524
2. Baltopoulos P, Tsintzos C, Papadakou E et al (2008) Hydroxyapatite-coated total hip arthroplasty: the impact on thigh pain and arthroplasty survival. Acta Orthop Belg 74:323–331
3. Bauer TW, Geesink RCT, Zimmerman R et al (1991) Hydroxyapatite-coated femoral stems. Histological analysis of components retrieved at autopsy. J Bone Joint Surg Am 73:1439–1452
4. Bloebaum RD, Merrel M, Gutske K et al (1991) Retrieval analysis of a hydroxyapatite-coated hip prosthesis. Clin Orthop Rel Res Jun(267):97–102
5. Bloebaum RD, Zou L, Bachus KN et al (1997) Analysis of particles in acetabular components from patients with osteolysis. Clin Orthop Rel Res May(338):109–118
6. Boldt J (2009) Bone remodeling in cementless HA-coated stems after 20 years. 10th EFFORT. Vienna, 2009
7. Campbell D, Mercer G, Nilsson KG et al (2011) Early migration characteristics of a hydroxyapatite-coated femoral stem: an RSA study. Int Orthop (SICOT) 35:483–488
8. Chambers B, St Clair SF, Froimson MI (2007) Hydroxyapatite-coated tapered cementless femoral components in total hip arthroplasty. J Arthroplasty 22:71–74
9. Chatelet JC, Setiey L (2004) Femoral component revision with hydroxyapatite-coated revision stems. In: Epinette JA, Manley MT (eds) Fifteen years of clinical experience with hydroxyapatite coatings in joint arthroplasty. Springer, Paris
10. Coathup MJ, Blunn GW, Flynn N et al (2001) A comparison of bone remodeling around hydroxyapatite-coated, porous-coated and grit-blasted hip replacements retrieved at post-mortem. J Bone Joint Surg Br 83:118–123
11. Crawford CH, Malkani AL, Incavo SJ et al (2004) Femoral component revision using an extensively hydroxyapatite-coated. J Arthoplasty 19:8–13

12. Devane PA, Horne JG, Martin K et al (1997) Three-dimensional polyethylene wear of a press-fit titanium prosthesis. Factors influencing generation of polyethylene debris. J Arthroplasty 12:256–266

13. Engh CA, Bobyn JD, Glassman AH (1987) Porous-coated hip replacement; the factors governing bone-ingrowth, stress-shielding and clinical results. J Bone Joint Surg Br 69:45–55

14. Epinette JA, Manley MT (2008) Uncemented stems in hip replacement – hydroxyapatite or plain porous: does it matter? Based on a prospective study of HA Omnifit stems at 15-years minimum follow-up. Hip Int 18:69–74

15. Figved W, Opland V, Frihagen F et al (2009) Cemented versus uncemented hemiarthroplasty for displaced femoral neck fractures. Clin Orthop Relat Res 467(9):2426–2435 [Epub 2009 Jan 7]

16. Froimson MI, Garino J, Machenaud A, Vidalain JP (2007) Minimum 10-year results of a tapered, titanium, hydroxyapatite-coated hip stem: an independent review. J Arthroplasty 22:1–7

17. Geesink RG (2002) Osteoconductive coatings for total joint arthroplasty. Clin Orthop Relat Res 395:53–65

18. Geesink RGT (1999) HA coatings in orthopaedic surgery. Raven Press, New-York

19. Hardy DCR, Frayssinet P, Guilhem A et al (1991) Bonding of hydroxyapatite-coated femoral prostheses: histopathology of specimens from four cases. J Bone Joint Surg Br 73:732–740

20. Havelin LI, Espehaug B, Vollset SE et al (1995) Early aseptic loosening of uncemented femoral components in primary total hip replacement. A review based on the Norwegian Arthroplasty Register. J Bone Joint Surg Br 77(1):11–17

21. Karachalios T, Tsatsaronis C, Efraimis G et al (2004) The long-term clinical relevance of calcar atrophy caused by stress shielding in total hip arthroplasty: a 10-year, prospective, randomized study. J Arthroplasty 19:469–475

22. Kärrholm J, Malchau H, Snorrason F et al (1994) Micromotion of femoral stems in total hip arthroplasty: a randomized study of cemented hydroxyapatite-coated and porous-coated stems with roentgen stereophotogrammetric analysis. J Bone Joint Surg Am 76:1692–1705

23. Kelly SJ, Robbins CE, Bierbaum BE et al (2007) Use of a hydroxyapatite-coated stem in patients with Dorr type C femoral bone. Clin Orthop Relat Res 465:112–116

24. Paulsen A, Pedersen AB, Johnsen SP et al (2007) Effect of hydroxyapatite coating on risk of revision after primary total hip arthroplasty in younger patients: findings from the Danish hip Arthroplasty Registry. Acta Orthop 78:622–628

25. Philippot R, Delangle F, Verdot FX et al (2009) Femoral deficiency reconstruction using a hydroxyapatite-coated locked modular stem. A series of 43 total hip revisions. Orthop Traumatol Surg Res 95:119–126 [Epub 2009 Mar 17]

26. Pinaroli A, Lavoie F, Cartillier JC et al (2009) Conservative femoral stem revision: avoiding therapeutic escalation. J Arthroplasty 24:365–373 [Epub 2008 Apr 11]

27. Rajaratnam SS, Jack C, Tavakkolizadeh A et al (2008) Long-term results of a hydroxyapatite-coated femoral component in total hip replacement: a 15- to 21-year follow-up study. J Bone Joint Surg Br 90:27–30

28. Reikeras O, Gunderson RB (2006) Excellent results with femoral revision surgery using an extensively hydroxyapatite-coated stem. Acta Orthop 77:98–103

29. Restrepo C, Lettich T, Roberts N et al (2008) Uncemented total hip arthroplasty in patients less than twenty-years. Acta Orthop Belg 74:615–622

30. Sanchez-Sotelo J, Lewallen DG, Harmsen WS et al (2004) Comparison of wear and osteolysis in hip replacement using two different coatings of the femoral stem. Int Orthop 28:206–210 [Epub 2004 Apr 29]

31. Shah NN, Edge AJ, Clark DW (2009) Hydroxyapatite-ceramic-coated femoral components in young patients followed-up for 16 to 19 years: an update of a previous report. J Bone Joint Surg Br 91:865–869

32. Søballe K, Gotfredsen K, Brockstedt-Rasmussen H et al (1991) Histological analysis of a retrieved hydroxyapatite coated femoral prosthesis. Clin Orthop 272:255–258

33. Søballe K, Toksvig-Larsen S, Gelinek J et al (1993) Migration oh hydroxyapatite coated femoral stems: a roentgen stereophotogrammetric study. J Bone Joint Surg Br 75:681–687

34. Tian H, Zhang K, Liu Y (2007) Long-term clinical and radiological results of entirely hydroxyapatite-coated femoral components. Zhonghua Yi Xue Za Zhi 87:3200–3202; Chinese

35. Vidalain JP (2004) Corail® stem long-term results based upon the 15-year ARTRO Group experience. In: Epinette JA, Manley MT (eds) Fifteen years of clinical experience with hydroxyapatite coatings in joint arthroplasty. Springer, Paris

36. Vidalain JP (2004) Hydroxyapatite and infection: results of a consecutive series of 49 infected total hip replacements. In: Epinette JA, Manley MT (eds) Fifteen years of clinical experience with hydroxyapatite coatings in joint arthroplasty. Springer, Paris

37. Wangen H, Lereim P, Holm I et al (2008) Hip arthroplasty in patients younger than 30 years: excellent ten to 16-year follow-up results with a HA-coated stem. Int Orthop 32:203–208 [Epub 2007 Feb 15]

4.2.2 10-Year USA Results: Taking It to the New World

Mark I. Froimson, Jonathan Garino, and Gurion Rivkin

The Corail® hip implant has proven to be a successful implant that yields reliable and consistent outcomes. Following a long delay after its introduction and use by the designing surgeons, adoption in the North American market was slow. The fixation philosophy of this implant differed significantly from the prevailing concepts that were popular, particularly in the USA, so widespread use did not occur until the results achieved in the European populations became known and were validated. Despite this slow acceptance, the success of this implant and technique has been reproduced by a number of US surgeons. The clinical data presented in this chapter documents the consistent results obtained with this technique at two US centres. These results confirm the intermediate-term success of this device.

Introduction

The Corail® total hip system was developed and introduced by the ARTRO Group in 1986, but was unavailable for widespread use in North America until 1998. Following a detailed programme of prospective data collection with assiduous attention to follow-up and documentation, the ARTRO Group began to report consistent and reproducible clinical outcomes rivalling or exceeding those of other implants [7]. The intramedullary design coupled with the biologically active HA coating proved to be extremely reliable in obtaining osseous integration of implant to bone that could serve as the foundation for a durable hip replacement construct. The results, increasingly reported in France and among congresses in Europe, were virtually unknown and certainly unappreciated in North America. The essential concepts espoused by the ARTRO Group, that is, the use of a titanium-tapered wedge with a hydroxyapatite (HA) coating to enhance fixation, implanted into a compacted bed of cancellous bone, were not widely employed among available implants in the American market. In fact, the competing and contrary concepts of fit and fill and diaphyseal, cortical purchase were considered essential to success in cementless femoral stem fixation. In addition, there was some scepticism about the results reported by the designing surgeons for the Corail® implant.

Depuy Purchases Landanger

As the success of the Corail® became increasingly apparent, Landanger became an attractive acquisition target for Depuy and in 1998 Depuy purchased Landanger and took possession of one of the most successful implants available in the European market. Depuy's prior success in the hip replacement market, particularly in North America, was due to implants that were in sharp contrast to the newly acquired Corail® implant. The mainstays for the company at that time were the AML® and the S-ROM®, both of which called for machining of the femoral canal to accept the diaphyseally purchased implant. The concept of fit and fill was widely discussed with the theory that success of a cementless femoral component rested on the ability to fill the femoral canal and establish direct cortical contact [1]. In the case of the AML® this was through a scratch fit of the porous coating with the endosteal surface of the canal, whereas the S-ROM® gained purchase, in part, through engagement of its distal splines into the endosteum. In both cases the concept was to maximise canal fill of the implant to prevent subsidence and to ensure osteointegration. Given this philosophical and theoretical basis for the success of DePuy's most successful hip stems, the broach-only, HA-coated, non-porous stem designed to engage a compacted bed of cancellous bone seemed difficult to reconcile. Consequently, no immediate marketing plan in North America was established and the stem was not featured prominently, or for that matter at all, in the company's educational and promotional efforts.

Early Adopters

Against this backdrop, the appeal of the stem, and the outstanding clinical heritage that had propelled it to success in Europe, was noticed by a number of American surgeons looking for a more physiologic, bone-sparing approach to hip arthroplasty. After attending an early learning centre in Annecy, and being introduced to the work of the ARTRO Group, these surgeons elected to embrace the philosophy espoused by the French and began to adopt the Corail® into clinical practice. During 1998, a small but dedicated group of American surgeons had begun to acquire experience with the stem, referring to it affectionately, with reference to its 10-year data, as a new 'old' stem. Utilising the ARTRO techniques, the early acceptance was bolstered by an ease of use and excellent clinical performance that appeared to match or exceed the more canal-filling alternatives that had been considered state of the art. In addition, these early users also were committed to patterning their approach to clinical follow-up after their French colleagues and developed strategies to collect clinical data on the long-term performance of the device.

As early clinical results were being collected by the American users, there was a desire to review the results reported by the ARTRO Group. The perception that pervaded the introduction of the stem to the US market was that, as compelling as the data appeared, there was, as yet, no independent validation of the ARTRO results. To address that need, Dr. Jonathon Garino and Dr. Mark Froimson set out to independently review the original series by updating the clinical and radiographic follow-ups. As expected, the results were validated and in the process of collecting the data and publishing the results [2] the American surgeons confirmed the ability of this implant to achieve durable and lasting results over the long term.

Clinical Success

The clinical success of the Corail® femoral stem in the North American market has been, as expected, quite the same as that seen in other populations and centres. Given the ability of multiple surgeons at multiple sites around the world to obtain success with this implant, it came as no surprise that a similar experience would be realised with the introduction of this stem to the US and Canadian market. There were, however, some technical issues that had to be overcome.

Having been accustomed to a more vigorous insertion technique that was demanded by canal-filling stems, some US surgeons had to learn to adapt to the more gentle, bone-preserving Corail® technique. In the process, some early stems were left proud due to oversizing and some femurs were cracked in the process.

Surgeons who had been to Annecy and had become ardent supporters of the compaction technique were dispatched to advocate a more physiologic technique of stem insertion. Gradually, surgeons came to appreciate the 'small mallet' technique and the tendency to overstuff the canal diminished.

A second challenge posed by the Corail® design required a different solution, involving redesign of the extramedullary portion of the implant. The original stem, when properly inserted, was able to consistently achieve osseous integration, but restoring the anatomy was not uniformly assured. The source of this challenge rested in the uniform neck length and angulation that required precise placement in the canal to assure restoration of the anatomic hip centre. Some femurs, especially those of smaller women, posed a considerable challenge in this regard, with the annoying risk of leg length inequality in a small but consistent cohort of patients. The Corail® Articul/eze® Mini-Taper (AMT) addressed this issue with several variations in the neck geometry that allowed more precise reconstruction of the kinematics of the hip. In addition to more reproducible kinematics, the new design featured a favourable neck geometry that allowed increased range of motion prior to impingement. Following the introduction of the high offset and coxa vara options for the Corail® implant, acceptance by the US surgical community was assured. In fact, with its reintroduction following redesign, it was the most rapidly growing implant in Depuy's portfolio for many years running. In addition, it was seen by many surgeons as versatile in a variety of surgical exposures, including the increasingly popular anterior approach and other 'minimally invasive surgical' techniques.

Results

We have been able to achieve clinical results with the Corail® stem that equal or surpass those achieved with any comparable stem. Beginning in 1998, following the introduction of the stem to the US market, we converted our primary hip replacement practice from a diaphyseal purchasing stem – the Replica, an AML® family stem – to the Corail® femoral component for all cementless total hip arthroplasties (THAs). At 10-year minimum follow-up, the results in this prospective cohort of patients were compelling and consistent with those that we reported in our independent review of the

ARTRO Group data. Two centres in the USA gained considerable experience with this stem and allow confirmation of its performance at an average follow-up of over 10 years. Data from the Cleveland Clinic include 169 hips implanted in 158 patients and data from the University of Pennsylvania included an additional 188 hips in 170 patients with follow-up averaging 10.5 years (range 9–12). Patients ranged in age from 31 to 90, with a mean of 63.6 years. Female patients constituted 46% of the cohort. The most common diagnosis was osteoarthritis, accounting for 85% of the patients treated.

The peri-operative protocols and surgical techniques at the two centres were similar. All patients were admitted on the day of surgery and 95% underwent a regional anaesthetic. Our protocol consisted of a modified posterolateral approach to the hip with small, but not minimal, incision, and meticulous repair of the posterior soft tissues, both capsule and piriformis, to the trochanter. We allowed immediate full weight bearing, even on the day of surgery if possible. Anticoagulation in this cohort was achieved with adjusted dose of warfarin or enoxaparin, with use consistent with ACCP guidelines and combined with portable calf compression pumps. More recently we have switched to aspirin as pharmacologic prophylaxis, except in the high-risk population where we use Lovenox or Coumadin. Patients usually were discharged on post-op day 3, with 60% of the cohort discharged directly home and the remainder receiving care at a rehabilitation facility. The demographics are outlined in Table 4.7.

At a minimum of 10-year follow-up (10–12 years) we had no cases of aseptic loosening. Re-operations were required in nine patients, including three for infection in which all components were removed, three for acetabular osteolysis requiring acetabular component revision with retention of the femoral component

and two for instability requiring polyethylene (PE) exchanges to anteverted liners with larger diameter heads and longer neck lengths. In only three cases, the infected cases, were the femoral components removed. When these data are combined, the composite outcomes of both groups combined comprise 357 hips at 10-year follow-up with a survival rate of 100% for aseptic loosening as the end point, 99.1% for stem retention as the end point, and 97.7% with no re-operations as the end point (Fig. 4.3). Overall, these results compare favourably with those of the ARTRO Group and those reported in the Norwegian Registry [3, 7].

Two groups of patients have been the subject of considerable interest in cementless hip arthroplasty: the younger patients who are under 50 at the time of arthroplasty, with concern about durability of the construct; and the older, osteoporotic patients who are over 75, who have been considered below-average candidates for osseous integration. In both groups, the results mirror the group at large. In fact, in a subgroup of 62 patients younger than 50 comprising 17% of the cohort, with 10 patients (2.9%) younger than 40, there was only one re-operation for infection and three re-operations for polyethylene wear, giving a stem survival of 98%, and a 96.2% survival without re-operations for any reason. These results in our cohort validate the assumption that cementless fixation will perform as well as, or better than, cemented femoral stems even in the younger, more active group of patients.

On the other extreme of the spectrum are the patients in their eighth decade and beyond who tend to have a higher incidence of osteoporotic, fragile, type C femora. Among our patients in this study, we evaluated 87

Table 4.7 Demographic distribution of Cleveland Clinic and University of Pennsylvania patients

Number of patients	357
Mean age	63.6
Male	54%
Female	46%
Age >80	32 (9%)
Age <50	63 (17%)

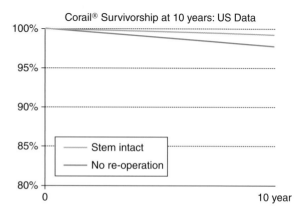

Fig. 4.3 Corail® survivorship at 10 years: US data on 357 cases

hips in 83 consecutive patients over age 75 with type C bone into which a Corail® femoral stem was implanted during primary hip arthroplasty. Although we currently advocate the use of a collared implant in this patient population, in the series evaluated, both collared and collarless prostheses were used. Biologic fixation occurred in all patients without any cases of aseptic loosening or late subsidence. Two patients in whom no collar had been used had early subsidence of 3–4 mm which then stabilised. There was no subsidence when a collared device was used. None of these suffered a peri-prosthetic fracture; nor was there subsidence necessitating revision. One patient dislocated, requiring closed reduction. There were no re-operations and no cases of failure of femoral fixation. Collared stems were used in all cases. No failures occurred. As an aside, six additional patients in this elderly age group were treated with Corail® hemiarthroplasty for femoral neck fractures. All collared stems were used. No failures occurred.

Discussion

Our results are comparable with the reported results of the Corail® stem in Europe by the ARTRO Group [7] and other investigators [4–6], as well as the Norwegian registry [3], with no aseptic loosening at 10-year follow-up and overall survivorship of 97.7%. This implant appears to perform well across a wide spectrum of patient characteristics and bone types without evidence of increased failure in any discernible subgroup. We continue to utilise this device as it enters its 25th year of clinical history and have, through our experience, continue to refine techniques to ensure success. Perhaps most important among these is the increasing recognition that the physiologic method of implantation that occurs with compaction broaching requires proper implant sizing. The most important error to avoid when one makes the transition to this stem is oversizing the implant.

Successful total hip arthroplasty requires, among other considerations, the reliable fixation of the prosthesis to the host bone. Current implant systems must accomplish this goal reliably and reproducibly in order to eliminate pain and restore function in a diseased hip for both the short and long terms. The Corail® stem can routinely be used to reliably obtain rigid biologic fixation in bone of a variety of shapes and densities including those that have been previously thought to be unsuitable for cementless applications. Together with modern bearing options this system represents the state of the art and for us it is the implant of choice in all bone types and anatomic variants. Surgeons choosing this implant will provide a time-tested and reproducible reconstruction for their patients that is compatible with rapid return to function and durable functional outcomes.

References

1. Engh CA, Claus AM, Hopper RH (2001) Long-term results using the anatomic medullary locking hip prosthesis. Clin Orthop Relat Res Dec(393):137–146
2. Froimson MI, Garino J, Machenaud A et al (2007) Minimum 10-year results of a tapered, titanium, hydroxyapatite-coated hip stem an independent review. J Arthroplasty 22(1):1–7
3. Hallan G, Lie SA, Furnes O et al (2007) Medium- and long-term performance of 11,516 uncemented primary femoral stems from the Norwegian arthroplasty register. J Bone Joint Surg Br 89(12):1574–1580
4. Reikeras O, Gunderson RB (2003) Excellent results of HA coating on a grit-blasted stem, 245 patients followed for 8–12 years. Acta Orthop Scand 74(2):140–145
5. Røkkum M, Reigstad A (1999) Total hip replacement with an entirely hydroxyapatite-coated prosthesis: 5 years' follow-up of 94 consecutive hips. J Arthroplasty 14(6):689
6. Vedantam R, Ruddlesdin C (1996) The fully hydroxyapatite-coated total hip implant. Clinical and roentgenographic results. J Arthroplasty 11(5):534
7. Vidalain JP (2004) Corail® stem long term results upon 15 years ARTRO Group experience. In: Epinette JA, Manley MT (eds) Fifteen years of clinical experience with hydroxy-apatite coating in joint arthroplasty. Springer, France, p 217

4.2.3 The Radiology of the Bone/Stem Interface: A Time-Tested Couple

Jean-Christophe Chatelet

Insertion of a fully hydroxyapatite (HA)-coated Corail® stem in the upper femur rapidly stimulates homogeneous osseointegration on the whole implant surface. Secondarily, according to the amount of load applied to the bone by the stem, radiographic evidence of bone bridges demonstrates the occurrence of bone remodelling under normal loading conditions. This biological fixation helps to stabilise the Corail®. The amount of stabilisation depends on various factors such as femoral shape, quality of cancellous bone, surgical technique and stem positioning within the femur.

Introduction

The cohabitation between the Corail® stem and the host bone of the upper femur has proven efficient over time, with 25 years of clinical and radiographic follow-up. After insertion of a cementless prosthesis such as the Corail® stem, the living elastic bone continuously rebuilds its structure around the hydroxyapatite (HA)-coated metal prosthesis. The biological response from loads exerted on the femoral cortices can be observed radiographically. These images should be obtained and evaluated to obtain good-quality cementless implant follow-up and fast detection of abnormal radiographic findings which could help predict failure of the osseointegration process, infection or loosening.

Radiographically, this biological fixation is not a single event but evolves through three stages: initial stem insertion within the compacted cancellous bone envelope, the subsequent osseointegration process and continued bone remodelling under load-bearing.

The author has closely observed and documented the osseointegration and remodelling of bone around the Corail® femoral stem. This observational study will discuss and explain the subjective radiographic appearances and changes that have been observed around a series of Corail® femoral stems over a 25-year period.

Stage 1: Insertion of the Corail® Stem

After insertion of a cementless femoral stem prosthesis, the mechanical load equilibrium in the proximal femur is disturbed. The presence of a metal prosthesis inside the medullary canal increases the stiffness of the whole construct. The trabecular pattern in the upper femur reflects the stress to which the bone is subjected according to the amount of load-bearing and muscle tractions. The natural femur exhibits stress patterns and trajectories: the compact sub-axial cervical lamina joining the inner cortex, the cephalic beam runs towards the outer cortex, forming with the former trajectory, the keystone of the ogival system. The third line that runs towards the greater trochanter is a compact sub-cervical lamella joining the trochanteric trajectory which runs down the inner and outer cortices. Depending on the level of the neck cut during surgery, some of these stress lines may disappear. Moreover, cancellous bone impaction will disrupt the ogival system and create a sleeve of lamellar compact bone around the stem.

Post-operative radiographic appearance is thus dependent upon the thickness of the cancellous tissue, its compaction strength, the thickness of the cortices and the size of the implant. Post-operative radiographic appearance after implantation of a Corail® stem should demonstrate the absence of any cortical contact with the stem due to the presence of a 1–2 mm thick cancellous bone bed (biological cement). At this stage, the ideal radiographic image should not reveal any stress or strain trajectory, as this is a clear image demonstrating no evidence of radiolucent line, condensation or bone remodeling. An intimate contact between the prosthesis and the cancellous bone bed is observed.

The degree of medullary canal filling by the stem can be post-operatively evaluated at this stage by measuring the width of the medullary canal, the femur and the implant at a level 1 cm from the tip of the stem. This measurement thus indicates the degree of medullary canal filling (Fig. 4.4).

Stage 2: Osseointegration

Microscopic evaluation during the first 6 post-operative weeks reveals a secondary osseointegration phenomenon which provides definitive stem fixation in the host bone. There is no macroscopic or radiographic change evident during that period of time. The

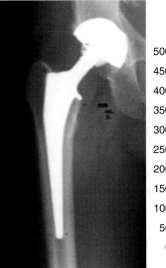

Fig. 4.4 Analysis of the stem size in the series of 2,143 Corail® stems (the mean size was 12)

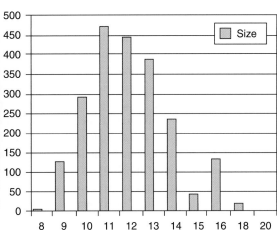

radiographic image is similar to that obtained during the post-operative implantation period with clear evidence of good filling around the implant by a cancellous bone sheath. Up to that phase, fixation is homogeneously performed and radiographic appearance is non-specific: the image is identical whatever the femur, the prosthesis and its size; the thickness and mechanical quality of cancellous bone are the only variables.

At this stage, the occurrence of a radiolucent line may be predictable of a poor-quality osseointegration. This rare image corresponds to a technical error associated with undersizing of the stem, which did not apply sufficient compression to the cancellous bone. If the Corail® stem is collarless, the stem may subside and reposition, thus inducing a shortening phenomenon. If the Corail® stem is collared, the stem will hang loose, unstable and poorly fixed: it does not correspond to a stem-loosening phenomenon but to poor osseointegration, therefore leading to an increased incidence of early revision requiring implantation of a larger stem.

Stage 3: Bone Remodelling under Load-Bearing Conditions

From the 6th to the 8th post-operative months, the first signs of bone remodelling can be observed according to Wolff's law, stimulated by the mechanical strain applied by the Corail® femoral stem to the surrounding bone. There is radiographic evidence of persistent bone bridging at the cortex–implant interface, demonstrating a progressive adaptation over a 25-year period according to the external factors such as bone ageing, reduced patient activity, bone quality, osteoporosis or even mal-position of the stem. These modifications, with respect to the natural state, cause the bone to adapt to the new conditions according to the variation in stress distribution. The patient's level of activity is a contributing factor: a regular walker will induce more compression strain than a weightlifter who possesses a higher tensile force.

Radiographic assessment of cementless prostheses is different from that performed with cemented implants. Two classification systems help evaluate the cementless stem behaviour and may help predict loosening: 'The ENGH and MASSIN score and ARA femoral score' [1, 2].

The radiographic changes to be assessed include endosteal modifications, reactive lines, bone pedestal, cortical hypertrophy, calcar remodelling, stem subsidence, osteolysis, stress-shielding and infection.

Endosteal Remodelling

It refers to the bony bridges described by Engh which develop within the space between the HA coating of the metal implant and the cortico-endosteal surface. Radiographic images of bone bridges may be different according to their location relative to the prosthesis (Gruen zones) [3]. These positive signs radiographically confirm the stresses and strains applied to the bone.

At the level of the greater trochanter and in zone 1, the muscular tensile stress has priority (gluteus medius). No compressive stress is observed in this zone (1a-1b) but only sliding and tensile stresses. Long trabeculae rise from the greater trochanter and run up to the prosthesis, thus illustrating the gluteus muscle tensile stress applied to the greater trochanter, which resists and remains connected to the prosthesis via its hydroxyapatite coating. (Fig. 4.5)

Zone 1c: Different observations can be made in this zone since the shape of the Corail® stem at the level of

its shoulder compresses the metaphyseal cancellous bone.

Zones 2–6 and 1c: In these zones true compressive forces are applied to the cancellous bone. There is radiographic evidence of bony bridges developing in lines orientated 45° downwardly (Fig. 4.6). These bridges persist around the Corail® stem.

Zone 7: This is a compressive zone from the stem. Compression is increased by the step macrostructure of the stem (7a). The lines of compressive stress run downwardly, extending along the macrostructure towards the inner cortex. However, no compressive force is observed under the collar (7b). The calcar does not undergo any stress, taking a blunt rounded aspect. Therefore, the collar does not have any long-term

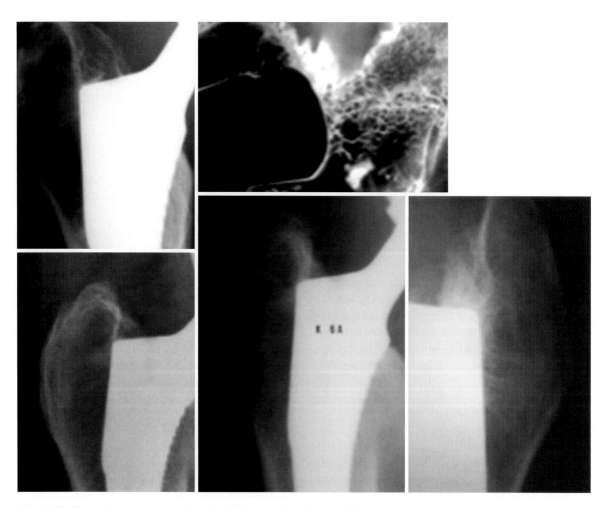

Fig. 4.5 Radiographic appearance and histological aspect of bone ingrowth in zone A

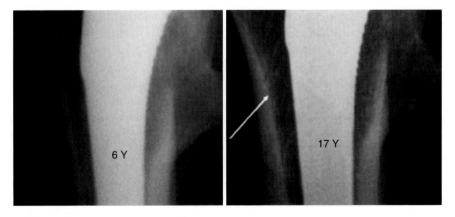

Fig. 4.6 Bone bridge formation in the metaphyseal region

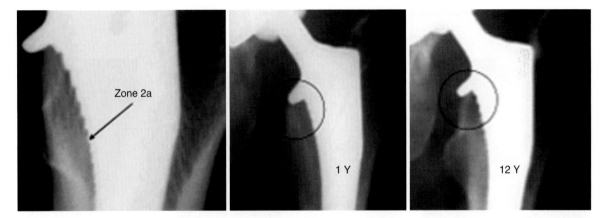

Fig. 4.7 Evolution of zone 7: bone bridge formation in (**a**) under load-bearing conditions and resorption in (**b**) with calcar rounding

effect and acts as a primary stabilising element while contributing and reinforcing implant stability for enhanced secondary osseointegration. In collarless implants, deep insertion and post-operative dynamic compaction should not be the objective but rather to achieve simple intra-operative stability (Fig. 4.7).

Zones 6, 2, 9 and 13: In the diaphyseal portion of the femur, bone bridges become more horizontal. These radiographic signs predominate in zones 2 and 6 on both sides but are more discreet on the anterior and posterior aspects (zones 9 and 13). However, maximum stress is typically observed on the prosthesis angles and confirmed in the histological analysis according to Hardy (Sect. 2.1.3.3); these radiographic

images reveal rounded trabeculae on the stem macrostructure corresponding to rotational strains (standing up from a chair). The Corail® stem macrostructure is of great interest in this case since it acts as a stress elevator at the level of the grooves, unlike smooth stems.

Distal zones 3, 5 and 4: The radiographic images are more diversified according to the stem positioning (valgus or varus) and the amount of cortical contact. When the Corail® stem is ideally centred, transition from the quadrangular to the thin conical shape allows a decreasing gradient of stiffness, thus avoiding distal fixation, which could lead to stress-shielding and thigh pain (Fig. 4.8). If stem positioning in varus or valgus does not have any clinical effect, some radiographic consequences have been observed: if the stem is placed in varus, outer cortical contact may induce a hemi-circumferential or hemi-ogival osteogenic reaction. However, there is no radiographic evidence of bone pedestal, a pejorative radiographic image described by Engh et al. [1] which corresponds to the fixation of the distal portion of the stem with a cortical bone.

Reactive Lines and Radiolucent Lines

Hydroxyapatite around the whole surface of the Corail® stem prevents the occurrence of fibrous encapsulation. An intimate contact is achieved between bone and prosthesis and is radiographically illustrated by the absence of any radiolucent line in normal condition.

The radiolucent line is a bright line (black on the radiograph) in contact with the stem, revealing the absence or disappearance of bone contact, and is over 2–3 mm thick. There is the impression of bone gap, therefore illustrating a failed osseointegration process. It has been observed in cases of infection (with an irregular or scalloped aspect) or poor fixation.

The reactive line is a rare radiographic image located in zone 1 of bone network densification at a few millimetres from the implant but with bone formation detected on both sides of this thin border. It is not recognised as a pejorative prognostic factor but only illustrates a solicitation localised in this zone which has neither macrostructure nor compressive force. This area of the Corail® prosthesis is the only part which is not subjected to compressive stress but rather to tensile/sliding stress.

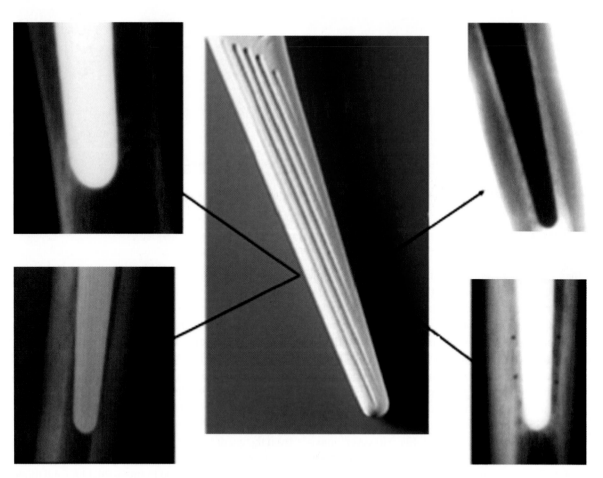

Fig. 4.8 Appearance of radiograph of the distal stem, which is centred or in varus (Copyright DePuyInternational Limited)

Cortical Hypertrophy

This is a bad predictive image, which is rarely seen due to the distal and full HA coating of the prosthesis. This phenomenon commonly occurs in cementless prostheses with proximal coating only, thus illustrating a change in stress distribution.

Cortical hypertrophy may occur when the Corail® stem has been implanted in a straight femur featuring thin cortices (champagne-flute femur), the stem being fixed distally. This technical mistake associated with an early-stage stress-shielding must be avoided intraoperatively through distal reaming of the femur, thus enhancing metaphyseal compression of cancellous bone by an increase in the diaphyseal canal diameter.

Stress-Shielding

The shape of the Corail® stem featuring a refined distal portion helps avoid the occurrence of stress-shielding in champagne-flute femurs if an 11 mm distal reaming is performed (Fig. 4.9). However, pseudo-images of stress-shielding in osteoporotic stove pipe femurs (type 3 according to the DORR classification) may be observed. Actually, it is osteopenia affecting the whole femur but the Corail® stem is fixed on its entire coating. Bone bridges of false pedestal–type structure are seen, thus increasing stem fixation and bonding to the cortices, the cancellous proximal fixation becoming elastic after 20 years, but the whole prosthesis remains stable (Fig. 4.10).

Osteolysis

A proximal femoral granulomatous osteolytic lesion may appear secondary to polyethylene wear debris. Release of polyethylene particulate debris induces a macrophage activation through phagocytosis. Such reaction depends on the size of the particles and the degree of particles per gram of tissue. Phagocytosis induces the release of inflammatory cytokine which

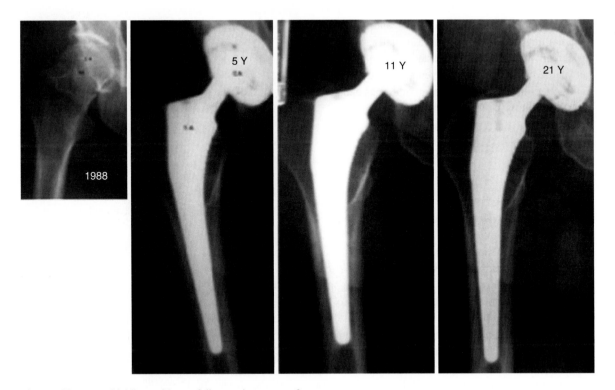

Fig. 4.9 No stress-shielding at 21-year follow-up in a narrow femur

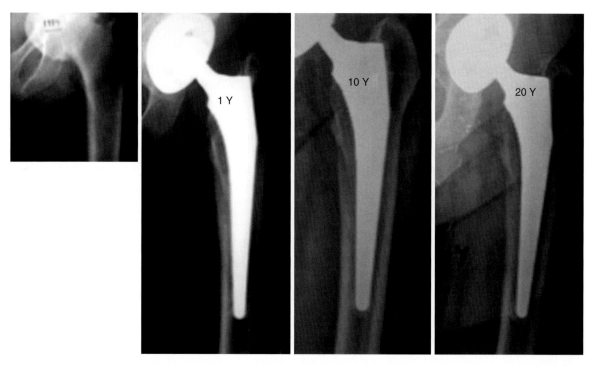

Fig. 4.10 No stress-shielding at 20-year follow-up in a cavernous femur

leads to osteoclastic bone resorption. Granuloma formation occurs in the proximal zone 1 and zone 7 but does not migrate down the stem as usually seen along the cement mantle of cemented stems. Intimate contact between bone and implant prevents particle migration and the presence of voluminous granulomas enhances distal fixation for better stem stability.

Conclusion

In conclusion, the radiographic image of the Corail®–host bone cohabitation has been evolving over a 25-year period but fixation remains stable.

Such fixation radiographically demonstrates lines of stress that develop during bone remodelling and depends on the amount of stress distributed to the bone.

During a period of 25 years, the ageing host bone will weaken, the patient will reduce his or her activities, thus modifying the stresses exerted by the prosthesis, but bone remodelling will adapt these changes and keep on maintaining the stem according to the amount and pattern of the compressive, tensile, shear and rotational forces transmitted.

Key Learning Points

> The radiographic images, which appear after implantation of a Corail® stem, illustrate the histological phenomenon occurring at the cancellous tissue-hydroxyapatite coating interface: osseointegration.
> This osseointegration is dependent upon the amount of stress transmitted to the bone by the prosthesis: this is bone remodelling under load-bearing conditions.
> Radiographic persistence of bone bridges due to the elasticity of the fixation in cancellous bone.

References

1. Engh CA, Massin P, Suthers KE (1990) Roentgenographic assessment of the biologic fixation of porous surfaced femoral components. Clinl Orthop Relat Res 257:107–127
2. Epinette JA, Geesink RGT (1995) Radiographic assessment of cementless hip prosthesis: ARA a proposed new scoring system. In: L'expansion scientifique (ed) Cahiers d'enseignement de la sofcot: hydroxyapatite coated hip and knee arthroplasty. Paris, France, p 114–126
3. Gruen TA, McNeice GM, Amstutz HC (1979) Modes of failures of cemented stem type femoral components. A radiographic analysis of loosening. Clin Orthop Relat Res 141:17–27

4.2.4 Long-Term Bone Remodelling: Reading Between the Lines

Jens Boldt

Femoral stress-shielding in cementless total hip arthroplasty (THA) is a potential complication commonly observed in distally loading press-fit stems. This study describes long-term femoral bone remodelling with cementless fully hydroxyapatite (HA)-coated Corail® stems at a mean of 17 years (range 15–20) in 209 consecutive patients with a complete clinical and radiographic history. All THAs were performed by one group of surgeons between 1986 and 1991. The concept of surgical technique included impaction of metaphyseal bone utilising bland femoral broaches until primary stability was achieved without distal press-fit. Radiographic evaluation revealed a total of five (2.4%) stems with peri-prosthetic osteolysis, which were associated with eccentric polyethylene (PE) wear. They were either revised or awaiting revision surgery. The remaining 97.6% stems revealed biologic load transfer in the metaphysis alone (52%) or in both metaphysis and diaphysis (48%). Stem survival of 97.6% after 15–20 years without stress-shielding was considered to be related to impaction of metaphyseal bone, bland broaches, full and thick HA coating, and unique prosthetic design.

Introduction

Cementless femoral stems have been successfully used since the very beginning of total hip arthroplasty (THA) and excellent long-term outcomes have been reported with survivorship of 80% and more after 20 years [2, 4]. The challenge facing the long-term success of cementless stems begins with obtaining primary stability of all components during and immediately after surgery.

The majority of cementless stems do not obtain primary stability in the proximal metaphysis, but instead are designed for distal diaphyseal interlocking and press-fit. Many metaphyseal locking cementless stems do not provide sufficient primary stability with the result that early subsidence, aseptic loosening and inadequate fixation occur, ultimately leading to medium-term failure.

In the long term, femoral stress-shielding in cementless THA is a potential complication commonly observed in all distally loading press-fit stems. The intrinsic conflict when using distally loading cementless stems comes with the fact that loading is reduced proximally, potentially causing stress-shielding and resorption of the proximal bone, and is increased distally causing thigh pain. Some clinical data report femoral stress-shielding with anterior thigh pain in over 10% of the cases, requiring various forms of treatment, both conservatively and surgically [5].

Physiological hip joint biomechanics is a complex process in which the patient's body weight is gradually transferred to the patient's proximal femur. The orientation of bone trabeculae follows a natural principle, namely Wolff's law (1891), which states that every change in form and function of a bone is followed by certain definite changes in its internal architecture and equally definite secondary changes in its mathematical laws. Thus bone is deposited and resorbed in accordance with the stresses placed upon it. On the femoral side cementless THA requires neck resection and a rigid femoral stem inserted into the medullary canal. Indisputably this procedure causes significant alterations of proximal load transfers and internal femoral stress-shielding. Following stem implantation the inferior (medial) cortex carries less load than it did before, which leads to bone resorption, whereas the metaphyseal cancellous bone carries more load, leading to cancellous bone deposition, remodelling and densification. Radiographic long-term follow-up studies in THA can provide extensive information on the natural history and continuous changes within the bone tissues involved.

The Corail® stem has been designed with a double taper and has proximal horizontal grooves to promote metaphyseal load transfer prior to loading the diaphyseal region. The proximal cancellous bone is compacted to allow efficient load transfer from the stem to the cortical bone. This loading pattern avoids proximal stress-shielding and reduces diaphyseal overloading. In addition, the Corail® stem is extensively hydroxyapatite (HA)-coated, which facilitates diaphyseal osseous integration without the need for extensive press-fit forces. Ideally, osseous fixation occurs predominantly within the metaphysis only.

This prospective study reports an in-depth radiographic analysis of a consecutive series of 209 Corail® cementless HA femoral stems in primary THA. The mean follow-up was 17 years (range 15–20 years). The analysis focuses on bone remodelling, osseointegration, stem subsidence and potential peri-prosthetic osteolysis around Corail® HA-coated stems. Furthermore, emphasis was placed on long-term alterations of metaphyseal and diaphyseal bone architecture, especially the observation of signs of proximal load transfer.

Materials and Methods

Surgery was performed between 1986 and 1991 in two centres by three experienced arthroplasty surgeons utilising the Corail® stem. All diagnoses were included and all patients were prospectively followed up by a strict regime including clinical and radiographical evaluations. Surgical technique for preparation and insertion of the Corail® stem was standardised and identical to the present technique. From a cohort of 584 primary THAs, 375 patients were either deceased or had their primary implant still in situ and were unable to attend clinical appointment for other reasons; 209 patients had a complete clinical and radiographic history and were available for review in this study. Ninety (33%) stems were collarless and 119 (67%) stems had an HA-coated collar on the medial side. Post-operative rehabilitation regime followed an identical protocol in both centres.

The acetabulum was addressed according to pathology using cementless cups in 199 cases and cemented all-polyethylene (PE) cups in 10 cases. In 49 cases (24%) one or more acetabular cup screws were used to enhance primary fixation. Various acetabular liners and heads with different articulating couples in different sizes were used: 196 (94%) ceramic on non-cross-linked polyethylene (CoP), 7 (3%) metal on polyethylene (MoP), and 6 (3%) ceramic on ceramic (CoC). The head diameter was 28 mm (28%) and 32 mm (72%).

Available radiographs included standard plain radiographs of an anteroposterior (AP) pelvis and the femur in two planes. Immediate post-operative, 6-week, 1-year and latest films were examined. All radiographs were reviewed by the author, an independent consultant orthopaedic surgeon with extensive experience in reading joint replacement radiographs [1].

Radiographic features were examined over time including major implant details, linear wear, stem alignment, calcar resorption, heterotopic ossification,

femoral canal fit, subsidence and stem–host bone interface. Signs of biological bone responses were evaluated in each of the 14 Gruen zones. These signs included presence and thickness of radiolucent lines, peri-prosthetic osteolysis and bone remodelling or alteration over time. Special interest was paid to evidence of stress-shielding, cortical thickening, thinning of the femoral cortex, both metaphyseal and diaphyseal. Trabecular orientation, lines and microstructure in relation to altered loads and stresses following neck resection and stem implantation were evaluated. Evidence of stem osseointegration and bone densification was evaluated. Immediate post-operative appearance of direct stem to cortex contact was documented according to Gruen zones on both AP and lateral views.

All radiographs were additionally digitized to accommodate magnification and contrast adjustments utilising DICOM Anonymizer v1.1.2. software. This technique allows improved identification of altered bone microanatomy, trabecular response and cancellous lines representing mechanical stresses and loads.

The magnification was determined for each radiograph so that accurate measurements of subsidence and poly wear could be made. For example, a 28 mm metal head that measures 32 mm in its largest diameter on the plain film leads to a magnification factor of 32/28 or 1.143 or 114%. Each distance measured was then corrected back to a 100% magnification in order to give 'true' millimetres.

Stem subsidence was measured in millimetres using a ruler and pencil and then calculated into 'true millimetres' as described. Polyethylene wear was measured on plain film using the immediate and latest follow-up radiographs. Wear was stated to be 'linear' when the femoral head approximated the middle of the acetabular cup without altering the centric location and vice versa. Wear was stated to be 'eccentric' when the femoral head changed its centric position within the acetabular component. Polyethylene cup wear was specified in true millimetres using the magnification factor.

Radiographic Results

All cases included in this study had at least a 15-year follow-up. The longest follow-up was 20 years (Fig. 4.11). Femoral stem alignment on antero-posterior views revealed 196 (94%) cases in neutral stem

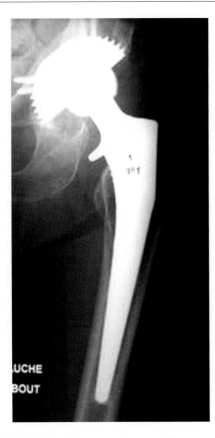

Fig. 4.11 First Corail® stem ever implanted 20 years ago showing successful osteointegration

alignment (within 2°) to the femoral shaft axis, no stem was in valgus alignment and 13 (6%) cases in varus alignment (range 3–10°). Overall the mean stem alignment was 0.6° of varus to the femoral shaft axis. Of these 13 varus stems, 3 had contact with the lateral diaphyseal cortex from within the medullary canal. One stem perforated the lateral cortex in a previously fractured and deformed femur. No stem altered its alignment at latest follow-up by more than 2°. Cases with considerable varus or valgus mal-positioning were successful despite poor alignment (Fig. 4.12a, b). Mean stem subsidence within the medullary canal was 0.1 mm (range 0–2 mm) with a standard deviation of 0.3 mm. There was no visible radiolucent line at the proximal metaphyseal bone–stem interface. Isolated radiolucent lines (RLL) larger than 2 mm were visible in 12 cases. In three cases these lines were evident in three or more Gruen zones, indicating possible loosening. One stem was revised for septic loosening. Three stems (1.4%) showed aseptic loosening and were revised and two stems (1%) showed aseptic loosening

and are awaiting revision surgery. Eight stems (3%) showed isolated proximal peri-prosthetic osteolysis larger than 2 mm, but diaphyseal stable osseous fixation. These eight stems were associated with the following significant radiographic findings:

1. Increased polyethylene wear of 4.6 true millimetres (the mean for the entire group was 2.6 mm)
2. Head diameter of 32 mm in all cases
3. More frequent acetabular failure (40% as opposed to 15% for the entire group)
4. Significantly increased contact of stems to inner cortex
5. A mean subsidence of 0.2 mm (twice the mean for the entire group)

These findings are considered to influence peri-prosthetic osteolysis and will be discussed in depth. In summary, 203 (97.6%) stems were still in place and showed stable osseous fixation at a mean follow-up of 17 years (Figs. 4.13 and 4.14). Five stems showed fixation failure, of which three were revised and two are awaiting revision surgery, giving an overall success rate of 97.6%. Desired metaphyseal bone remodelling in terms of bone densification or re-trabeculation was observed in 97.6% of Corail® stems (203 of 209). Radiographic appearance of long-term stable osseointegration at the metaphysis was noted in 98.1% (204/209) and osseointegration at the diaphysis in 99.6% (209/209). Those cases that lacked signs of re-trabeculation were associated with either septic or aseptic loosening, peri-prosthetic osteolysis and/or excessive polyethylene wear. Combined metaphyseal and diaphyseal osseointegration and stem incorporation were visible in 100 stems (48%). Predominant metaphyseal osseointegration and radiographic signs of load transfer were noted in all except five cases (97.6%). One hundred cases exhibited remodelling of cortical bone into cancellous bone without increasing the overall diameter of the femur. Eight (3.8%) cases showed increased diaphyseal bone remodelling, indicating predominant distal load transfer. Diaphyseal stress-shielding and cortical thickening was observed in three stems (1.4%).

Exact quantitative bone density changes are not measurable on plain radiographs except in extreme cases as suggested by the Singh index. The orientation of bone trabeculae had changed in all femora following Corail® implantation and followed the altered stresses and loads employed within the proximal metaphyseal femur. Stem implantation altered the

Fig. 4.12 Undersized Corail®
stem placed in severe valgus
shown at 19-year follow-up
(**a**) and undersized Corail®
stem in severe varus at
17-year follow-up (**b**). Note
successful and sound
long-term osteointegration in
both cases

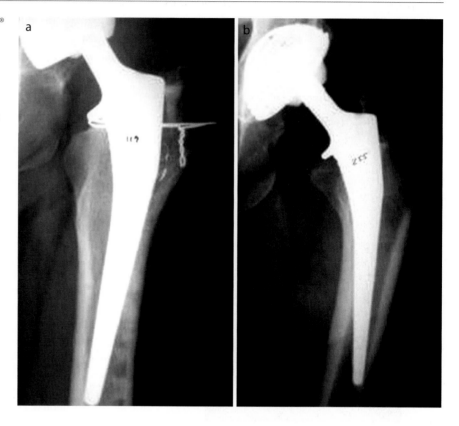

normal physiologic pattern of the proximal bone trabeculae to accommodate the new prosthetic load situation. Trabeculae reoriented according to increased
compressive loads at the cancellous part of the entire
metaphysis including the greater trochanter (Wolff's
law). The proximal part of the greater trochanter often
showed less trabeculation as a sign of decreased
loads. This behaviour was observed at the earliest at 6
weeks post-operatively, but more impressively at the
10-years follow-up. This indicated stable osseointegration and desired proximal load transfer. One hundred femora showed diaphyseal cortical remodelling
and development of cancellous bone as a sign of additional diaphyseal load transfer without measurable
femur thickening.

The mean eccentric polyethylene cup wear was
2.7 mm; however, this was not associated with the
development of radiolucent lines and peri-prosthetic
osteolysis. The eight cases with proximal 'moth damage'-like osteolytic lesions were associated with significant polyethylene wear and 32 mm large heads
articulating against non-cross-linked polyethylene
cups. Heterotopic ossification according to the Brooker
classification showed two (1%) cases with grade IV

and four (1.9%) cases with grade II ossification. Absent
or very mild heterotopic ossification was noted in the
remaining 202 (98%) cases (Fig. 4.15).

Discussion

Modern THA should have a survivorship of 80% or
more after 20 years as suggested by Branson and
Goldstein in 2003 [2]. There are a number of cementless stems that match these requirements such as the
Corail® stem, porocoated AML® stem, Zweymuller®,
CLS® and other stems. The highest published survivorship for the Corail® stem is 100% at 15 years and for
the AML® stem it is 99% at 15 years [4]. All existing
and future femoral stems will have to compete against
these reported outcomes. However, the longevity of
the femoral stem is only one of many considerations.

Further radiographic and clinical factors are equally
important such as function, thigh pain, stress-shielding, bone remodelling, cortical thickening, bone density and load transfer. In general, predominant
metaphyseal fixation is desired as opposed to combined metaphyseal and diaphyseal fixation. Moreover,

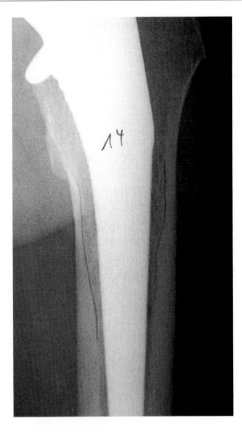

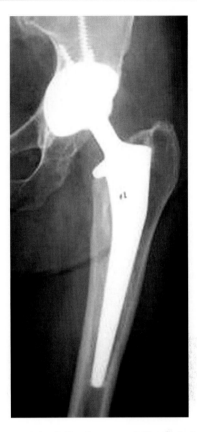

Fig. 4.13 Bone remodelling from cortex to cancellous bone at the diaphyseal part of Corail® stem 18 years post-operatively as a sign of combined metaphyseal and diaphyseal stem incorporation and load transfer

Fig. 4.14 Example of silent bone remodelling at the junction of metaphysis and diaphysis at 18-year follow-up. There is gradual remodelling of cortical bone into cancellous bone without increase of the overall outer diameter of the femoral bone. Thus, no ballooning, no stress-shielding, no thigh pain

diaphyseal press-fit with consequent stress-shielding and potential thigh pain should be avoided [3]. Clinical data seem to suggest that more proximally loaded stems lead to decreased thigh pain and vice versa. Females and to a lesser extent males have a high chance of developing osteopenia or osteoporosis within two decades following THA. This fact has implication on the stem life expectancy due to the decreasing bone quantity and quality with time.

The microanatomy at the bone–stem interface is increasingly challenged to carry normal physiological body loads and runs the risk of ultimate fixation failure [4]. Increasing age leads often to decreasing activity and muscle strength, which leads to suboptimal joint reaction forces and increasing stress in all THA implants. Kaplan–Meier survivorship analyses have generally shown non-linear survival with increasing follow-up time. Survivorship seems fairly constant until 10 years post-operatively, decreases rapidly after

15 years and gets significantly worse after a 20-year follow-up [3]. Since the femoral metaphysis has less bone mass compared to the diaphysis, it is just a question of time before the distal cortex plays an increasing role in THA stem fixation. Femoral implants that are designed for diaphyseal press-fit from the time of surgery carry the advantage of using the distal part of the femur more efficiently, but the disadvantage of stress-shielding and thigh pain as, for instance, with the CLS® Spotorno® stem [6].

An ideal stem would therefore use the metaphyseal bone as long as possible before loading and using up the diaphysis by remodelling cortical bone to cancellous bone. Data from this study suggested that the Corail® stem seems to behave in this way.

This long-term radiographic analysis revealed excellent survivorship of 97.6% after a mean follow-up of 17 years. One case even represented Paget's

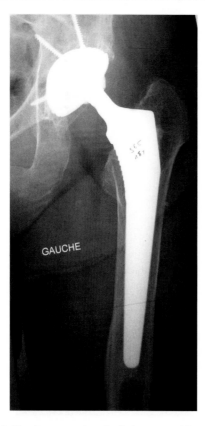

Fig. 4.15 Massive eccentric polyethylene wear 18 years post-operatively with a 28 mm ceramic head in a gamma in air-irradiated conventional polyethylene liner. The Corail® stem shows no osteolysis and no loosening despite excessive amounts of polyethylene wear particles

components and that they commonly represent osteoporosis rather than the presence of a fibrous membrane at the cement–bone interface. Data from various studies indicated that solid stem fixation is associated with good radiographic outcomes irrespective of the amount of biologically active polyethylene wear particles generated. So, it is as if the adjacent stem–bone interface builds a watertight barrier to prevent the ingress of biologically active wear particles (Fig. 4.17).

Secondary fixation of THA stems is a result of repair and bone remodelling during the healing process comparable to fracture healing. Calcar resorption was noted in the vast majority of cases and was expected as a biological response by the metaphyseal bone to the altered biomechanical loads and stresses within the proximal femur. This resorption occurred in stems both with and without a collar. Remodelling of bone occurs in response to physical stresses or to the lack of them in that bone is deposited in sites subjected to stress and is resorbed from sites where there

disease and was successful at 18 years (Fig. 4.16). Eight femora showed cystic osteolysis at the proximal stem–bone interface and this was interpreted as wear-induced bone resorption. However, seven of eight stems showed radiographic criteria for solid stem–bone fixation despite proximal osteolysis. Only three stems out of 209 revealed radiographic signs of loosening with 1–2 mm radiolucent lines in more than 50% of the Gruen zones coupled with 2 mm subsidence. All cases with femoral osteolysis were associated with significantly high linear polyethylene wear rates. Another noteworthy finding was the fact that peri-prosthetic osteolysis was not observed despite the presence of a mean 2.7 mm eccentric polyethylene wear. When present, radiolucent lines were observed at the proximal pole of the stem–bone interface and were more spherical and cystic rather than linear. Harris et al. demonstrated that radiolucent lines can occur with well-fixed

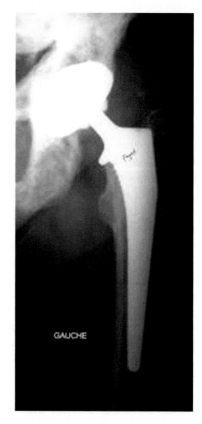

Fig. 4.16 Well-fixed Corail® stem implanted in a Paget's disease bone 18 years ago

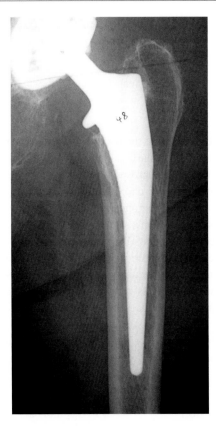

Fig. 4.17 Twenty-year follow-up of a collarless Corail® stem in a female patient with a hollow and osteoporotic femur demonstrating a combined metaphyseal and diaphyseal load transfer without femoral stress-shielding

occurred in stems with larger filling of the medullary canal. This demonstrates that the optimal stem size should be at least one size smaller than the maximum fill of the medullary canal. Extensively coated cementless stems faced criticism because of their tendency for diaphyseal remodelling. The Corail® stem did not cause cortical thickening or diaphyseal stress-shielding in 98.6% of cases after a mean follow-up of 17 years. This indicates that bone fixation in the metaphysis is sufficient and does not require further distal fixation. A potential reason for this behaviour is the orientation of the grooves on the stem which run horizontally at the metaphyseal and vertically at the diaphyseal part of the stem. Radiographic analyses of the trabecular architecture and orientation revealed increased apposition of load-bearing trabeculae at the groove edges and decreased ingrowth at the distal part of the stem.

Conclusions

Radiographic long-term analysis of the extensively HA-coated Corail® stem revealed excellent secondary bone fixation without subsidence and only 1.4% stress-shielding in 209 cases. Radiographic outcomes in this series suggested increased proximal bone remodelling and osseointegration as a sign of successful implant design and osseous incorporation. Histological specimens taken from the metaphyseal area during revision surgery confirm re-trabeculation of metaphyseal cancellous bone microstructures indicating the occurrence of proximal femoral loading. The Corail® stem uses the metaphyseal bone as long as possible before loading the diaphysis by remodelling cortical bone to cancellous bone. The Corail® stem performed well, with metaphyseal fixation being the predominant fixation even after 20 years of implantation and even in cases with osteopenia, suboptimal surgical technique or elderly patients with decreasing activity and bone quantity. The extensively HA-coated Corail® stem is a safe long-term implant in THA. In a population of 209 hips in which all indications were included, the 20-year survivorship was 97.6% excluding septic loosening [7]. The long-term survival of the Corail® stem that showed no stress-shielding after 20 years is considered to be related to five major contributing factors:

is little stress. The Corail® revealed remodelling of the metaphyseal bone in over 99% of cases as a sign of the altered biomechanics and cementless stem osteointegration.

Three (1.4%) cases showed diaphyseal cortex thickening after a mean follow-up of 17 years as a response to increased distal femoral load transfer. This study demonstrated that Corail® stems remain primarily fixed within the metaphyseal part of the femur despite its stem being extensively HA-coated. Radiographic data from this study showed that the micro-architecture of the cancellous bone trabeculae follows the pattern of proximal load transfer only in 55% of the cases after a 20-year follow-up. The remaining 45% showed combined metaphyseal and diaphyseal bone fixation with remodelling of cortical bone to cancellous bone at the stem–bone interface. Distal load transfer was noted in 1.4% of cases. It was interesting to observe that this cortical remodelling

1. Impaction and enhancement of metaphyseal bone
2. Blunt broaches
3. Full and thick layer of HA coating
4. Sound primary fixation with and without collar
5. Narrow stem in all dimensions

References

1. Boldt JG, Dilawari P, Agarwal S et al (2001) Revision total hip arthroplasty using impaction bone grafting with cemented nonpolished stems and charnley cups. J Arthroplasty 16(8):943–952
2. Branson JJ, Goldstein WM (2003). Primary total hip arthroplasty. AORN J 78(6):947–953, 956–969; quiz 971–974
3. Hallan G, Lie SA, Furnes O et al (2007) Medium- and long-term performance of 11,516 uncemented primary femoral stems from the Norwegian arthroplasty register. J Bone Joint Surg Br 89(12):1574–1580
4. Kwong LM, Jasty M, Mulroy RD et al (1992) The histology of radiolucent line. J Bone Joint Surg Br 74(1):67–73
5. Lavernia C, D'Apuzzo M, Hernandez V, Lee D (2004) Thigh pain in primary total hip arthroplasty: the effects of elastic moduli. J Arthroplasty 19(7 suppl 2):10–16
6. Müller LA, Wenger N, Schramm M et al (2010) Seventeen-year survival of the cementless CLS Spotorno stem. Arch Orthop Trauma Surg 130(2):269–275
7. Vidalain JP (2010). Twenty-year results of the cementless Corail® stem. Int Orthop 35(2):189–194

4.2.5 Clinical and Radiological Aspects of the Collar: To Be or Not to Be

Laurent Jacquot and Jean-Charles Rollier

The authors present the results of two selected groups of collared and collarless Corail® femoral stems taken from a continuous prospective series of patients operated between 1986 and 2007. This chapter compares the results and complications during the first postoperative year and in a separate group the outcome at a minimum of 5 years. The authors prefer to use a collar because of the theoretical advantages of improved stability and reproduction of the preoperative plan. Moreover, the results confirm that the use of collared stems does not induce any long-term negative radiological effects (stress-shielding), and that the clinical results are similar for the two cohorts – collared and collarless.

Introduction

The Corail® stem was originally designed with and without collar, in order to offer two options to the surgeon, considering the personal choice of the surgeon. Hence, the surgeon may opt for a collared or collarless stem as a function of both a biomechanical choice and the patient's bone quality.

A collared stem offers numerous theoretical advantages: reduced subsidence, better rotational stability, implantation as preoperative planning and lower risks of calcar fracture propagation.

This paper reports the results of two historically selected groups of patients with collared and collarless Corail® stems taken from a continuous prospective series of 2,712 stems implanted over a period of more than 20 years (Table 4.8).

Material and Method

Between 1986 and 2007, 2,712 total hip prostheses (THP) have been implanted in Annecy, France, by two

Table 4.8 Global cohort and groups

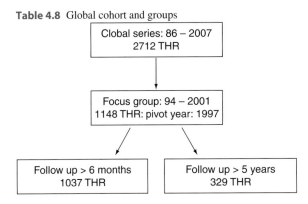

surgeons (Mr. Vidalain and Mr. Machenaud) who used the same technique and the same approach (Watson–Jones antero-lateral). Until 1997, most of the stems implanted were collarless (initial choice of the surgeons). As of 1997, most of the stems implanted were collared stems. This shift did not result from technical failures but from the choice of the implantation technique (cf. collar mechanical basis). The year 1997 was selected as the pivot year in order to compare the two cohorts of patients who received collared or collarless Corail® stems. The selection of the patients operated on between 1994 and 2001 made it possible to determine a cohort of 1,148 patients, with 720 collared stems (KA) and 428 collarless stems (KS).

The mean follow-up of the last examination is 2.44 years (KA) and 4.01 years (KS). A total of 1,037 patients (620 KA–417 KS) were followed up at least 6 months post-operatively. These early follow-up examinations have made it possible to compare the clinical and radiological post-operative evaluation, as well as the complications observed in each group.

The selection of patients reviewed at more than 5 years has enabled two cohorts to be compared: 171 KA (mean follow-up 6.99 years) and 158 KS (mean follow-up 8.93 years). The long-term clinical and radiological data of the two groups have been compared.

Patients' mean age at the time of the surgery was 66 years (18–94), with 578 males (51%) and 570 females (49%). Thirteen percent of the patients exhibited contralateral damages (Charnley B) and 16% general damages (Charnley C) before the surgery. The pre-op mean body mass index (BMI) was 27.8 (13–37), indicating global overweight, with 21% of obese patients (BMI >

30). Eighty-two patients (7%) had already undergone hip surgery before the implantation of the prosthesis. The pre-op mean Harris score was 40.9 (2–93), essentially penalised by the pain score. Arthrosis was the main aetiology (71%) of the operated hips, followed by aseptic osteonecrosis of the femoral head (8%) and dysplasia (7%). All patients received a fully HA-coated collared or collarless Corail® stem. The suprajacent acetabular component implanted was a cementless HA-coated screw cup (Tropic), with a lipped polyethylene (PE) insert (up to 2000). Nine percent of the patients received an HA-coated press-fit acetabular component with a ceramic insert (Lagoon) (since 2000). Post-operative follow-up visits took place at 3 months, 1 year and then every 3 years.

Patients were submitted to clinical evaluation using the Harris score preoperatively and during the follow-up examinations. Radiological evaluations comprised hip anteroposterior (AP) and LM x-rays and pelvis AP x-rays.

Results

Early Clinical and Radiological Follow-Up: 1,037 Patients Followed Up During the 6-Month Post-Operative Period
A reliable and significant interpretation of data was possible owing to the very high rate of patients (99.1%) for whom operative and post-operative data are available (Table 4.9).

Surgical Data

Thirty-nine stems were observed as proud (9%) in the collarless group, versus one stem (0.13%) in the collared group. This very significant difference ($p < 0.001$) is most likely due to the fact that with collarless stems, although rotational stability has been achieved, the quest for perfect vertical stability leads to using a larger-sized broach. This, in turn, leads to closer contact with the cortical walls and to additional risk of having the stem remaining slightly proud.

Table 4.9 Results of the collarless and collared groups: postoperative period, and more than 5-year follow-up

	Collar	Collarless
Results FU < 6 months	*n* = 620	*n* = 417
Harris score	88.2 (36–93)	87.3 (21–93)
Per op complications		
Proud	1 (0.1%)	39 (9%)
Cracks	98.31%	23 (5%)
Cables	98.31%	6 (1%)
Complications before day 21		
Dislocation	6 (1%)	6 (1.5%)
Subsidence	0	1 (0.2%)
Complications after day 21		
Dislocation	1 (0.1%)	2 (0.4%)
Infection	1 (0.1%)	
Results FU > 5 years	*n* = 171	*n* = 158
Harris score	88 (39–93)	87 (21–93)
X rays lucent lines	0	4 (Zone 1)
Calcar		
Calcar demineralisation	10 (6%)	3 (2%)
Calcar remodeling	19 (11%)	109 (38%)
Calcar bone loss (1–5 mm)	1 (0.5%)	1 (0.6%)
Complications		
Infection	2 (1%)	0
Dislocation	0	2 (1%)
Loosening	1 (0.5%)	2 (1%)
Survival rate	98.34% (93.2–99.6)	100%

During the broaching process 44 cracks (6%) occurred in the collared group versus 23 cracks (5.3%) in the collarless group. There is no significant difference between the two groups for this parameter. The cracks occurred in a similar percentage of cases during the broaching process using a similar technique regardless of the type of stem – collared or collarless.

Post-operative Data

The Harris scores at 6 months post-operatively were comparable in the two groups. The mean score was 88.25 (36–93) for the collared group and 87.34 (21–93) for the collarless group. The Charnley A patients (no contralateral or general damages) exhibited similar scores: 89.93 (45–93) for the collared group and 87.78 (36–93) for the collarless group.

Radiologically, no case of secondary subsidence has been observed after 3 weeks and no visible radiolucent lines (RLLs) on the AP and profile x-rays (Fig. 4.18). Less than 5% of reactive lines have been observed in zone 1 on the shoulder of the prosthesis (non-progressive lines without pathological values).

The surgical complications were as follows: 7 (1%) dislocations (6 early, 1 after 21 days), 2 sepses (0.3%) (lavage) in the collared group and 8 (2%) dislocations (6 early, 2 after 21 days); 1 radiological subsidence unrevised in the collarless group. These complications did not lead to revision surgery.

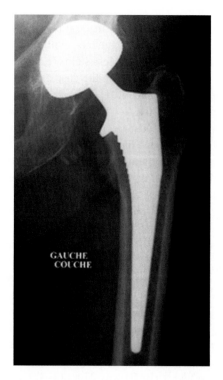

Fig. 4.18 Under-dimensioned collared Corail® stem: perfect osseointegration; no subsidence (D + 6 months)

Late Clinical and Radiological Follow-Ups: 329 Patients with at Least 5 Years of Follow-Up

Clinical Results

No significant difference has been evidenced in the Harris score between the two groups with a follow-up longer than 5 years: 88.81 (39–93) for the collared group, 87.03 (21–93) for the collarless group. The results obtained with isolation of the Charnley A groups with unilateral damage are similar: 89.26 (39–93) for the collared group versus 88.62 (32–93) for the collarless group. No thigh pain has been reported in the groups (collared or collarless).

Radiological Results

In spite of the PE wear measured on the x-rays, – 22 cases (12%) in the collared group versus 37 (24%) in the collarless group – only 4 radiolucencies (2%) have been noted in the collarless group in zone 1 (prosthesis shoulder), without any clinical impacts (Fig. 4.19).

Specific radiological study of the calcar is relevant. Simple demineralisation has been noted in ten cases (6%) for the collared group versus three cases (2%) in the collarless group. As to calcar remodelling, it should be noted that while only 19 cases (11%) have been observed in the collared group, 109 cases (68%) have been evidenced in the collarless group. This significant difference ($p < 0.001$) is very clear between the two groups. It is not the case for substance losses between 1 and 5 mm, since only one case had been observed in each group. This confirms the medium-term innocuousness of the collar, the absence of stress-shielding in zone 7 as well as the preservation of the calcar below the collar (Figs. 4.20–4.22).

Complications

In the collared group, lavage was necessary due to two late haematogenous infections. In the collarless group, two late dislocations and two potential loosenings caused by polyethylene granulomas have been reported.

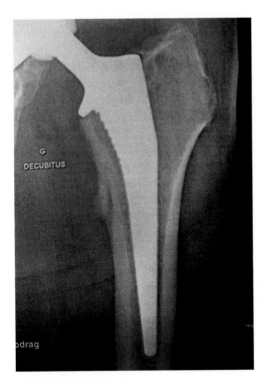

Fig. 4.19 Reactive line in zone 1

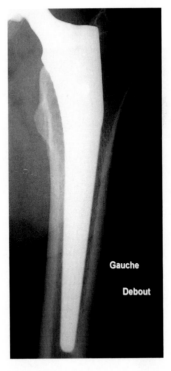

Fig. 4.20 Collared Corail® stem placed in varus. No radiolucent line, no stress-shielding (D + 16 years)

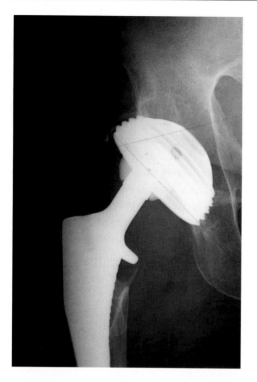

Fig. 4.21 Collared Corail® stem. PE wear–induced granuloma. No stress-shielding (D + 18 years)

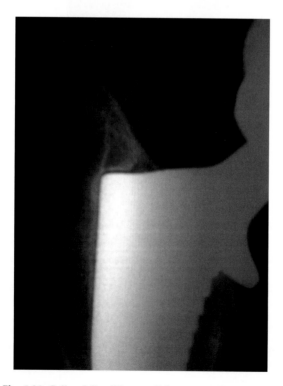

Fig. 4.22 Collared Corail® stem. Calcar remodelling. No radiolucent line (D + 19 years)

Survival Curves

In the collarless group, there has been no revision with replacement of component. Hence the Kaplan–Meier survival rate is 100% (100–100) at 9.57 years of follow-up. In the collared group, (mean follow-up 7.01 years), there have been two revision cases with replacement of components: one replacement of cup due to loosening and one replacement of stem due to peri-prosthetic fracture. The Kaplan–Meier survival rate is 98.34% (93.2–99.6) at 12.3 years of follow-up (Fig. 4.23).

Discussion

The utilisation of a collar for cementless stems in general is not frequent [8]. There is a lack of data in the literature on hydroxyapatite (HA)-coated cementless collared stems [3, 5, 7, 9]. The follow-up of this series enables taking stock of the possible long-term consequences of the collar.

The collar offers several theoretical and technical advantages: increased primary stability; precise position of the stem at the cut height; elimination of the need to increase the size of the stem in order to increase primary stability (therefore less risk of cracks perioperatively propagating). Moreover, the collar is assumed to 'seal' the femur. This limits the penetration of PE wear debris into the femoral canal, hence preventing the formation of granulomas. However, bearing in mind the fact that the use of a collar for cemented stems may have deleterious effects, there is a legitimate reluctance to use cementless collared stems because of the lack of results [1, 4, 7].

The present study provides preoperative and postoperative data on a selected group of more than 1,000 patients with more than 99% of the patients in the follow-up cohort (6 months post-operative period). Since patients have been selected from a larger continuous prospective series without patients being interviewed again specifically for the study, the rate of patients at more than 5 years follow-up is lower, although more than 300 patients are included in the follow-up results. As to the rationale for the collared versus collarless stem, this was essentially a technical choice made by the surgeons in 1986 and again in 1997, and as such this series is considered a historical comparative study.

The operating data analysis shows an equivalent rate of cracks (occurring during femur preparation) in the two cohorts. This preparation must comply with

Fig. 4.23 Survival curve of the global Corail® series. Patients with longer than 5-year follow-up

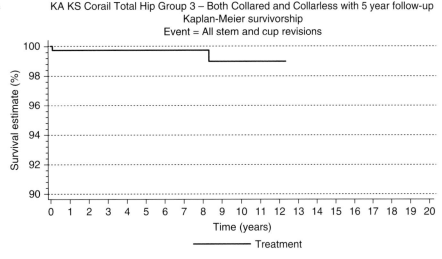

the principle of cancellous bone compaction, without seeking maximum filling using the largest possible stem. The preoperative planning gives an idea of the size, and the broach that provides proper rotational stability must be the last one in the broaching process. Collared stems theoretically prevent post-operative subsidence and hence minimise the risk of cracks as there is no need for maximum filling intended to prevent secondary subsidence. Moreover, the use of a stem with 'optimum' filling enables the reaming to be minimised during femoral preparation in the case of a flared femur associated with early distal locking.

More stems remained proud in the collarless cohort without consequence or need for explantation and rebroaching. This moderate protrusion (<3 mm) is probably related to the need for more filling to prevent subsidence when collarless stems are being used. Currently, collared stems are almost systematically used. Optimal filling is not sought. The broaching process ends once rotational stability has been achieved. This enables the number of cracks to be minimised. However, there was no significant difference between the two groups in this study.

It should be noted that there has been no subsidence after the 21st day post-operatively, which confirms that the definitive stability of the implant is achieved before the end of the first month post-operatively; this has also been demonstrated in other studies [2, 10]. Radiographic examination has shown the occurrence of reactive lines, sometimes early in zone 1, on the prosthesis shoulder. These reactive lines which have always been stable have never been associated with clinical signs. This radiographic specificity could be explained by the

absence of macrostructures at the prosthesis shoulder. In the absence of clinical signs, progressive or real radiolucent lines, we consider this parameter as non-pathological. Besides these radiolucent lines in zone 1, we must insist on the radiological silence of these stems (collared or collarless), with the almost total absence of radiolucent lines over time.

The analysis of zone 7 – and more specifically the calcar – has confirmed that the collar does not have any deleterious effects, especially no stress-shielding [6, 7], and that calcar reshaping is observed mostly with collarless stems, whereas it is not observed in the first 10 years post-operatively with the collared stems.

The complications that led to surgical revision without replacement of component are non-specific (infection, dislocation, wear). The two revisions with replacement of prosthetic component (cup loosening, peri-prosthetic fracture) are independent of the presence or absence of a collar.

Key Learning Points

> The fully HA-coated Corail® stem confirms the quality of its long-term outcomes with and without a collar, especially the lack of thigh pain in both cases.
> The collar offers surgical technical advantages in terms of the precision of the implantation level without any risk of post-operative subsidence by resetting, which is a form of additional safety.

> ❯ This study found no clinically significant difference concerning radiological and clinical data, and survival rate between collared and collarless Corail® femoral stems.
> ❯ The collar has no deleterious radiological effect (radiolucent line or stress-shielding). Calcar remodelling was even less frequent than with the collar stem in this study.

References

1. Berend KR, Lombardi AV Jr (2010) *Intraoperative femur fracture is associated with stem and instrument design in primary total hip arthroplasty.* Clin Orthop Relat Res 468(9):2377–2381
2. Campbell D, Mercer G, Nilsson KG et al (2009) Early migration characteristics of a hydroxyapatite-coated femoral stem: an RSA study. Int Orthop Dec 13 http:\www.ncbi.nlm. nih.gov/pubmed/20012862.
3. Froimson M, Garino J, Machenaud A et al (2007) Minimum 10-year results of a tapered, titanium, hydroxyapatite-coated hip stem. An independent review. J Arthroplasty 22(1):1–7
4. Karachalios T, Tsatsaronis C, Efraimis G et al (2004) The long-term clinical relevance of calcar atrophy caused by stress shielding in total hip arthroplasty: a 10-year prospective randomized study. J Arthroplasty 19(4):469–475
5. Mandell JA, Carter DR, Goodman SB et al (2004) A conical-collared intramedullary stem can improve stress transfer and limit micromotion. Clin Biomech (Bristol, Avon) 19(7):695–703
6. Markolf KL, Amstutz HC, Hirschowik DL (1980) The effect of calcar contact on femoral component micromovement. J Bone Joint Surg 62:1315
7. Meding JB, Ritter MA, Keating EM et al (1997) Comparison of collared and collarless femoral components in primary uncemented total hip arthroplasty. J Arthroplasty 12(3):273–280
8. Vidalain JP (2004) Corail® stem long-term results based upon the 15-years ARTRO group experience. In: Epinette JA, Manley MT (eds) Fifteen years of clinical experience with hydroxyapatite coatings in joint arthroplasty. Springer, France, pp 217–224
9. Whiteside LA, Easley JC (1989) The effect of collar and distal stem fixation on micromotion of the femoral stem in uncemented total hip arthroplasty. Clin Orthop Relat Res Feb(239):145–153
10. Whiteside LA, Amador D, Russell K (1988) The effects of the collar on total hip femoral component subsidence. Clin Orthop Relat Res Jun(231):120–126

4.2.6 Restoration of Biomechanics: Extramedullary Fine-Tuning

Michel-Henri Fessy and Michel Bonnin

One of the purposes of total hip arthroplasty (THA) is to reconstruct the bony anatomy of the hip joint and restore the functional lever arm of the abductor muscles. The lateralised or high offset Corail® stem range has been designed in addition to the standard range to serve this purpose. In this article, the authors assess the outcome of a lateralised (high-offset) range in restoring hip anatomy and function.

Introduction

Restoring the biomechanics of the hip joint has been shown to reduce wear and improve stability in hip arthroplasty [1, 2, 4–8, 12, 13, 16, 17, 20, 22, 24]. We believe it is important to restore the lever arm of the abductor muscles to improve functional recovery and restore physiological stress to the bone in the proximal femur. With this objective in mind, the ARTRO Group decided to design a range of high-offset femoral stems in addition to the standard range of Corail® stems. Currently the Corail® total hip arthroplasty (THA) system comprises three ranges of femoral stems:

Standard range: 135° neck angle, sizes 8–20, with collar (KA) and collarless (KS).
High-offset range: 135° neck angle, offset (+7 mm), sizes 9–20, collarless (KHO).
Coxa vara range: 125° neck angle (−5 mm vertical height), offset (+7 mm), sizes 9–20, with collar (KLA).

To assess the introduction of the extended range of Corail® stems, we performed a retrospective clinical and radiographic evaluation of a cohort of patients who received a lateralised (either a coxa vara or high-offset) Corail® stem. The primary objective of this study was to determine if the selective use of lateralised stems restored hip joint biomechanics. The secondary objective was to carry out a clinical evaluation of this population and a radiological analysis of bone remodelling taking place around the femoral stem during the first year after implantation compared to the previously documented data for the standard range of stems.

Material and Methods

Between January 2007 and December 2008, 407 consecutive THAs with a primary diagnosis of osteoarthritis or osteonecrosis received a Corail® THA by the same surgeon (M-HF). Based on the preoperative planning using plain radiographs and templates, 106 THA in 103 patients were templated as needing a high-offset stem to restore hip joint biomechanics (KLA stem = 34, KHO stem = 72). The aim of the preoperative x-ray planning was always to obtain equal leg lengths and restore the combined femoral and acetabular offset of the hip (global offset).

The mean age was 65 years [range 30–93 years]. Surgery was performed through the posterolateral approach according to the preoperative plan. Based on the age of the patients, the following acetabular components were implanted: Pinnacle™ cup (ceramic–ceramic bearing) in patients <70 years: $n = 60$ and dual mobility cup (ceramic or metal–polyethylene (PE) bearing) in patients >70 years: $n = 46$.

Patients were assessed at a minimum follow-up of 13 months (range 13–32 months). Clinical assessment was with pre- and post-operative Postel-Merle d'Aubigné (PMA) and Harris hip score [14, 18], pain location assessment and documentation of complications. Digitized anteroposterior (AP) pelvis radiographs were taken with the patient standing and the patella pointing forwards in the frontal plane. Radiographs were analysed preoperatively and at the last follow-up visit by two independent observers. The following biomechanical, extramedullary and endomedullary parameters were recorded (Figs. 4.24 and 4.25):

1. Caput–collum–diaphyseal (CCD) angle: neck shaft angle.
2. Abductor lever arm (ALA): horizontal distance between centre of femoral head and lateral cortex of femur at level of greater trochanter.
3. Femoral offset: horizontal distance between centre of femoral head and anatomical axis of femur.
4. Gluteus medius action angle (GMAA): angle between vertical line dropped from anterior superior iliac spine (ASIS) and line between ASIS and lateral greater trochanter.
5. Acetabular offset, which is equivalent to the weight lever arm (WLA): horizontal distance between centre of femoral head and midline symphysis pubis.
6. Proximal and distal endofemoral diameter: transverse femoral diameter at the level of neck resection (proximal) and 10 cm below (distal).
7. Femoral flaring [19].

The term global offset defines the sum of two measurements: (a) the weight lever arm (acetabular offset) and (b) the abductor lever arm, i.e. the distance – on the pelvic x-ray – between the pubic symphysis and the

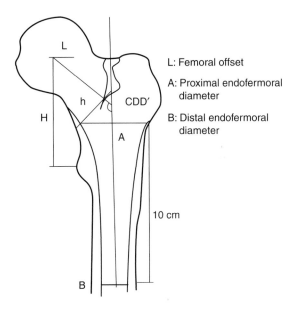

Fig. 4.24 Lateralisation and endomedullary and extramedullary parameters

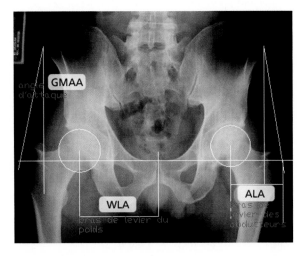

Fig. 4.25 Weight lever arm, abductor lever arm, gluteus medius angle of action

most lateral point of the greater trochanter – (a) and (b) meet at femoral head centre.

In addition, bone remodelling was analysed on all the patients (AGORA Roentgenographic Assessment [ARA] score and Engh and Massinet score) [9, 10] around the stem with the longest follow-up.

The statistical analysis was carried out using the software JMP 7.0. The comparison tests between the two groups for the continuous variables were Mann and Whitney and Kruskall and Wallis non-parametric tests. For the categorical variables, the authors used the exact Fisher test to compare the intergroup percentages. The correlations between continuous variables were measured using the Spearman rhô coefficient. The significance threshold selected was $p < 0.05$.

Results

The Postel Merle d'Aubigné score changed from 9.1 preoperative to 17.1 post-operative; two thirds of the patients exhibited excellent results [9] at 1 year. The Harris score was 30 preoperative and 91 post-operative. This is a clinically significant improvement of 60 points. No thigh pain was reported; two patients complained of pain at the attachment of the gluteus medius on exertion. No post-operative infection was observed in this series. There was one isolated dislocation at 3 months without recurrence at the time of 1-year follow-up.

Descriptive data for the radiographic parameters is reported in Table 4.10, differences in Table 4.11 and a further sub-group assessment in Table 4.12.

Table 4.10 Evolution of intra- and extramedullary parameters between the preoperative x-ray and the last follow-up measurements

	Preoperative	Last F.U.	p
CCD angle	126.5° [108.5; 139.7]	129.9° [118; 140.6]	<0.0001
GMAA	11.1° [5.5; 18]	11.3° [7; 18]	NS
ALA	57.5 mm [46.4; 77]	59.3 mm [48; 72]	0.02
Femoral offset	46.9 mm [35.6; 67.4]	49.8 mm [37; 64.1]	<0.0001
Acetabular offset	90.1 mm [73.5; 108]	82.5 mm [68; 97.4]	<0.0001
Global offset	137 mm [118; 149]	132.3 mm [115.6; 142.8]	0.004

Table 4.11 Variation of intra- and extramedullary parameters between the preoperative values and the last follow-up values

	Variation, in mm	Variation, in %
ALS	2.1 mm [−13.5; 17.2]	4.5% [−19.96;32.4]
Femoral offset	2.9 mm [−11;21]	7.4% [−17.5;50]
Acetabular offset	−7.6 mm [−23.7; 11.8]	−8.2% [−23.2;13.8]
Global offset	−4.7 mm [−28; 24]	−3.2% [−19;19.3]

Preoperatively, global offset was on average 137 mm ± 11.5, femoral offset 46.9 mm ± 6.3, acetabular offset 90.1 mm ± 6.7 and GMAA 11.1° ± 2.3. The mean ALA was 57.5 mm ± 6.7 and the flaring was 0.28 ± 0.05.

The femoral offset was correlated with the ALA ($p < 0.0001$) and to the GMAA ($p < 0.006$), but did not correlate with the flaring ($p = 0.7$).

At the last follow-up, global offset was on average 132.3 mm ± 12.5, femoral offset 49.8 mm ± 4.7, acetabular offset or WLA 82.5 mm ± 6.8 and GMAA 11.3° ± 2. The mean ALA was 59.3 mm ± 5.

Femoral offset increased by 3.1 mm (7.8%). Acetabular offset was reduced on average by 7.4 mm (8%); the cup was therefore medialised by 7.4 mm, with a maximum of 11.8 mm (Table 4.11).

Femoral offset and ALA increased post-operatively ($p < 0.0001$), but acetabular offset and global offset diminished ($p < 0.0001$). GMAA remained stable ($p = 0.8$).

Thus, if we look at the results (Table 4.10):

- There is a significant acetabular medialisation post-operatively.
- The abductor lever arm increased significantly post-operatively.
- There is no difference between the gluteus medius action angle pre- and post-operatively at 11°.

A strong correlation is observed between the value of the hip global offset and the gluteus medius action angle.

The mean ARA score was 5.7 (respectively 5.3 for KLA and 5.8 for KHO stems, note differences between the two stems $p = 0.2$), and the mean Engh and Massin score was 23.4 (respectively 23 for KLA and 23.5 for KHO stems, note differences between the two stems $p = 0.5$).

Table 4.12 Preoperative femoral lateralisation subgroup values

	Group 1			Group 2			Group 3		
	Femoral offset <40 mm			40 mm < femoral offset < 45 mm			Femoral offset > 45 mm		
	n = 14			n = 34			n = 60		
	KLA = 5/ KHO = 7			KLA = 12/ KHO = 22			KL = 17/ KHO = 43		
	Preop	Postop	p	Preop	Postop	p	Preop	Postop	p
GMAA	12.5° [10; 16]	11.1° [8.7; 14.1]	NS	11.7° [5.5; 18]	11.7° [8.2; 18]	NS	10.5° [6.5; 16.3]	11.1° [7; 15.9]	NS
ALA	52.4 mm [47.2; 57.4]	59.6 mm [53.3; 67]	0.0003	55.05 mm [46.4; 68.8]	58.7 mm [47; 69]	0.01	60 mm [48.2; 77.1]	59.7 mm [49.6; 72.1]	NS
Femoral offset	37.7 mm [35.6; 39.9]	45.9 mm [39.3; 54]	<0.0001	43 mm [40.2; 45]	48.8 mm [37.7; 64.2]	<0.0001	50.9 mm [45.1; 67.4]	51.1 mm [39.5; 62.9]	NS
Acetabular offset	87.2 mm [81.7; 94.5]	81.7 mm [77.6; 97.4]	0.02	87.8 mm [78.6; 100.7]	80.5 mm [72.8; 90.2]	<0.0001	91.9 mm [73.4; 108]	83.8 mm [68; 95]	<0.0001
Global offset	124.9 mm [1178; 134]	127.7 mm [117.4; 137]	NS	130.9 mm [121.8; 142.8]	129.3 mm [125.6; 145.7]	NS	142.9 mm [0.8; 46.3]	134.9 mm [116.4; 154.9]	<0.0001

Discussion

The use of high-offset femoral stems led to a moderate increase of the femoral offset and of the ALA, without affecting the GMAA. The independent nature of the femoral offset and of the endomedullary parameters reinforces our opinion for the use of stems with non-homothetic neck. In other words, the dimensions of the neck geometry do not increase in direct proportion to the size of the femoral canal.

During the design phase of the high-offset femoral stems the ARTRO Group performed an anatomical study and predicted that 30% of cases would benefit from a high-offset stem. In this study, high-offset implants were used in 106 hips (103 patients) part of a cohort of the 407 THAs implanted over the same period. Hence the surgeon used a high-offset implant in just over 25% of the cases. Thirty-four KLA Corail® stems (125° varus high-offset) have been used versus 72 KHO Corail® stems (high-offset 135°). The varus implants were used in 30%

of the cases, and the high-offset implants in 70% of the cases when a high-offset implant was indicated.

Bone remodelling around a lateralised implant is comparable to that achieved with a standard implant, assuming that the same implantation technique is used [15]. In our study, there was no difference between KLA and KHO stems for the ARA and Engh and Massin scores.

The gluteus medius action angle (GMAA) remained stable after the prosthetic reconstruction. This demonstrates that the method used with high-offset implants has made it possible to respect the mechanics of the gluteus medius. However, global offset was slightly reduced; therefore it could be argued that the mechanics of the gluteus medius were not totally respected. However, it has been reproduced as closely as possible without any apparent clinical consequence to date.

This suggests that global offset provides a more discriminatory measure of hip biomechanics than the gluteus medius action angle alone.

In fact, global offset has been quite effectively restored changing by only 4.7 mm from 137 mm on average (preoperative) to 132.3 mm on average (postoperative). This preservation of the global offset was achieved at the cost of an increase of the abductor lever arm due to the reduction of the weight lever arm (acetabular offset). During the arthroplasty, with the technique used, we observed a medialisation of the prosthetic centre of the hip relative to the anatomical centre of the native hip. On average, there was a medialisation of 7.6 mm of the prosthetic centre of the hip. This medialisation of the centre of rotation reached a maximum of 11.8 mm in this series. It can therefore be said that placing the cup on the floor of the acetabular fossa leads to the automatic medialisation of the acetabulum by 7.5 mm on average (12 mm maximum). In order to compensate for this medialisation of the centre of rotation so as to respect the mechanical function of the gluteus medius, the authors decided to increase the abductor lever arm by increasing the femoral offset. This increased the abductor lever arm by 4.5% and the femoral offset by 7.5%. This increase of the femoral offset would appear to have no obvious clinical impact.

There are, however, two cases in which pain was reported and was attributed to tendinopathy at the attachment of the gluteus medius. This pain could be explained by an excessive post-operative global offset in each of the patients of +8 and +15 mm, respectively. This occurred in two female patients who had a preoperative coxa vara with a femoral offset of less than 40 mm. The use of a coxa vara stem with 125° CCD angle (KLA) was justified to avoid an increase in leg length. This, however, led to excessive tension of the gluteus medius and a short neck range had to be used to overcome this problem. There was only one case of increased global offset of the same amplitude without gluteal pain.

The respect of the integrity of the gluteus medius is a necessary prerequisite in achieving a successful THA (pain-free normal function with an unrestricted walking range without the aid of a stick). The gluteus medius application force must be restored, respected and maintained both in terms of attachment and direction. It is therefore necessary to respect the relative position of its attachment, i.e. the relative position of the femur (greater trochanter) vis-à-vis the pelvis. Ideally this force should be submitted to a three-dimensional (3D) analysis [16, 21], but in routine practice the analysis is made using an AP x-ray of the pelvis. The force of the gluteus medius expressed on an AP x-ray of the pelvis can be characterised by:

The action angle of the gluteus medius
The global offset

The surgical procedure creates a prosthetic hip centre of rotation which modifies the centre of rotation of the native hip as well as the femoral offset.

Steinberg and Harris [23] postulated the biomechanical advantages of increased femoral offset because of the resultant increased abductor lever arm. This reduces the abduction force and thus the resulting force applied to the joint is reduced. Furthermore the stability of the prosthesis is increased due to the increased tension applied to the gluteal muscles, and the risk of femur–pelvis impingement is also reduced. Hence the increase of the abductor lever arm is favourable since it enables the intra-articular constraints to be lowered. Acetabular medialisation is favourable too, since it enables the weight lever arm – hence the intra-articular constraints – to be reduced [11, 14].

The restoration of the gluteus medius angle of action permits the optimal function of the hip abductors to be restored.

In one preliminary study [3], we identified two distinct causes that can result in poor restoration of the gluteus medius action angle and from this we postulate three causes of potential hip limping:

1. Acetabular cause with excessive medialisation of the cup despite correct restoration of the femoral offset
2. Femoral cause with femoral offset restored to less than 75% of its preoperative value associated with correct acetabular medialisation
3. Mixed cause combining inadequate restoration of the femoral offset with an excessive acetabular medialisation; these two errors become additive

This study made it possible to re-evaluate our method of preoperative x-ray planning. Therefore we no longer focus on femoral offset alone but also on acetabular offset, which in turn makes us consider the global offset. Yet, questions remain as to the minimum restoration value of the gluteus medius angle of action.

The analysis in Table 4.12 makes it possible to specify the indications.

When preoperative femoral offset exceeds 45 mm, a lateralised stem should be used. This enables the abductor lever arm to be restored and respected, yet it does not necessarily reproduce global offset because of the potential decrease in offset or medialisation of the acetabular component.

When the preoperative femoral offset ranges from 40 to 45 mm, using a lateralised stem compensates for the fact that the native hip centre has been medialised because of the acetabular component placement. Thus the abductor lever arm is increased by using a femoral component with a higher offset but the global offset is respected.

When the preoperative femoral offset is less than 40 mm a high-offset implant should only be used in the case of excessive medialisation of the acetabulum in order to preserve global offset. This group includes the two observations of gluteus medius tendinopathy as well as an excessive increase of the global offset.

Therefore, the authors recommend the mandatory use of a lateralised Corail® stem whenever femoral offset is greater than 45 mm. In all other cases, careful preoperative planning optimizes the offset needed to respect the function of the gluteus medius.

Key Learning Points

> Insufficient restoration of offset can lead to hip limping due to suboptimal function of the gluteus medius.

> Due to the routine medialisation of the cup, if at least 75% of the offset cannot be restored there will be hip limping due to compromised function of the gluteus medius.

> In 25% of our arthroplasties, a high-offset femoral component was required (1/3 Corail® 125° Coxa Vara and 2/3 Corail® 135° High Offset).

> The global offset of the hip must be respected. Any increase in global offset is always detrimental.

> A *lateralised Corail® stem* must always be used when preoperative femoral offset is greater than 45 mm.

> Careful preoperative planning ensures the choice of the optimum femoral offset so as to respect the function of the gluteus medius.

References

1. Amstutz HC, Sakai DN (1975) Total joint replacement for ankylosed hips. J Bone Joint Surg Am 5:619–625
2. Asayama I, Naito M, Fujisawa M et al (2002) Relationship between radiographic measurements of reconstructed hip joint position and the Trendelenburg sign. J Arthroplasty 17:747–751
3. Béguin L, Limozin R, Demangel et al (2002) Boiterie et défaut de latéralisation dan les arthroplasties de hanche. Rev Chir Orthop Oct 88(6):25
4. Bourne RB, Rorabeck CH (2002) Soft tissue balancing: the hip. J Arthroplasty 17(suppl 1):17–22
5. Charles MN, Bourne RB, Davey JR et al (2004) Soft tissue balancing of the hip: the role of femoral offset restoration J Bone Joint Surg Am 86:1078–1088
6. Davey JR, O'Connor DO, Burke DW et al (1993) Femoral component offset: its effect on strain in bone-cement. J Arthroplasty 8:23–26
7. Devane P, Home G, Winemaker M et al (1997) The effect of restoring femoral offset during THR on 3D volumetric wear J Bone Joint Surg Br 79(suppl):385
8. Dolhain P, Tsigaras H, Bourne R et al (2002) The effectiveness of dual offset stems in restoring offset during total hip replacement. Acta Orthop Belg 68:490–499
9. Engh CA, Massin P, Suthers KE (1990) Roentgenographic assessment of the biologic fixation of porous-surfaced femoral components. Clin Orthop Relat Res Aug(257):107–128
10. Epinette JA, Geesink R et al Etude radiologique des prothèses de hanche non cimentées. Proposition d'un nouveau système d'évaluation: le score ARA. In: Duparc J (ed) Cahier d'enseignement de la SOFCOT. Elsevier, Paris, pp 107–119
11. Fessy MH, N'Diaye A, Carret JP et al (1999) Locating the center of rotation of the hip Surg Radiol Anat 21:247–250
12. Frain P (1978) Moyen fessier et appui unipodal. Variations géométriques sur le thème des ostéotomies fémorales et pelviennes Rev Chir Orthop 64:445–458
13. Girard J, Touraine D, Soenen M et al (2005) Mesure de la pénétration céphalique sur des radiographies numérisées: reproductibilité et précision. Rev Chir Orthop 91:137–142
14. Harris WH (1969) Traumatic arthritis of the hip after dislocation and acetabular fractures: treatment by mold arthroplasty. An end-result study using a new method of result evaluation. J Bone Joint Surg Am 51:737–755
15. Kärrholm J, Garellick G, Herberts P (2005) The Swedish hip arthroplasty register, Annual Report 2005
16. Lecerf G, Fessy MH, Philippot R et al (2009) Femoral offset: anatomical concept, definition, assessment, implications for preoperative templating and hip arthroplasty. Orthop Traumatol Surg Res. 95(3):210–219
17. McGrory BJ, Morrey BF, Cahalan TD et al (1995) Effect of femoral offset on range of motion and abductor muscle strength after total hip arthroplasty J Bone Joint Surg Br 77:865–889
18. Merle d'Aubigné (1990) Cotation chiffrée de la fonction de la hanche. Rev Chir Orthop 76:371–374
19. Noble PC, Lindahl LJ, Jay JL et al (1986) Femoral anatomy and the design of total hip replacements. Trans Orthop Res 11:335

20. Ramaniraka NA, Rakotomanana LR, Rubin PJ et al (2000) Prothèse totale de hanche sans ciment: influence des paramètres extramédullaires sur la stabilité primaire et les contraintes à l'interface os–prothèse. Rev Chir Orthop 86:590–597

21. Rubin PJ, Leyvraz PF, Aubaniac JM et al (1992) The morphology of the proximal femur. A three-dimensional radiographic analysis. J Bone Joint Surg Br 74:28–32

22. Spalding TJ (1996) Effect of femoral offset on motion and abductor muscle strength after total hip arthroplasty J Bone Joint Surg Br 78:997

23. Steinberg B, Harris WH (1992) The offset problem in total hip arthroplasty. Contemp Orthop 24:556–562

24. Yamaguchi T, Naito M, Asayama I et al (2004) Total hip arthroplasty: the relationship between posterolateral reconstruction, abductor muscle strength, and femoral offset. J Orthop Surg 12:164–167

4.3 Hip National Registers: The Three Tenors

4.3.1 The Voice from Norway: 15-Year Results

Helge Wangen

The Norwegian Arthroplasty Register is one of the oldest in the world, founded in 1987. From 1987 to 2008, 137,414 hip replacements have been registered. The compliance rate is close to 100%. Corail® is the most used uncemented stem in Norway. Since 1987 the Register has registered the outcome of 10,331 Corail® stems. The 2007 Annual Report gave long-term results for Corail®. Defining failure to be revision for whatever cause the 15-year survival was 97%.

Introduction

The Norwegian Arthroplasty Register was founded in 1987. The Register is owned and operated by the Norwegian Orthopaedic Association. The register is located at Haukeland University Hospital in Bergen. In 1994 the register expanded from just reporting hip replacements to reporting all joint replacements. The register is designed to identify prostheses with inferior results as early as possible. The published annual report now mainly gives general statistics. Comparative results, for example, of different types of prosthesis or surgical techniques, are published in the form of scientific lectures, posters or articles. In addition, in-depth data on specific prostheses or techniques is available on request.

The Norwegian Arthroplasty Register believes that the results comparing different brands of prosthesis must be presented together with the explanation for selection of patient material and statistical methods, along with a discussion of how the results should be interpreted. This is slightly different from other registries such as the Australian one, where results for different prostheses are presented and discussed in the annual report.

The value of a register is entirely dependent on a high compliance from all orthopaedic surgeons who are supposed to report to the register. It has been shown through scientific publications that this is close to 100% in the Norwegian register [1]. The strength of a register is that it reports the outcome of a large number of patients. All levels of surgeons report to the register and the results therefore reflect what the average surgeon can expect when using a specific implant. The Norwegian register records all re-operations with replacement of one or more components including exchange of liners. What is not recorded is re-operations where no components are changed, for example dislocation treated with closed reduction or soft tissue revision without exchange of some of the components.

From 1987 to 2008, 137,414 hip replacements have been registered. Norway has about 4.5 million inhabitants. The annual number of total hip arthroplasties (THAs) is about 8,000 and has been unchanged during the last 10 years. Approximately 7,000 are primary arthroplasties and about 1,000 are revisions. In the Norwegian register the majority of hip prostheses are still cemented, but since 2003 the proportion has declined. Today about 69% are cemented, 16% reversed hybrids, 14% uncemented and 1% hybrids (Fig. 4.26). The main approach is the straight lateral (Hardinge) and this is used in 63.8%. The posterolateral approach is used in 28%.

Corail® Outcome from the Norwegian Arthroplasty Register

Corail® was introduced into the Norwegian market in 1987 as was the first country outside France to use the

stem and report on the outcome. The prosthesis was first used in patients below 50 years of age and initially was coupled with a cementless cup and polyethylene (PE) liner. Between 1987 and 2008 the Norwegian register has registered the outcome of 10,331 Corail® stems. About two thirds have been inserted with various types of cementless cups and one third have been implanted with a cemented cup, a so-called reverse hybrid. Both stainless-steel and ceramic femoral heads have been used.

The number of Corail® stems implanted annually has increased every year and since 2005 there has been a sixfold increase from about 500 to about 3,000 (Fig. 4.27). The number of Corail® stems used in fracture treatment has also increased since 2005, and has almost doubled during this period. Today 16% of the hemiarthroplasties in Norway are cementless and the stem most frequently used is Corail®.

In the early years, the tropic hydroxyapatite (HA)-coated screw cup and Atoll grit-blasted HA-coated press-fit cup were the uncemented cups most frequently used together with Corail®. These two cups are no longer on the market because of inferior results compared to modern contemporary cementless cup designs. Because the register had reported poor results with cementless cups there was also a general scepticism towards cementless stems as a general concept among major orthopaedic departments in Norway. The register initially encouraged caution in the use of cementless prostheses waiting for long-term results.

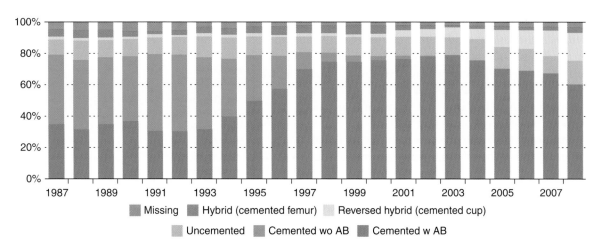

Fig. 4.26 Fixation of hip prostheses has changed in Norway from 1987 to 2008 (With permission from Norwegian Arthroplasty Register, 2009 Annual Report, p. 20, Fig. 5)

Femur	1987-2002	2003	2004	2005	2006	2007	2008	Total
Charnley	34,911	1,723	1,525	1,308	1,077	699	368	41,611
Exeter	7,909	997	1,062	1,235	1,349	1,674	1,614	15,840
Titan	8,521	686	557	657	571	452	446	11,890
Corail	5,441	445	491	573	805	1,086	1,490	10,331
Spectron-EF	2,788	1,451	1,240	1,236	1,044	1,011	903	9,673
ITH	3,659	26	28	10	–	–	–	3,723
SP II	999	99	88	177	279	488	500	2,630
FILLER	737	252	211	246	249	210	255	2,160
BIO-FIT	1,990	2	1	–	–	–	–	1,993
MS-30	995	217	149	154	152	97	50	1,814

Fig. 4.27 The ten most commonly used stems in Norway from 1987 to 2008 (With permission from Norwegian Arthroplasty Register, 2009 Annual Report, p. 30, Table 23)

	Number of hips	Age of patient (years)	Aged <60 years (%)	Males	OA	RA	Sequelae fracture	Squelae DDH	Squelae high DDH	Perthes/ epipyseolysis	Other
Corail	5,456	54	78	38	45	6.9	6.6	21	5.4	5.4	9.3

Fig. 4.28 Demographics of Corail® used in Norway from 1987 to 2007 (From Hallan et al. [2]. Reproduced with permission and copyright © of the British Editorial Society of Bone and Joint Surgery)

In 2007 the first publication from the register on the long-term results of cementless stems in primary total hip arthroplasty was published [2]. Fourteen different primary stem brands were included and 11,516 hips operated on between 1987 and 2005 were available for analysis. The Corail® was the most frequently used stem with a number of 5,456 hips. For all the stems the mean age of the patients increased during the study period. For Corail® the mean age was 54 years. Seventy percent of the patients receiving Corail® were less than 60 years, percent of which 38% were males. The primary diagnosis for patients who received Corail® hips was 45% OA, 21% developmental dysplasia of the hip (DDH), 5.4% high DDH, 6.9% RA, 6.6% fracture and 5.4% Perthes/epiphyseolysis (Fig. 4.28).

Survival of the Corail® stems was studied for different end points. When the end point was revision for any reason the 10-year survival was 98% and the 15-year survival was 97% (Fig. 4.29). The causes of revision for Corail® stems were the same as for the other cementless stems. Infection and dislocation were the most frequent causes of revision. Revision for aseptic loosening was less frequent when using Corail® compared to other cementless stems.

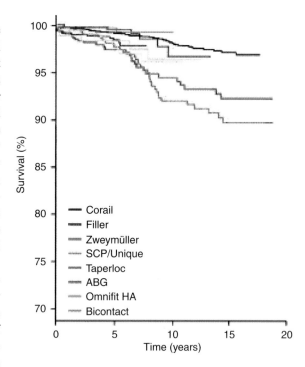

Fig. 4.29 Stem revisions for uncemented stems in the Norwegian Arthroplasty Register, all causes (From Hallan et al. [2]. Reproduced with permission and copyright © of the British Editorial Society of Bone and Joint Surgery)

In 2002, Havelin et al. published results from the Norwegian arthroplasty Register regarding the Tropic and Atoll uncemented cups compared with Charnley all-poly cemented cups [3]. In this study the risk of revision beyond 4 years was increased 3.4 times for the Tropic compared with the Charnley when used in combination with stainless-steel heads. When used with ceramic heads the results were better. The Atoll cup had an increased risk of revision of 3.8 when used with alumina heads and an increased risk of revision of 6.1 times when used with stainless-steel heads.

This publication together with some other reports was one of the main reasons why many Norwegian surgeons stopped using uncemented cups. Instead they started to do Corail® as a reversed hybrid prostheses; in other words, with an uncemented stem and an all-poly cemented cup. Today 16% of hips in Norway are reversed hybrids and Corail® represents about 80% of these cases. Long-term results for the reversed hybrids are until now not published.

Looking at the mid-term results of Corail® in reversed hybrids from the Norwegian register, it seems that Corail® with a cemented cup performs as well as Corail® with an uncemented cup with highly cross-linked polyethylene. At the same time when the register published inferior results for the uncemented cups, other Norwegian surgeons reported very good results for the Corail® [4, 5]. Because of this, Norwegian surgeons continued to believe in the Corail® as a stem.

especially Corail®. The Corail® stem is used for all types of diagnoses and the average age of the patients is increasing. It is not just a stem reserved for ordinary osteoarthritic (OA) hips in young patients. This is confirmed by figures from the register.

Until now there is no tradition for using bearings other than ceramic or metal on polyethylene in Norway. For this reason the Norwegian register cannot tell us if the new hard-on-hard bearings together with Corail® are better than old polyethylene or highly cross-linked polyethylene. Other registers such as the Australian or UK one may provide this information in the future.

The main value of a register is to get results from a large number of prostheses from surgeons of varying ability. The weakness is that there is no information about cases not being revised. Measures of quality of life (QoL), function and radiological data are not registered in the Norwegian register. Another weakness is that patients not revised because of comorbidity or long waiting lists are not registered. Nevertheless, a survival of 97% after 15 years gives us a clear picture of a very well-functioning hip prosthesis even when used by many different orthopaedic surgeons with varying degrees of competence. In order to improve the results in the future one has to look at the main reasons why the Corail® is revised today. Looking at register results, dislocation and deep infection are the most frequent reasons for revision. That is why these are the most important single factors to improve, in order to achieve even better results with the Corail® in the future.

Discussion

The Norwegian Arthroplasty Register plays a central role in Norwegian hip arthroplasty surgery. The annual reports and the many publications have had and still have a great impact on Norwegian hip arthroplasty. We see this clearly when studying what kind of hip prostheses Norwegian orthopaedic surgeons choose in their daily practice. Because the register has reported poor results for uncemented cups, cemented cups have dominated the market. Now that there have been very good results of Corail® reported in several publications and these have been confirmed by the register report, we can now see how this is about to change Norwegian hip surgery in the direction of using more and more uncemented stems,

Conclusion

Even though Corail® was introduced to Norwegian orthopaedic surgeons as early as 1987 it is still the fastest-growing stem based on recent figures from the Norwegian Arthroplasty Register. This corresponds to what is reported from other registers worldwide such as the Australian and UK ones. The Norwegian register has the longest follow-up of Corail® and the 2007 report shows that 5,456 were implanted. The 15-year survival rate for Corail® was 97% taking into account all causes of revision. This rate was superior to that for all other stems studied in the register.

Key Points

> Corail® is the most used uncemented stem in Norway
> Used for all diagnoses
> Fifteen years follow-up in the Norwegian register
> Ninety-seven percent femoral stem survival at 15-year follow-up, all causes of stem revisions included

References

1. Espehaug B, Furnes O, Havelin LI et al (2006) Registration completeness to the Norwegian arthroplasty register. Acta Orthop 77:49–56
2. Hallan G, Lie SA, O Furnes et al (2007) Medium- and long-term performance of 11516 uncemented primary femoral stems from the Norwegian arthroplasty register. J Bone Joint Surg Br 89-B(12):1574–1580
3. Havelin LI, Espehaug B, Engesæter LB (2002) The performance of two hydroxyapatite- coated acetabular cups compared with Charnley cups. From the Norwegian arthroplasty register. J Bone Joint Surg Br 84:839–845
4. Reikerås O, Gunderson RB (2003) Excellent results of HA coating on a grit-blasted stem: 245 patients followed for 8–12 years. Acta Orthop Scand 74(2):140–145
5. Røkkum M, Reigstad A (1999) Total hip replacement with an entirely hydroxyapatite-coated prosthesis: 5 years' follow-up of 94 consecutive hips. J Arthroplasty 14(6): 689–700

4.3.2 The Voice from Australia: 7-Year Results

Scott Brumby

The Australian National Joint Registry is now in its tenth year of operation. Data has been collected on over 8,781Corail® total hip arthroplasties (THAs). The Corail® femoral stem is the most commonly used cementless stem in Australia. The outcome is dependent on the age of the patient and the type of acetabular component used. There is a small increased risk of femoral peri-prosthetic fracture in patients aged greater than 75 years. When used in combination with a Pinnacle™ acetabular cup the early to mid-term results are excellent, with only 2.6% cumulative percent revised at 5 years.

Introduction

The Australian Orthopaedic Association National Joint Replacement Registry (AOANJRR) was established in 1993 and started collecting data in 1999. The registry has been able to collect complete data for all of Australia since 2003. The Australian Orthopaedic Association (AOA) maintains ownership of the registry and the Australian Government funds the registry with cost recovery from the orthopaedic industry. The University of Adelaide is contracted to provide independent data analysis. Hospitals around Australia provide data to the registry on specific forms that include patient demographic details, diagnosis and prosthetic components implanted. The data is validated and entered by the registry staff.

A report is compiled annually that describes and discusses the outcome of joint replacement in general using a standard approach, which includes a review process by a panel of orthopaedic surgeons who are members of the Arthroplasty Society of Australia. Individual prosthesis performance is also assessed and poorly performing prostheses are identified by the registry. In each report a list of prostheses with a higher than anticipated rate of revision is created. Surgeons and other stakeholders can request specific and more detailed data, if needed.

The 2009 report is the tenth report from the registry and is available on the Web site www.dmac.adelaide. edu.au/aoanjrr/publications.jsp. The report is released in October each year, to coincide with the annual scientific meeting of the AOA. The 2009 report documents the outcome on 472,966 primary and revision hip and knee joint replacements. Demographic data is available online but not included in the report. The primary outcome is time to first revision surgery. The annual report analyses outcome based on age, sex, diagnosis and implant type.

Outcome is reported as revisions per 100 component observed years as well as cumulative percent revised. Statistical analysis includes hazard ratios, which are calculated to quantify comparative risk of revision between groups. This year hazard ratios are calculated for various time periods to help explain how risk of revision varies with time. Confidence intervals are also reported to assist in interpreting results with small numbers. As the registry is still young, the outcomes only reflect the early and mid-term results of joint replacement. Early revision is most likely due to dislocation, infection, fracture and failure to achieve initial fixation. Over time we will see differences due to bearing type, osteolysis and late aseptic loosening in addition to the early causes.

Primary Total Hip Arthroplasty

The majority of primary THA in Australia is performed for a diagnosis of osteoarthritis (88.7%); other common diagnoses include avascular necrosis (3.7%), fractured neck of femur (3.2%), developmental dysplasia (1.4%) and rheumatoid arthritis (1.3%). Conventional THA is used in 92.3% and total resurfacing hip replacement in 7.6%. The use of resurfacing has decreased over the last 3 years. Cementless fixation accounts for 62% of all primary conventional THA and continues to increase: hybrid 31% and cemented 7%.

The outcome of conventional THA has been assessed for age, gender, diagnosis, fixation method, bearing surface and also for individual prosthesis brands. The many combinations of these variables make the analysis complicated. For females, the risk of revision decreases with increasing age. There is no apparent relationship between risk of revision and age for males. There is an early increased risk of revision with cementless fixation; this is most apparent in patients 75 years and older.

Revision data is reported for the first revision of a known primary THA recorded by the registry. These revisions are of primaries with a maximum follow-up of 9 years, the majority have a considerably shorter follow-up. The most common reasons for early and mid-term revision are loosening or osteolysis 31%, dislocation 24%, infection 15%, fracture 17%.

The registry has started to report outcome on bearing surface and head size. Caution should be taken when interpreting these early results. Without taking head size into consideration, metal-on-metal bearing surface has a higher revision rate than other bearing surfaces. For each of the bearing surfaces, larger head size is associated with a lower risk of revision (except for metal on metal).

The results of specific THA stem and cup combinations vary. The outcome may be dependent on many factors such as the combination of stem, cup, bearing and head size. The outcome of the most commonly inserted resurfacing, cementless, hybrid and cemented THA combinations are presented below. The results are very early and do not show any major clinical differences. There is a small increased early revision of the Corail® stem, mainly due to femoral shaft fracture, which is seen more often in the elderly age group (Fig. 4.30).

Corail® Stem

The Corail® femoral stem is the most commonly used cementless stem and the second most commonly used stem overall in Australia. The number implanted each year continues to increase. Data has been collected on over 8,781 Corail® stems. Corail® has a similar demographic usage to all other conventional THAs in Australia (median age of 67 years, 52% are female and diagnosis of osteoarthritis in 89.8%). The Corail® stem is used with a variety of acetabular cups (Fig. 4.31).

Revision of the Corail® femoral stem for any reason is very low (1.9% at 7 years). Albeit low, these early revisions were mainly due to peri-prosthetic femoral fractures and failure to achieve initial stability. Surgical education for the Corail® hip system in Australia has since focused on correct templating and intra-operative sizing, correct and careful compaction technique and treatment of intra-operative calcar fractures with a single wire and a collared stem. It is hoped that these measures will result in a further reduction of this already very low revision rate.

CPR	1 Yr	3 Yrs	5 Yrs	7 Yrs	8 Yrs
BHR Resurfacing	1.4 (1.2, 1.7)	2.4 (2.1, 2.8)	3.3 (2.8, 3.8)	4.5 (3.9, 5.3)	4.7 (4.0, 5.6)
Corail/Pinnacle	1.7 (1.3, 2.2)	2.1 (1.7, 2.7)	2.6 (1.9, 3.5)		
Exeter V40/Contemporary	1.2 (0.9, 1.5)	2.3 (1.9, 2.9)	2.9 (2.4, 3.6)	4.1 (3.1, 5.6)	
Exeter V40/Trident	1.1 (1.0, 1.3)	1.8 (1.6, 2.1)	2.6 (2.3, 3.1)	3.2 (2.7, 3.8)	

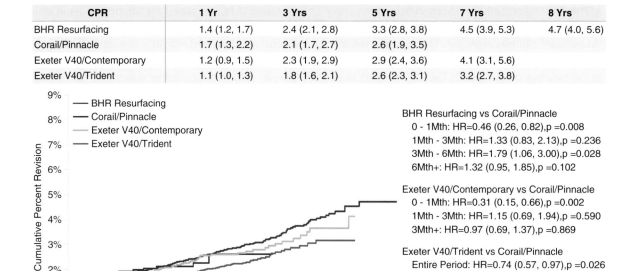

BHR Resurfacing vs Corail/Pinnacle
0 - 1Mth: HR=0.46 (0.26, 0.82),p =0.008
1Mth - 3Mth: HR=1.33 (0.83, 2.13),p =0.236
3Mth - 6Mth: HR=1.79 (1.06, 3.00),p =0.028
6Mth+: HR=1.32 (0.95, 1.85),p =0.102

Exeter V40/Contemporary vs Corail/Pinnacle
0 - 1Mth: HR=0.31 (0.15, 0.66),p =0.002
1Mth - 3Mth: HR=1.15 (0.69, 1.94),p =0.590
3Mth+: HR=0.97 (0.69, 1.37),p =0.869

Exeter V40/Trident vs Corail/Pinnacle
Entire Period: HR=0.74 (0.57, 0.97),p =0.026

Note: Adjusted for age and gender

Fig. 4.30 Cumulative percent revision for the most commonly used resurfacing, cementless, cemented and hybrid THAs in Australia

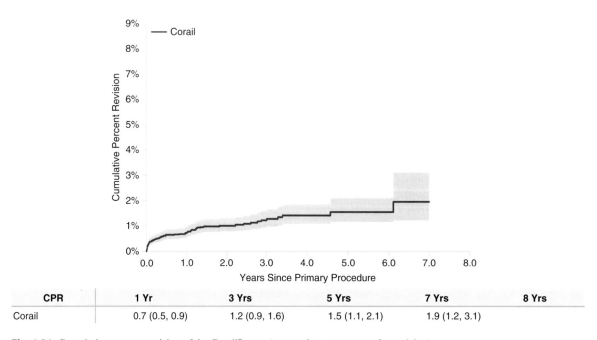

CPR	1 Yr	3 Yrs	5 Yrs	7 Yrs	8 Yrs
Corail	0.7 (0.5, 0.9)	1.2 (0.9, 1.6)	1.5 (1.1, 2.1)	1.9 (1.2, 3.1)	

Fig. 4.31 Cumulative percent revision of the Corail® stem (stem only – any reason for revision)

Femoral	Acetabular	1 year	3 years	5 years	7 years	8 years
Corail	ASR	1.9 (1.4, 2.6)	5.4 (4.1, 7.0)			
Corail	Duraloc	1.3 (0.7, 2.3)	1.9 (1.1, 3.0)	2.5 (1.6, 4.0)	3.7 (2.1, 6.4)	
Corail	Elite Plus LPW	2.6 (0.4, 16.8)	2.6 (0.4, 16.8)	2.6 (0.4, 16.8)		
Corail	Option	1.5 (0.5, 4.6)	2.0 (0.8, 5.2)	3.5 (1.7, 7.3)	4.4 (2.2, 8.7)	4.4 (2.2, 8.7)
Corail	Pinnacle	1.7 (1.3, 2.2)	2.1 (1.7, 2.7)	2.6 (1.9, 3.5)		
Corail	Trident	0.0 (0.0, 0.0)				
Corail	Other (20)	2.4 (0.8, 7.2)	3.7 (1.4, 9.8)	10.1 (2.8, 32.9)		

Note: Only prostheses with over 20 procedures have been listed.

Fig. 4.32 Yearly cumulative percent revision of primary THA using theCorail® stem by acetabular component

When revision of any component for any reason is analysed, the outcome of the Corail® THA is dependent on the type of acetabular component used and the age of the patient. The Corail® – Pinnacle™ – is the most common combination and also the most successful. This has a low rate of revision (2.6% at 5 years) and is comparable with the most commonly used cemented and hybrid THAs in Australia. The most common reasons for revision are dislocation, infection and femoral peri-prosthetic fracture. Surgical education has also focused on acetabular component position, bearing and head size selection. It is hoped that use of the transverse acetabular ligament to position the acetabular component and selection of a head size between 32 and 36 mm will result in a further reduction of revision procedures (Fig. 4.32).

Corail® has been used with the ASR® acetabular component and an XL head over the last 5 years. The theoretical advantage of this combination using a large-diameter metal-on-metal articulation was a reduced incidence of dislocation, greater range of motion and lower wear rates. However, the Corail® ASR® combination has been shown to have a higher than anticipated revision rate and the ASR® cup has since been withdrawn from the Australian market. The main reason for revision was acetabular loosening, infection and metal sensitivity. There was also a small increased incidence of femoral stem revision due to fracture and loosening. This early detection of higher than anticipated rate of revision demonstrates one of the strengths of registry data.

Conclusion

The Corail® femoral stem is the most commonly used cementless stem in Australia. When used in combination with a Pinnacle™ acetabular cup the early to mid-term results are excellent – 2.6% cumulative percent revised at 5 years.

It is important to recognise that the risk of revision is due to multiple factors including patient selection (age, gender, diagnosis) and component type (stem, cup, bearing, head size), which are recorded in the registry, and surgeon-specific factors such as surgical experience, surgical approach and technique, which are not recorded. Many of the small differences we see may be due to these unknown factors. Assessment of these other factors with clinical trials and review of the known literature is equally important.

The AOANJRR is a work in progress. Each report provides a snapshot of the outcome of joint replacement surgery in Australia. It is hoped that this will assist surgical education and prosthesis selection.

Recommended Reading

Australian Orthopaedic Association National Joint Replacement Registry. Annual Report. Adelaide:AOA; 2009 www.dmac.adelaide.edu.au/aoanjrr/publications.jsp
Data requested by SA Brumby to AOA NJRR September 2009
Data request by SA Brumby to AOA NJRR April 2010

4.3.3 The Voice from the UK: 5-Year Results

Henry Wynn Jones, Andrew G. Sloan, and Martyn L. Porter

The National Joint Registry (NJR) for England and Wales was established in 2002 and started collecting data in 2003. The Corail® stem is currently the most commonly used uncemented stem in the UK. In June 2010, data had been collected on 48,988 Corail® stems. The majority of Corail® stems were used in combination with a Pinnacle™ uncemented acetabular component. The early results are good, with an overall cumulative revision rate of 2.6% (95% confidence interval: 2.3–3.0%) at 3 years reported in the NJR sixth annual report.

Introduction

A national joint registry was first proposed by Sir John Charnley. The Trent Arthroplasty Register and the North West Arthroplasty Register were established and collected local regional data. It was not until strong recommendations for the establishment of a national joint registry came from the National Audit Office and National Institute for Clinical Excellence (NICE), with the Royal College of Surgeons' report on the investigation into the failure of the 3M Capital Hip, that finally plans were made to establish a national joint registry. The National Joint Registry (NJR) for England and Wales was established in 2002, and data for total hip arthroplasty (THA) and total knee replacement (TKR) was first collected in April 2003. The first annual report was published in 2004. Subsequently annual reports have been published.

The NJR is funded by a levy that is placed on the sale of implants. The levy applies to the acetabular component for hip replacements, the femoral component for knee replacements and the talar component for ankle replacements (with effect from 1 July 2010). Companies supplying joint prosthesis collect levies from the purchasing hospital. The NJR Centre then collects the levies from the suppliers and forwards them on to the Department of Health to cover the costs of the ongoing operation and development of the NJR.

The NJR is managed by an independent company (Northgate Information Solutions (UK) Ltd) under a contract with the Healthcare Quality Improvement Partnership (HQIP), which took over responsibility for the overall management of the NJR from the Department of Health on 1 April 2008. The activities of the NJR are overseen by a Steering Committee that is an advisory non-departmental public body. The steering committee is made up of members from the orthopaedic profession, a patient representative, industry members, National Health Service (NHS) management, an epidemiologist and an orthopaedic practitioner. There are a number of other representatives from other stakeholder groups such as the Department of Health and the Medicines and Healthcare products Regulatory Agency.

Institutions submit data to the NJR on a voluntary basis. The period 2008–2009 saw 160,027 submissions of hip and knee joint replacement operations, which represent 92.5% of all operations carried out in England and Wales, in both the NHS and independent healthcare sector, in a 12-month period. Overall compliance with reporting to the NJR at the time of publication of the sixth report was 78%. The total number of records submitted to the NJR from 1 April 2003 to 31 March 2009 was 742,706.

Data is submitted to the NJR using a minimum data set form. Submitting institution, patient demographics, indication, procedure type, anaesthetic type, surgeon and grade, implant details, thromboprophylaxis type and intra-operative complications are entered. Patient consent and patient identifier numbers are required to facilitate longitudinal linkage of primary to revision procedures. Linkage of the NJR data to data from the Hospital Episode Statistics (HES) database enables an increased detection and linkage rate for primary procedures to revision procedures.

Primary Total Hip Arthroplasty in the NJR

A total of 64,722 primary hip replacement operations were undertaken in 2008, of which 38% were cemented total hip replacements, 33% cementless THAs and 14% hybrid THAs. Of the remainder, 8% were resurfacing and 7% were large-head metal-on-metal procedures.

Analysis of revision rates in the sixth annual report was performed using data on the 157,232 patients who had a first primary hip replacement procedure in the NHS or who were NHS-funded in the independent sector, between 1 April 2003 and 30 November 2008 in England and for whom there was an NJR-HES-linked record.

The overall revision rate following primary hip replacement was 1.0% (95% CI: 0.9–1.0%) at 1 year, 2.0% (95% CI: 1.9–2.1%) at 3 years and 2.8% (95% CI: 2.7–3.0%) at 5 years.

The majority of femoral stems included in the revision analysis in the sixth annual report were cemented (86,524) with an overall revision rate at 3 years of 1.3% (95% CI: 1.2–1.4%). The 45,100 uncemented stems had an overall revision rate at 3 years of 2.6% (2.4–2.8%).

Reasons for revision are recorded by the NJR. However, interpretation of these results should be done with caution as multiple reasons can be listed, without the major cause being identified. The number of causes of revision may therefore be greater than the number of revisions.

The Corail® Stem

The Corail® stem was market leader in uncemented stems in 2008 with a market share of 46%, and it continues to lead the market in 2010. Of the 18,905 Corail® stems reported upon in the NJR sixth annual report, the revision rate at 3 years was low at 2.6% (2.3–3.0%).

Further detailed analysis specific to the Corail® stem was not available in the sixth annual report. NJR data are available on request to permit independent analysis. In order to present additional Corail® data for the purpose of this chapter, a download of NJR-linked data was obtained by DePuy from the NJR Centre in June 2010 for analysis by DePuy's biostatistician. It is important that readers are aware that this data does not include HES data linkage. This means that it is likely that revisions are under-reported. The reason for this is that some revisions may not have been reported or linkable within the NJR, but would be detected by HES data analysis. HES data linkage is only performed for preparation of the annual NJR report. It is estimated that without HES data linkage, revision rates are underestimated by approximately 15%. However, it is anticipated that the underestimation of revisions is probably equal across groups, so comparison of relative revision rates between groups is still valid within the same data set. It is not valid to use these revision rates as absolute values for comparison with other data sets, or studies.

Up to June 2010 data was available on 48,988 Corail® stems. Forty-two percent of patients were male, and the mean age was 66 years (range 14–104). Osteoarthritis (93%) was the most common indication for surgery. The overall survival rate at 7 years was 96.8% (96.3–97.3%) (Table 4.13).

Multiple reasons for revision of a Corail® stem were recorded. The most common causes were dislocation (approximately 17%), followed by infection (16%), aseptic stem loosening (16%) and peri-prosthetic femur fracture (10%).

Acetabular Components and Articulations

The Corail® stem has been used with a variety of acetabular components and bearing surfaces, from a number of different manufacturers. The Corail® stem

Table 4.13 Overall survival of the Corail® stem based on data downloaded from the NJR in June 2010

	Overall Corail® survival						
	Survival (%)	Standard error	LCI (%)	UCI (%)	Number at start	Failures	Number at end
1 year	at end	0.000396	99.22	99.38	48,988	316	35,758
2 years	98.72	0.000594	98.60	98.84	35,758	488	23,020
3 years	98.16	0.000819	98.00	98.32	23,020	588	12,746
4 years	97.66	0.00109	97.45	97.87	12,746	637	6,409
5 years	97.17	0.00157	96.86	97.48	6,409	657	2,524
6 years	96.96	0.00205	96.56	97.36	2,524	660	717
7 years	96.79	0.00267	96.27	97.31	717	661	66

LCI Lower Confidence Interval, *UCI* Upper Confidence Interval

was used with a DePuy acetabular component in the majority of cases (93%). Data is available for 45,128 cases where the Corail® stem was used with a DePuy acetabular component. The following analysis has been performed using the data available for a Corail® stem with a DePuy acetabular component.

Acetabular Fixation

The majority of stems were used with an uncemented acetabular component (92.3 %). A smaller number were used as a reverse hybrid with a cemented ultra-high-molecular-weight (UHMW) polyethylene (PE) cemented cup (7.7%). The Pinnacle™ uncemented acetabular component was used in the majority of cases (75.7%). The effect of acetabular fixation method on Corail® stem with an uncemented DePuy cup showed the 5-year survival rate was 97.6% (97.3–97.9%)

(Table 4.14), compared to 98.2% (97.1–99.3%) with a cemented cup (Table 4.15).

Articulation

Thirty-two percent of cases had a metal-on-, ultrahigh molecular weight polyethylene (UHMW) PE (MoP) articulation (either cemented or uncemented), 22% metal-on-metal (MoM), and 22% ceramic-on-ceramic (CoC). The remainder were ceramic against UHMW polyethylene or were not specified. Comparison of the survival of the Corail® stem with a metal on UHMW polyethylene (MoP) (Table 4.16), ceramic on ceramic (CoC) (Table 4.17) and a metal on metal (MoM) (Table 4.18) articulation has been performed.

The NJR data available confirm that the Corail® stem appears to be performing well at 5–7 years, with the majority of acetabular components. It appears that at 5

Table 4.14 Corail® stem survival with a DePuy uncemented acetabular component (Pinnacle™, Duraloc, Duraloc Option)

	Corail® stem survival with an uncemented cup						
	Survival (%)	Standard error	LCI (%)	UCI (%)	Number at start	Failures	Number at end
1 year	99.29	0.000446	99.20	99.38	38,942	256	28,016
2 years	98.81	0.000636	98.69	98.93	28,016	368	18,026
3 years	98.39	0.000839	98.23	98.55	18,026	426	10,234
4 years	98.08	0.00105	97.87	98.29	10,234	451	5,326
5 years	97.61	0.00162	97.29	97.93	5,326	467	2,088
6 years	97.35	0.00231	96.90	97.80	2,088	470	570
7 years	97.13	0.00317	96.51	97.75	570	471	57

LCI Lower Confidence Interval, *UCI* Upper Confidence Interval

Table 4.15 Corail® stem survival with a DePuy cemented polyethylene acetabular component (Elite Plus, Ogee, Charnley®, Ultima, Marathon™, Wroblewski)

	Corail® stem survival with an cemented cup						
	Survival (%)	Standard error	LCI (%)	UCI (%)	Number at start	Failures	Number at end
1 year	99.58	0.00117	99.35	99.81	3,467	13	2,491
2 years	99.09	0.00194	98.71	99.47	2,491	23	1,502
3 years	98.87	0.00251	98.38	99.36	1,502	25	578
4 years	98.21	0.00561	97.11	99.31	578	27	167
5 years	98.21	0.00561	97.11	99.31	167	27	60
6 years	98.21	0.00561	96.11	99.31	60	27	25

LCI Lower confidence interval, *UCI* Upper confidence interval

Table 4.16 Corail® stem survival with a metal-on-polyethylene articulation

	Survival (%)	Standard error	LCI (%)	UCI (%)	Number at start	Failures	Number at end
1 year	99.31	0.00084	99.15	99.47	10,417	67	7,100
2 years	99.00	0.00111	98.78	99.22	7,100	86	4,578
3 years	98.73	0.00143	98.45	99.01	4,578	95	2,679
4 years	98.51	0.00173	98.17	98.85	2,679	100	1,267
5 years	98.31	0.0026	97.80	98.82	1,267	101	310
6 years	98.31	0.00264	97.79	98.83	310	101	50

LCI Lower confidence interval, *UCI* Upper confidence interval

Table 4.17 Corail® stem survival with a ceramic on ceramic articulation

	Survival (%)	Standard error	LCI (%)	UCI (%)	Number at start	Failures	Number at end
1 year	99.14	0.00102	98.94	99.34	9,477	72	5,982
2 years	98.69	0.00142	98.41	98.97	5,982	93	3,268
3 years	98.29	0.00192	97.91	98.67	3,268	103	1,432
4 years	97.96	0.00278	97.42	98.50	1,432	106	564
5 years	97.96	0.00278	97.42	98.50	564	106	128

LCI Lower confidence interval, *UCI* Upper confidence interval

Table 4.18 Corail® stem survival with a metal on metal articulation

	Survival (%)	Standard error	LCI (%)	UCI (%)	Number at start	Failures	Number at end
1 year	99.27	0.000853	99.10	99.44	10,677	73	8,619
2 years	98.62	0.00127	98.37	98.87	8,619	120	5,746
3 years	98.03	0.00173	97.69	98.37	5,746	146	3,066
4 years	97.66	0.00219	97.37	98.09	3,066	154	1,275
5 years	97.20	0.00299	96.61	97.79	1,275	159	270
6 years	97.20	0.00299	96.61	97.79	270	159	17

LCI Lower confidence interval, *UCI* Upper confidence interval

years a metal on polyethylene articulation has the most favourable results, either cemented or uncemented. As the data set becomes larger and follow-up duration increases it will be interesting to analyse whether this trend continues, or whether the contemporary hard-on-hard bearing begins to outperform the metal on polyethylene articulations. It will also be interesting to observe whether highly cross-linked polyethylene has a survival advantage over conventional UHMW polyethylene. Hopefully in the future it will also be possible to use NJR data to perform an analysis of the Corail® stem with a ceramic-on-polyethylene articulation.

Conclusion

Since its conception in 2002, the NJR for England and Wales has grown rapidly, and now contains data on over one million lower limb arthroplasty procedures. The data quality has also been steadily improving, with a compliance rate for procedures entered in 2009 of over 92.5%. Linkage with HES data has also improved the accuracy of reporting of survival analysis.

The Corail® stem is the market leader in uncemented femoral stems in the UK. Early results reported in the sixth annual report are good. Independent analysis of data downloaded in June 2010 confirms that the stem is continuing to perform well up to 7 years.

A femoral stem does not function in isolation, and the choice of bearing surface and acetabular fixation will have an effect on the survival. Analysis of the available data in June 2010 suggests that a polyethylene acetabular bearing surface has the most favourable survival at 5 years. Future analysis will help to determine the optimum bearing and acetabular fixation combination for the best long-term survival, and to determine whether contemporary bearing options confer any long-term survival advantage over metal on polyethylene.

As the NJR continues to grow, and the data quality improves, it is hoped that it will be possible to perform a more in-depth analysis of the many patient-, implant-, peri-operative- and surgeon-related factors that may affect implant survival.

Recommended Reading

National Joint Registry for England and Wales. 6th Annual Report 2009, http://www.njrcentre.org.uk/njrcentre/AbouttheNJR/Publicationsandreports/Annualreports

National Joint Registry for England and Wales. 1st Annual Report 2004

Data download request from the NJR, by DePuy, Leeds, United Kingdom, June 2010

4.4 Both Ends of the Age Spectrum: A Stem for All Seasons

4.4.1 Corail® in the Young: The Spring

Helge Wangen

It is well accepted that youth and high activity levels are among the most important factors that increase the risk of mechanical failure of total hip prostheses (THP). At the Rikshospitalet, Oslo, Norway, we have throughout the years treated very young hip patients with implantation of hip prostheses. Forty-four patients below 30 years of age at the time of surgery were treated with a total number of 49 Corail® prostheses at this hospital between 1989 and 1996. In this chapter the long-term results for these very young patients are presented and discussed.

Introduction

The excellent results of total hip arthroplasty (THA) in an elderly population may not be replicated in young and active patients. Reports on the outcomes of cemented implants in the younger patients vary widely. Wroblewski et al. [9] reported an overall revision rate of 6% at 10-year follow-up, increasing to 15% at 15 years. Dorr et al. [2] reported a revision rate of 33% in a series of 49 hips in patients below 45 years of age at a mean follow-up of 9 years.

In studies where age was not a criterion, excellent results have been reported using hydroxyapatite (HA)-coated stems. Hallan et al. [5] reported from the Norwegian Arthroplasty Register, 97% survival of the Corail® stem after 15 years including all causes of stem revision. These results have to a certain extent been repeated in younger patients. Capello et al. [1] reported a low failure rate of the stem in patients below 50 years of age when using a proximally HA-coated stem. Despite this it is still well accepted that young age and high activity levels are among the factors that increase the risk of mechanical failure of total hip prostheses (THPs) [4, 6].

This group of patients are especially demanding in terms of functional outcome and also regarding the survival of the hip prosthesis. Many of the patients have had previous operations during childhood and arthroplasty surgery may be technically demanding. Knowing this, we wanted to investigate the outcome of the Corail® stem in patients aged 30 years or younger.

Material and Methods

In Rikshospitalet, Oslo, Norway, we performed a retrospective follow-up 10–16 years after surgery [8]. Between 1989 and 1996 we inserted 49 primary Corail® THAs in 44 young adults. The age of the patients was between 15 and 30 years (mean age: 25 years). The diagnosis was secondary osteoarthritis due to congenital dislocation in 24 hips (Fig. 4.33), avascular necrosis in 6, coxitis in 4, acetabular fractures in 4, Calve Legg Perthes disease in 3, epiphyseal dysplasia in 2 and chondrodystrophia in 1.

In 36 cases a press-fit hemispherical HA-coated cup (Atoll, Landos) was implanted, in 7 cases an HA-coated screw cup (Tropic, Landos) and in 6 patients a press-fit fibre-mesh cup (Harris-Galante, Zimmer) was inserted. In all cases a polyethylene (PE) liner was used. The heads used were either alumina or stainless steel and all were 28 mm in diameter. Surgery was performed through either a posterior or direct lateral approach. Radiographic evaluation included assessments of bone remodelling, osteolysis and fixation of the stem. Clinical rating was according to the Harris hip score. The Western Ontario and McMaster Universities (WOMAC) score for osteoarthritis was used to evaluate functional outcome.

Results

At a minimum of 10 years after implantation, none of the 49 femoral stems had been revised for any reason. All stems were well integrated at follow-up, with no signs of radiological loosening. No stem had subsided. Radiolucent lines (RLL) were found around 7 stems in Gruen zone 1 and around 1 stem in zone 5. There was bone atrophy in Gruen zones 1 and 7 in 8 stems. Three stems had atrophy in Gruen zone 1 and 10 stems had atrophy in zone 7. Endosteal bone hypertrophy was found around 19 stems in zone 4 and around 2 stems in zone 5. Some osteolysis was observed in zone 1 and 7 in 9 prostheses.

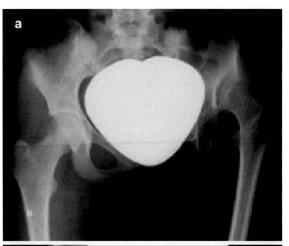
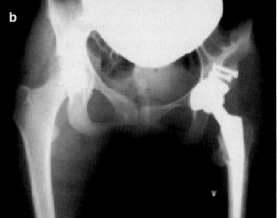
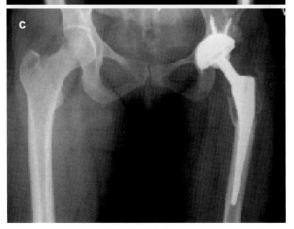

Fig. 4.33 (**a**) A 17-year-old girl with a high dislocation of the left hip. (**b**) Subtrochanteric resection and implantation of an HA-coated hemispheric cup and stem. (**c**) After 10 years the stem is fully incorporated, but due to polyethylene (PE) wear and medial detachment at the acetabular side, the cup has been revised

Table 4.19 Different cups used. Number used and reason for revision

Cup	n=	Revised	Loosening	Dislocation	Wear
Atoll	36	17	14	2	1
Tropic	7	4	0	0	4
Harris Galante 1	6	3	0	1	2

The average Harris hip score was 88 (range: 62–100) and the WOMAC score 80 (range: 37–100). There were no differences in clinical outcome scores between the revised and unrevised patients at review.

In contrast, 24 of the 49 cups had been revised (Table 4.19). Seventeen of the 36 HA-coated hemispheric press-fit cups were revised: 14 because of loosening, 2 because repeated dislocations and 1 because of PE wear. Four of the HA-coated screw cups were revised, all because of PE wear. Among the Harris Galante cups, 3 were revised: 2 because of PE wear and 1 because of dislocation.

Discussion

The age below 50 is often defined as young when talking about hip prostheses. However, there are very few reports of long-term results in the very young patients. Ekelinen et al. report on mid- to long-term follow-up studies of uncemented total hip arthroplasty for primary osteoarthritis in patients younger than 55 years of age [3]. All uncemented stems studied showed a survival rate of more than 90% at 10 years with the end point of stem revision for any reason. When end point was defined as any revision of any component, the 10-year survival rate was less than 80%. Capello et al. report 10-year results with a proximally HA-coated femoral component and press-fit uncemented cups in 111 hips in 97 patients less than 50 years old [1]. They found 95% 10-year survival of the stem for all reasons included and only a 65% acetabular component survivorship when end point was defined as any revision.

When Corail® was used in a very young population, below 30 years, all revisions were related to the acetabular component. The acetabular components used have in general shown a very high rate of failure that has been associated with a high degree of PE wear, osteolysis and subsequent loosening (Fig. 4.34). This

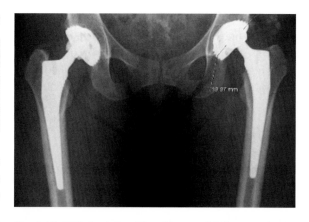

Fig. 4.34 Well-fixed Corail® at 10-year of follow-up, despite huge wear of the acetabular liner. The cup was revised with liner exchange only

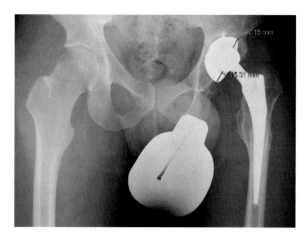

Fig. 4.35 Wear of the acetabular liner, loosening of the cup but the stem is still well integrated, with some osteolysis in zone 1

early generation of uncemented cups with poor polyethylene and locking mechanism is no longer used. The prevalence of osteolysis in uncemented prostheses has been reported to vary between 40% and 50% in the younger age groups [7]. What was quite remarkable with Corail® was that even in the presence of huge amounts of PE wear none of the stems were loose after 10–16 years (Fig. 4.35). Despite extensive acetabular osteolysis there was little or no femoral osteolysis. It seems that the fully coated stem withstands even the most demanding situations without loosening. It has been suggested that the full HA coating seals the femoral canal from wear particles causing osteolysis. We now use modern cemented and cementless cups and hard bearings in the young age group. We hope this will at least improve results at the acetabular side; however, it is difficult to improve on the 100% survival of the stem even in very young and active patients.

In our experience radiological appearance of the Corail® stem in the very young is the same as we find in older patients. Proximally we found little osteolysis and distally seldom hypertrophy of the cortex. Radiolucent lines were uncommon and if present almost always located to proximal Gruen zone 1. The central and distal zones of the prostheses were otherwise well integrated despite the huge amount of PE wear particles caused by excessive wear of the acetabular liners. These observations indicate that the design of the stem and the extensive coating provide reliable fixation even in very young patients.

Conclusion

Even though it is well accepted that youth and high activity levels are among the most important factors that increase the risk of mechanical failure of total hip prostheses, total hip surgery is not only for the elderly any more. The average age of the patients operated today is lower than it was 10–15 years ago, and their expectations and demands regarding functional outcome are also much higher than before. Because of this, the situation is far more challenging regarding design, quality and durability of the prostheses than it was when Sir John Charnley started up in the 1960s. In our experience, Corail® provides enough evidence to say that a fully HA-coated uncemented stem is the best solution for these patients. Corail® is documented to give very good and predictable results, both radiologically and clinically, even if the patients are younger than 30 years with high activity levels.

References

1. Capello WN, D'Antonio JA, Feinberg JR et al (2003) Ten-year results with hydroxyapatite-coated total hip femoral components in patients less than fifty years old. A concise follow up of a previous report. J Bone Joint Surg Am 85:885–889
2. Dorr LD, Kane TJ 3rd, Conaty JP (1994) Long-term results of cemented total hip arthroplasty in patients 45 years old or younger. A 16 year follow up study. J Arthroplasty 19:453–456
3. Eskelinen A, Remes V, Helenius I et al (2006) Uncemented total hip arthroplasty for primary osteoarthritis in young patients. A mid- to long-term follow up study from the Finnish arthroplasty register. Acta Orthop 77(1):57–70
4. Furnes O, Lie SA, Espehaug B et al (2001) Hip disease and the prognosis of total hip replacements. A review of 53,698 primary total hip replacements reported to the Norwegian arthroplasty register 1987–99. J Bone Joint Surg Br 83-B:579–586
5. Hallan G, Lie SA, Furnes O et al (2007) Medium- and long-term performance of 11,516 uncemented primary femoral stems from the Norwegian arthroplasty register. J Bone Joint Surg Br 89(12):1574–1580
6. Johnsen S, Sørensen HT, Lucht UT et al (2006) Patient-related predictors of implant failure after primary total hip replacement in the initial, short-, and long-terms: a nationwide Danish followup study including 36984 patients. J Bone Joint Surg Br 88:1303–1308
7. Kawamura H, Dunbar MJ, Murray P et al (2001) The porous coated anatomic total hip replacement. A ten to fourteen-year follow up study of a cementless total hip arthroplasty. J Bone Joint Surg Am 83:1333–1338
8. Wangen H, Lereim P, Holm I et al (2008) Hip arthroplasty in patients younger than 30 years: excellent ten to 16-year follow up results with a HA coated stem. Int Orthop 32(2):203–208
9. Wroblewski BM, Siney PD, Fleming PA (2002) Charnley low-frictional torque arthroplasty in patients under the age of 51 years. Follow up to 33 years. J Bone Joint Surg Br 84:540–543

4.4.2 Corail® in the Old: The Fall

Dominique C.R.J. Hardy

We present the clinical and radiological outcome of 204 Corail® bipolar hemiarthroplasties for femoral neck fractures in 196 unselected and consecutive patients with a mean age of 88.7 years at the time of operation and followed up to 5 years thereafter (no lost cases). Only 13 intra-operative difficulties related to the stem (11 calcar cracks, 1 trochanteric fracture, 1 diaphyseal fissure) were noted. One hundred twenty-one (61.7%) had died by the time of final follow-up (5 years) and there were no revisions for acetabular erosion or stem loosening.

All the stems were satisfactorily fixed at final x-ray, with limited subsidences of 1–6 mm usually occurring at early weight-bearing. No hip pain was noted during the entire follow-up.

Introduction

Hip fractures are undoubtedly a public health issue. Their prevalence rate is increasing, their management is essentially surgical and calls for substantial resources (implants, medical staff, hospital days, rehabilitation) and the recovery is marked by significant morbidity and mortality rates. Moreover, the socio-economic environment in which they occur is often unfavourable.

Among hip fracture patients, octogenarians (and older) are those whose risk to suffer a hip fracture increases with time (risk doubled between 1950 and 1980 [18]) with major risks of complication. Many such patients are in institutions – due to a lack of resources or various forms of infirmity – and for them hip fracture is a major problem prone to leading to early death or severe physical degradation.

Numerous articles may be found in the literature on post hip fracture prognosis in elderly patients. However, such material is rendered unusable by numerous statistical biases among which the following should be noted: incomplete patient follow-up, numerous variations in the therapeutical procedures and broad heterogeneousness of the economic, social and comorbidity parameters.

The controversy fuelled by the prosthesis choice is wide: total hip arthroplasty versus hemiarthroplasty, cemented versus uncemented, unipolar versus bipolar, hydroxyapatite (HA)-coated or non-coated implants.

With these questions in mind, but unresolved (or only partly resolved), the present body of work was initiated in order to determine whether an HA-coated implant, used systematically and continuously, without any specific selection, could be part of our therapeutic arsenal. This chapter does not discuss the choice between internal fixation and arthroplasty.

Equipment and Methods

A total of 204 unstable intracapsular hip fractures (type 3 or 4 as per Garden's classification [14]) in 196 consecutive patients have been included in the study. All patients were at least 80 years old (mean age 88.7, range 80–94), and 171 (83.8%) were female. The series was consecutive and only patients with a pathological fracture or suffering from osteoarthritis or rheumatoid arthritis were excluded. The functional status was registered prospectively in a computerised file.

Surgery was performed using a posterior approach under general (38/204) or spinal (166/204) anaesthesia. All the patients received a Corail® (DePuy) stem fitted with a bipolar head (BHP, Zimmer Inc.) (Fig. 4.36). Cezafoline (2 g IV) was administered during surgery and was followed by anti-DVT (deep vein thrombosis) prophylaxis (Fraxiparine 0.4 mL/day for 20 days) in the absence of any contraindication.

All the patients were mobilised post-operatively using a walking frame, then using crutches as their functional development improved.

All patients stayed at least 1 week in hospital and after being discharged most of them were referred to a geriatric rehabilitation service. They were reviewed at 3 months, 12 months and then every year for 5 years. The observations were recorded in the prospective file. Only six patients (= six fractures) were lost to follow-up.

The preoperative and post-operative mobility was evaluated using the Parker and Palmer score [26] (Table 4.20).

The Tinetti score was used post-operatively only in follow-ups longer than 1 year.

Mental state was evaluated using the Qureshi and Hodkinson score [29]. The patients were asked ten questions and received one point for each correct answer.

The autonomy level was evaluated using the Jensen index [17] (Table 4.21).

Osteoporosis was evaluated using the Singh index.

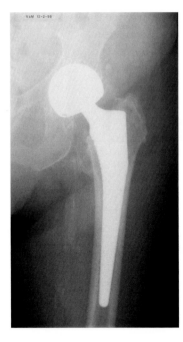

Fig. 4.36 Corail® prosthesis, with a bipolar head. AP view at 2 months

Table 4.20 Assessment of mobility in elderly patients. The Parker's score (0–9 points)

Walking ability	No difficulty	Alone, with an assistive device (stick, cane, …)	With help of another person	Not at all
Able to walk inside house	3 points	2 points	1 points	0 points
Able to walk outside house	3 points	2 points	1 points	0 points
Able to go shopping, restaurant, or to visit family	3 points	2 points	1 points	0 points

Late post-operative complications – such as dislocations, infections, femoral fractures, fractures of the contralateral hip – were recorded for all the patients, including those lost to follow-up. Radiological signs of loosening and the medical complications that occurred during the first 3 months were recorded at each review, which was carried out either in the hospital or in a geriatric institution upon the initiative of the author.

Table 4.21 Assessment of autonomy in elderly patients. The Jensen's index (1–4 points)

Independent	Manages everything. Possible working	1
Slightly independent	Manages household. Meals-on-wheels, home-help ≤ 4 hours/week	2
Moderately dependent	Home-help ≥ 5 h/week. Possible district nurse	3
Totally dependent	Living in nursing home or long-term nursing at home	4

Statistical analyses were performed with an analysis of variance (ANOVA) one-way test, using Analyze-It Software (Analyze-It Ltd, Leeds, UK). A $p < 0.05$ was considered as significant.

Results

Demographics

The average age at time of surgery was 88.7 years (range 80–94 years); the mean body weight was 59.2 kg (SD 10.18, range 35–88 kg); and the female to male ratio was 171:25. The preoperative assessment is listed in Table 4.22.

Surgery

Surgery was performed under spinal anaesthesia in 189 cases on the day after admission, but occasionally

Table 4.22 Preoperative autonomy, mental and mobility scores in the 204 hips (196 patients)

		In cases: 204
Autonomy	I	34
	II	31
	III	36
	IV	103
Mental	0–4	111
	5–7	68
	8–10	25
Mobility score	0–3	82
	4–6	53
	7–9	69

up to 6 days after admission in cases where there were multiple medical problems. The average operative time was 58 min (SD 14 min; range 38–126 min). The six longest operations (90, 94, 100, 106, 115 and 126 min) were complicated by intra-operative femoral fractures in three cases, difficulty to obtain a stable implant due to excessive muscle weakness and despite a stable implantation of the stem in two cases and the impossibility to achieve stable implantation in one case, which required conversion to a KAR™ stem.

Eight incomplete and three complete cracks of the inner cortex were noted. The incomplete cracks were treated with a prophylactic cerclage in five cases and non-weight-bearing for 4 weeks. The complete cracks were treated with one or two cerclages. One fracture of the greater trochanter occurred during impaction of the definitive implant, possibly due to the impingement of the implant holder on the medial edge of the trochanter, and was fixed with two screws. One incomplete diaphyseal fissure was also seen on the immediate post-operative x-ray, preventing weight bearing for 4 weeks and healed uneventfully thereafter (Fig. 4.37a, b).

The mean intra-operative blood loss was 179 mL (SD 38 mL; range 125–490 mL). The breakdown of the stem sizes is shown in Fig. 4.38.

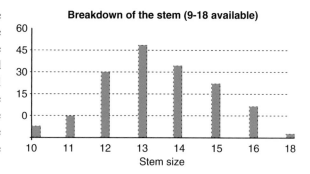

Breakdown of the stem (9-18 available)

Stem size

Fig. 4.38 Breakdown of the sizes of the stem (9–18 available)

The diameter of the bipolar cup varied from 44 to 58 mm and matched the diameter of the excised head.

Post-operative Course

Patients lost 219.9 mL (SD 42.6 mL; range 70–490 mL) in their drains. Eighty-two patients were transfused and 116 had at least one complication: urinary tract infection (52), bedsores (41), cardiac failure (16), pulmonary embolus (4), deep vein thrombosis (4), chest

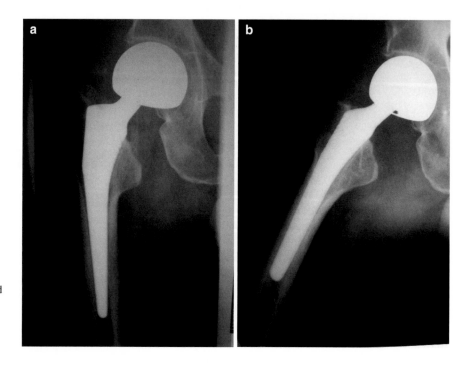

Fig. 4.37 (a) (AP view) and (b) (oblique view): Diaphyseal fissure on immediate post-operative oblique view

infection (9), acute renal failure (1) and thrombosis of the femoral artery (1). All patients were out of bed and in an armchair by the second post-operative day with the exception of those with an intra-operative calcar crack. All were allowed to walk full weight-bearing by the third or the fourth post-operative day. Fifteen (7.4%) were totally unable to walk, despite considerable effort and encouragement. This was attributed to mental impairment and muscle weakness, in the absence of orthopaedic complications.

Hospital stay averaged 12.5 days (SD 3.6; range 8–47 days). Ten patients died during their hospital stay. One hundred and seventy-eight (87.3%) patients were discharged to geriatric facilities. The other 26 went back to their own homes or to their relatives.

Mortality

Thirty-two (16.3%) patients died within 1 month of the operation and 57 (29.1%) during the first year. At 5-year review, mortality reached 61.7% (121/196).

There is a close relationship between the preoperative autonomy, as estimated with Jensen's score, and the length of post-operative survival (one-way ANOVA, $p < 0.0001$). Similarly, life expectancy correlated with the preoperative walking ability graded with Parker's mobility score (one-way ANOVA, $p < 0.0001$).

Local Early Complications

Five patients had a wound dehiscence, one of which required resuturing. One patient developed a deep infection on day 7. This was successfully treated with lavage and antibiotics. This patient died 2 years later.

Among the eight incomplete calcar splits, one, untreated during surgery, was displaced secondarily on the fifth day, producing a large haematoma of the thigh along with a compression of the deep femoral vein and subsequent non-fatal pulmonary embolism.

Twelve early dislocations were seen in this series, of which six were recurrent (respectively 2 – 2 – 2 – 3 – 3 – 4 episodes). In one of these cases, a femoral fracture occurred during difficult reduction manoeuvres, requiring surgical treatment (cerclage). The patient healed uneventfully, but died 4 months later after a third dislocation.

Radiographic Findings

All the prostheses implanted for a minimum of 6 months displayed visible signs of osseointegration. This was first seen in zones 3 and 5 with development of bridging trabeculae between the cortex and the implant. Later, long and thin radially oriented trabeculae crossing the greater trochanter area became visible (Fig. 4.39). At the level of the calcar, a slow remodelling process took place, rounding the shape of the inner cortex. After 1 year of implantation or more, bony trabeculae fixed on each groove of the medial aspect of the implant became visible.

It is notable that there was no radiological evidence of loosening or any signs of stress-shielding. Stem subsidence of 1–4 mm was recorded in 24 cases, 16 in type C femora and 8 in type B. This occurred within the first 3 post-operative months in all cases. There was no later subsidence. During the follow-up of these 24 cases all prostheses appeared stable and osseointegration took place uneventfully.

Radiolucent lines were seen in 13 cases, mostly in zone 1 (11 cases) and in zone 7 (3 cases). No signs of osteolysis were observed or any cortical hypertrophy or ballooning. Most of the radiolucent lines (RLL) in

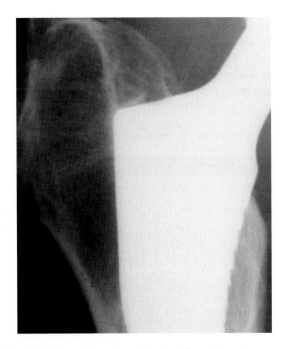

Fig. 4.39 Osteointegration of the Corail® prosthesis. Zoom on the trochanteric area (3 years post-op, 91-year-old woman)

zone 1 were seen in the stems that subsided at early weight-bearing.

Forty-one stems were placed in varus and one in valgus. This had no effect on the clinical outcome. None of these cases developed cortical thickening in zones 3 and 5, but the density of trabecular bone developed in these zones appeared higher in the compression area.

Thirty-three cases had peri-articular ossification of varying degrees (9 grade 1, 18 grade 2, 6 grade 3 and none grade 4), but these did not affect the functional result of the hemiarthroplasty.

Functional Results

The functional results for the 75 patients still alive 5 years after their fracture are summarised in Table 4.23. Among the 61 patients with a mobility score >2 before fracture occurred and still alive after 5 years, 54 patients recovered their preoperative mobility score. None complained of hip pain. Forty-eight patients recovered their preoperative autonomy, as assessed with Jensen's index.

Late Hip Complications

Two fractures of the femur occurred after 4 and 13 months. These fractures followed a second fall in each case and were treated by open reduction, internal fixation (ORIF). One case of recurrent dislocation required

Table 4.23 Autonomy, mental and mobility score among the 75 survivors after 5 years

		In cases: 75
Autonomy	I	7
	II	2
	III	25
	IV	41
Mental	0–4	20
	5–7	38
	8–10	17
Mobility score	0–3	22
	4–6	36
	7–9	17

revision surgery. The total re-operation rate was thus 3/204 (1.4%).

Discussion

Since the 1970s, the use of bipolar prostheses has become increasingly popular for the management of femoral neck fractures. Endoprosthetic replacement was pioneered by Judet in the 1940s, then the Vitallium stem from Austin Moore in the 1950s [23] and finally the unipolar cemented Thompson prostheses in the 1960s [15, 16]. These unipolar prostheses made it possible to treat these fractures with increasing reliability throughout the decades. But their intensive use has also outlined the limits of unipolar arthroplasties [21, 22]. The acetabular complications with these prostheses led Monk and Christiaensen [4] to insert a polyethylene (PE) cup between the bony acetabulum and the femoral head, a concept that then evolved towards the current bipolar prosthesis. More recent articles mention revision rates for these bipolar hemiarthroplasties, particularly in the less aged patients, and recommend instead the use of total hip arthroplasty as a primary surgery [13, 20, 29].

The choice of type of prosthesis to be used is marked by a total lack of consensus:

> Total arthroplasty versus hemiarthroplasty
> Cemented versus uncemented arthroplasty
> Unipolar versus bipolar hemiarthroplasty

In octogenarian patients, the following clinical parameters are likely to influence the therapeutical choice: (1) reduced physical activity, (2) high prevalence of mental deficiency, and (3) omnipresence of cortico-trabecular osteoporosis of the femur.

1. *Reduced physical activity* renders (almost) improbable the occurrence of acetabular erosion after hemiarthroplasty, unlike in patients who are far more active, in which the acetabular protrusion of the Thompson or Austin Moore prostheses has been frequently observed [1, 2, 10, 15]. This suggests that femoral hemiarthroplasty is undoubtedly the treatment of choice for octogenarian patients.

2. *Senile dementia* significantly reduces the involvement of the patient in his or her own rehabilitation. This compromises the application of anti-dislocation precautions due to the fact that these patients – whose muscle mass is often reduced – are significantly

confused. Yet, the incidence of dislocation after total hip arthroplasty exceeds that of dislocation occurring after hemiarthroplasty, which advocates for the use of the latter.

3. *Femoral osteoporosis*, which mainly affects trabecular bone, makes prosthetic fixation difficult, be it with cemented prostheses because of the reduced number of microdigitations in the trabecular bone [8, 9] or with cementless prostheses because primary stability is difficult to achieve.

The choice between cemented and cementless prostheses is hard in the absence of any clear-cut argument in favour of one or the other.

Those in favour of the cemented solution argue that it provides better mechanical stability. This observation results from experimental works that compared cemented Thomson versus uncemented Austin Moore prostheses [31, 32]. This observation is supported by the critical analysis of the randomised studies that compared the same implants [27]. The performance of the cementless Austin Moore implants appear to be worse and their follow-up is marked with numerous complications, such as a high number of peri-prosthetic radiolucent lines [10], prosthetic revisions [25] and a lower functional performance [10].

Those in favour of an uncemented solution argue that:

1. Elderly patients enjoy a significantly longer survival rate (cf. our own figures), and thus a 5-year outcome must be considered when making the choice of an arthroplasty.

2. Endosteal osteopenia can lead to cemented stem loosening and the need for stem revision. A prosthetic revision is difficult and is accompanied by a high mortality rate in octo- or even nonagenarian patients, in whom loosening is most frequently encountered.

3. It is widely accepted that cementless femoral fixation is a gold standard for hip arthroplasty in young patients because of its exceptional longevity. Nevertheless, uncemented implants, particularly those coated with HA, are reliable even in elderly patients. There is no biological evidence that an 'old' bone is unable to react adequately in the presence of an osteoconductive material. The same sequence of inflammatory process, followed by ossification and bone remodelling is thought to occur [12]. Intuitively, surgeons who have no experience with HA-coated implants fear that the

osteogenesis mechanisms will be impaired to such an extent that they will hinder the formation of bony bridges. An examination of 28 samples of bone marrow from men between 37 and 80 years of age showed an age-related decline in differentiation of osteoblasts in three-dimensional (3D) culture [24]. Whether this is due to a loss of progenitor cells, to a diminished capacity of the osteoblasts or to an increased potential to support osteoclastogenesis remains unknown. However, it has also been demonstrated that this loss of osteoblastogenic potential is only partial, without any significant reduction of the osteointegration potential. Animal experiments clearly demonstrated the positive role of calcium hydroxyapatite, leading to more intense and earlier osteogenesis compared to that observed with porous metallic implants. Clinical experience and radiographic examinations demonstrated that the osteointegration of implants – even within the difficult context of osteoporosis and lower ambulatory performance – occurred systematically in all subjects, and led to prosthetic fixation. The histological experience demonstrated that for femurs taken from patients operated between 10 and 15 days beforehand, there was systematic, convincing and reproducible osteointegration in all the patients. This therapeutic choice is validated by the constant satisfactory results and the absence of 'surprises' once the implant has been correctly implanted inside the femur.

4. There is a high incidence of intra-operative mortality during the cementing process – particularly in elderly patients with altered cardiac function [30], a still unsolved problem, despite the years and progress in resuscitation [3, 19]. This is due to the fall in stroke volume and cardiac output caused by embolism during cementation [6]. Christie et al. [5] have shown using transoesophageal echocardiography during cemented and uncemented arthroplasties that cemented arthroplasty caused greater and more prolonged embolic cascades than did uncemented procedures. An estimated rate of mortality attributable to the use of polymethylmethacrylate (PMMA) cement of 0.14% has been calculated by Weinrauch et al. [33].

5. There is a possible increase in the incidence of acetabular protrusion with cemented hemiarthroplasties [7, 15, 34].

Additional advantages in cementless fixation include shorter surgical times and substantial savings in health-care costs [11].

References

1. Baker RP, Squires B, Gargan MF et al (2006) Total hip arthroplasty and hemiarthroplasty in mobile, independent patients with a displaced intracapsular fracture of the femoral neck. J Bone Joint Surg Am 88-A:2583–2589
2. Blomfeldt R, Törnkvist H, Eriksson K et al (2006) A randomized controlled trial comparing bipolar hemiarthroplasty with total hip replacement for displaced intracapsular fractures of the femoral neck in elderly patients. J. Bone Joint Surg Br 89-B:160–165
3. Casteleyn PP, Melon C, Opdecam P (1977) Treatment of intracapsular femoral neck fractures by femoral prostheses. Acta Orthop Belg 43: 693–701
4. Christiaensen T (1969) A new hip prosthesis with trunnion-bearing. Acta Chir Scand 135:43–46
5. Christie J, Burnett R, Potts HR et al (1994) Echocardiography of transatrial embolism during cemented and uncemented hemiarthroplasty of the hip. J Bone Joint Surg Br 76-B:409–412
6. Clark DI, Ahmed AB, Baxendale BR et al (2001) Cardiac output during hemiarthroplasties of the hip. A prospective, controlled trial of cemented and uncemented prostheses. J Bone Joint Surg Br 83:414–418
7. D'Arcy J, Devas M (1976) Treatment of fractures of the femoral neck by replacement with the Thompson prosthesis. J Bone Joint Surg Br 58:279–286
8. Ding M, Dalstra M, Danielsen CC et al (1997) Age variations in the properties of human tibial trabecular bone. J Bone Joint Surg Br 79:995–1002
9. Ding M, Dalstra M, Linde F et al (1998) Mechanical properties of the normal human tibial cartilage-bone complex in relation to age. Clinic Biomech (Bristol, Avon) 13:351–358
10. Dorr LD, Glousman R, Sew Yoy AL et al (1986) Treatment of femoral neck fractures with total hip replacement versus cemented and noncemented hemiarthroplasty. J Arthroplasty 1:21–28
11. Dutton A, Rubash HE (2008) Hot topics and controversies in arthroplasty: cementless femoral fixation in elderly patients. Instr Course Lect 57:255–259
12. Engh CA, Glassman AH, Bobyn JD (1986) Surgical principles in cementless total hip arthroplasty. Tech Orthop 1:35–53
13. Figved W, Dybvik E, Frihagen F et al (2007) Conversion from failed hemiarthroplasty to total hip arthroplasty: a Norwegian arthroplasty register analysis of 595 hips with previous femoral neck fractures. Acta Orthop 78:711–718
14. Garden RS (1961) Low angle fixation in fractures of the femoral neck. J Bone Joint Surg Br 43:647–663
15. Gingras MB, Clarke J, Evarts CM (1980) Prosthetic replacement in femoral neck fractures. Clin Orthop 152:147–157
16. Hestermans Y, Amiri-Lamraski A, Bertrand P et al (1985) Traitement des fractures intracapsulaires du col fémoral du vieillard par prothèse de Thompson. Acta Orthop Belg 51:298–309
17. Jensen JS (1984) Determining factors for the mortality following hip fractures. Injury 15:411–414
18. Johnell O, Nilsson B, Obrant K (1984) Age and sex pattern of hip fracture – changes in 30 years. Acta Orthop Scand 55:290–292
19. Leighton RK, Schmidt AH, Collier P (2007) Advances in the treatment of intracapsular hip fractures in the elderly. Injury 38(suppl 3):S24–S34
20. Macaulay W, Nellans KW, Garvin KL et al (2008) Prospective randomized clinical trial comparing hemiarthroplasty to total hip arthroplasty in the treatment of displaced femoral neck fractures. J Arthroplasty 23(suppl 1):2–8
21. Maxted MJ, Denham RA (1984) Failure of hemiarthroplasty for fractures of the neck of the femur. Injury 15:224–226
22. Meyer S (1981) Prosthetic replacement in hip fractures: a comparison between the Moore and Christiansen endoprostheses. Clin Orthop Relat Res 160:57–62
23. Moore AT (1953) The Moore self-locking Vitallium prosthesis in fresh femoral neck fractures. A new low posterior approach (The Southern exposure). In: American Academy of Orthopaedic Surgeons Instructional Course Lectures, 3rd edn. vol 16.CV Mosby, Louis, pp 309–321
24. Mueller SM, Mizuno S, Glowacki J (1998) The effect of age on the osteogenic potential of human bone marrow cells cultured in three-dimensional collagen sponges. Bone 23:S536
25. Obrant KJ, Carlsson AS (1987) Survival of hemiarthroplasties after cervical hip fractures. Orthopedics 10: 1153–1156
26. Parker MJ, Palmer CR (1993) A new mobility score for predicting mortality after hip fracture. J Bone Joint Surg Br 75:797
27. Parker MJ, Gurusamy K (2006) Arthroplasties (with and without bone cement) for proximal femoral fractures in adults (review). Cochrane Database Syst Rev 3. Art. No.: CD001706. doi 10.1002/14651858. CD001706.pub3
28. Qureshi KN, Hodkinson HM (1974) Evaluation of a ten-question mental test in the institutionalized elderly. Age Ageing 3:152
29. Rogmark C, Johnell O (2005) Orthopaedic treatment of displaced femoral neck fractures in elderly patients. Disabil Rehabil 27:1143–1149
30. Sikorski JM, Millar AJ (1977) Systemic disturbance from Thompson's arthroplasty: a age-matched and sex-matched controlled retrospective survey. J Bone Joint Surg Br 59:398–401
31. Sonstegaard DA, Kaufer H, Matthews LS (1974) A biochemical evaluation of implant, reduction and prosthesis in the treatment of intertrochanteric hip fractures. Orthop Clin North Am 5:551
32. Wagner J, DeMarneffe R (1968) Mechanical study of the cemented Austin Moore hip prosthesis. Acta Orthop Belg 34:253
33. Weinrauch PC, Moore WR, Shooter DR et al (2006) Early prosthetic complications after unipolar hemiarthroplasty. ANZ J Surg 76:432–435
34. Whittaker RP (1972) Fifteen years experience with metallic endoprosthetic replacement of the femoral head for femoral neck fractures. J Trauma 12:799

The Corail Revision Family

Tim Board

5

Contents

J.-P. Vidalain et al. (eds.), *The CORAIL® Hip System*,
DOI: 10.1007/978-3-642-18396-6_5, © Springer-Verlag Berlin Heidelberg 2011

5.1 HA and Conservative Revision: A Philosophy

Tim Board and Helge Wangen

Revision hip surgery is a complex and challenging task. The frequency of revision surgery is increasing with time and the need for a conservative approach to preserve bone stock and load the femur as physiologically as possible is paramount. The various options for reconstruction of the femur are discussed in the following chapter. The benefits of a long, flexible, titanium, fully hydroxyapatite (HA) coated implant are simplicity of use, bone regeneration, proximal loading and an exceptionally low incidence of stress shielding and thigh pain.

Year	Number of revisions at Wrightington
2000	310
2001	333
2002	354
2003	424
2004	446
2005	449
2006	487
2007	539
2008	526
2009	514

Fig. 5.1 Represents the growing number of revisions performed at Wrightington Hospital over the last decade

The Problem

Revision hip arthroplasty is a complex, surgical challenge; the decision over when to operate on a loosening hip, the difficulty of removing implants without complication and the need to maintain maximum bone stock are perhaps more of a challenge than the actual reconstruction itself. Although more taxing surgically, the overall goals of revision hip arthroplasty are similar to primary surgery:

Restore the biomechanics and joint centre of the hip
Create a stable joint with a low-wear bearing
Preserve bone

The first two of these goals can be achieved with virtually any of the reconstruction systems available today; however to achieve the final goal of preserving bone we need to develop a consistent philosophy that allows us to choose the appropriate implant depending on the support available from the femur. We recommend using the least invasive revision implant that will provide adequate fixation in the femur without extending distally into the femur further than is necessary, but without exposing the patient to increased risk of complications. This philosophy of 'conservative revision' demands that the surgeon always thinks about the next revision and attempts to reduce the complexity of the reconstruction not increase it. A useful way to think about this approach is to aspire to make the revision look like a primary one. This will clearly not be achievable in every case, but often it is possible to reduce the length of the femoral stem using the Corail® family of implants as we will see in subsequent chapters. The importance of this philosophy becomes clear when analysing the growing number of revisions performed (Fig. 5.1).

Figure 5.1 shows the number of revision arthroplasties performed at Wrightington hospital over the last decade indicating almost a doubling of the revision burden. Furthermore, in an analysis of 4,382 revision hips performed at Wrightington, only 76% were first time revisions, 18% second time, 5% third time and 1% fourth time or more. These figures indicate the importance of planning for the next revision, as many patients will undergo multiple surgeries.

For a cementless revision implant to be successful in the long term it must achieve two objectives. The first is to be stable within the femur to allow ingrowth of host bone. The second is to allow proximal loading of the femur during gait. Many revisions systems easily achieve the first, but very few achieve the second. Particularly long, stiff stems that rely primarily on distal press-fit fixation actively offload the proximal femur, resulting in proximal bone loss, hardly an approach that will preserve bone and make any future revision easy.

The Potential Solutions

There is a huge variety of differing options for revision of a femoral component whether dealing with major bone loss or not. As in primary hip surgery, the solutions are broadly divided into two different techniques, that is with or without cement.

Cement Only

In the early experience of revision surgery it was commonplace to simply remove the stem and the cement and then re-cement a new implant in the sclerotic femur. Using this technique the early results were satisfactory, however the medium-term results were less so. Data from Wrightington Hospital showed a 5-year survival rate of 88% in 74 stems revised with a long-stemmed, cemented implant [3].The fundamental problem with purely cemented revision is that cement works by interlocking with exposed trabecular bone and this is often lacking in the revision situation. After removal of implants and cement, the femoral canal is often sclerotic with very little cancellous bone to allow cement micro-interlock.

Cement and Bone Grafting

Impaction cancellous allografting for revision of a femoral component is an excellent option that was initially described by Gie in 1993 [4] as a modification of a technique used for the reconstruction of acetabuli with protrusio. Of the many papers in the literature, the results from Exeter are probably the most favourable, citing a 10-year survivorship for revision for any reason of 90% [5]. Many other papers report survivorships between 92% and 97%, but at shorter follow-up times, typically between 2 and 6 years. Impaction allografting is a technically demanding process, which is reflected in the frequency of complications reported. The most frequent complication recorded in addition to infection and dislocation is periprosthetic fracture. These fractures usually occur during the vigorous process of impaction required to obtain a stable neo-endosteum. Postoperative fracture may also occur, usually around the tip of the stem. This may be related to unrecognised intraoperative femoral perforations or

fractures or to unappreciated areas of osteolysis. Even if this does not lead to re-revision, a postoperative fracture almost invariably leads to a re-operation. The rates of complications in some papers are as high as 30%. Impaction allografting requires a reliable supply of bone. Whilst in many places, such as the UK, bone is readily available, this is not the case everywhere. Rules governing the operation of Bone Banks have become increasingly stringent and the cost of bone has risen accordingly.

Whilst the results of impaction grafting are certainly better than those of purely cemented revision, this approach has not found universal acceptance, mostly due to the time taken to perform the procedure, the high rate of complications and the availability of bone.

Seth et al. presented an algorithm for femoral reconstruction in 1999 [10]. In this algorithm impaction allografting is reserved for the following types of patients:

1. Patients for whom standard distal fixation without cement is not suitable.
2. Patients in whom restoration of proximal bone stock is particularly important.
3. Patients in whom proximal stress shielding and thigh pain from modulus mismatch are major concerns.

These conditions are often seen in patients who have a large ectatic diaphysis and in whom less than 4 cm of bone is usable for the distal fixation of a large extensively coated stem. In these settings, an alternative to impaction allografting is replacement of the proximal aspect of the femur and reconstruction with an allograft-prosthetic composite. Allan et al published results on 78 proximal femoral allografts at an average follow-up of 3 years [1]. They showed that large grafts had a success rate of 85%, but also concluded that usage of calcar allografts less than 3 cm long had poorer results (81%) and should be abandoned and that cortical strut grafting seemed to be an effective method of bridging isolated cortical defects. Hugh et al. reported on 60 patients who had been revised with a proximal femoral allograft-prosthesis construct [2]. They found their results encouraging with a success rate of 78% after an average follow-up of 9 years. Whilst these results are less favourable than those shown above for purely cemented and impaction grafted revisions, the cases reconstructed with bulk allograft are certainly more complex and involved greater bone loss, and hence the results would be expected to be inferior to the more simple revisions.

Uncemented Stems

Registry data from different countries certainly demonstrates that uncemented femoral revisions are becoming more and more popular even in countries like Norway and Sweden, where impaction grafting has been widely used in the past [7, 11]. When using uncemented stems the traditional concept is to bypass the osteolytic areas or defects by using longer and bigger stems in order to achieve primary stability of the stem in the diaphyseal bone. Published results for such stems are satisfactory, for example a survivorship of 95.9% at 13.2 years in 170 stems was published by Paprosky [8] and similar results have been published in other studies [6]. However, the incidence of thigh pain associated with this type of stem is high. Of the 170 patients described above, 31% had thigh pain. This high incidence is confirmed in other series. The thigh pain is secondary to the distal fixation of the rigid stem and is also the herald of proximal bone loss due to stress transfer. Both the studies cited above quoted unacceptably high rates of radiographic stress shielding as shown in Fig. 5.2.

This type of stem does not fit the philosophy of conservative revision outlined above. Proximally loading stems such as the S-ROM® system allow proximal loading, but are not without their own problems of fretting at interfaces and thigh pain from the long smooth stem.

The Corail® Family of Revision Implants

The Corail® family of implants consists of the standard Corail® stem, the Corail® Revision Stem (Previously named the KAR™ stem) and the Reef® stem. All these

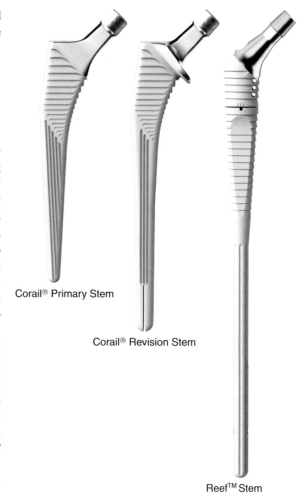

Corail® Primary Stem

Corail® Revision Stem

Reef™ Stem

Fig. 5.3 The Corail® family of implants (Copyright DePuy-International Limited)

implants (Fig. 5.3) are fully hydroxyapatite coated and made from titanium alloy. The Corail® Revision Stem is identical to the Corail® Primary Stem except for two differences: (1) each size of the revision stem is 40 mm longer than its primary counterpart and (2) the distal segment of the revision stem has crossed slots, which are intended to allow bending of the stem to conform to the bow of the femur and to allow three-point fixation

Fig. 5.2 Represents the rate of stress shielding of the femur in revision series carried out with long, porous-coated cobalt chrome stems

Stress shielding	Year Paprosky 1999 170 stems	Moreland 2001 137 stems
Mild	89%	14.2%
Moderate	15%	66.4%
Severe	6%	19.5%

of the stem. The Reef® stem is a modular system allowing a wide range of stem lengths and diameters, all with distal interlocking. This family of implants allows the surgeon to match the implant to the level of bone loss seen at revision and therefore to maintain the conservative revision philosophy. We will see in the chapters that follow in this section that the use of these fully hydroxyapatite coated revision stems not only produces excellent clinical results in terms of survivorship, but also allows proximal loading of the femur with protection against thigh pain and stress shielding [9]. Moreover, we will show many cases of significant bone regeneration without the need to resort to bone grafting of the femur.

Conclusion

Revision hip arthroplasty is a complex, technically demanding process and the number of hips needing revision is increasing significantly. In choosing a hip system for the reconstruction of the femur, it is of paramount importance that both, initial stability is achieved and the proximal femur is loaded by the stem. In this way stress shielding can be prevented and long-term bone regeneration can occur.

Key Learning Points

> Revision hip arthroplasty is an increasingly frequent problem
> Impaction bone grafting with cemented stems offers good results, but at the expense of high complication rates
> Long, porous coated, distal-fit stems offer good results in terms of survivorship, but at the expense of a high incidence of thigh pain and proximal stress shielding.
> A philosophy of 'conservative revision' is suggested, tailoring stem choice to bone loss, with the use of extensively hydroxyapatite coated titanium stems that achieve reliable fixation and allow proximal loading of the femur.

References

1. Allan G, Lavoie GJ, McDonald S et al (1991) Proximal femoral allografts in revision hip arthroplasty. J Bone Joint Surg Br 73:235–240
2. Blackley HRL, Davis AM et al (2001) Proximal femoral allografts for reconstruction of bone stock in revision arthroplasty of the hip. J Bone Joint Surg Am 83:346
3. Crawford SA, Siney PD, Wroblewski BM (2000) Revision of failed total hip arthroplasty with a proximal femoral modular cemented stem. J Bone Joint Surg Br 82(5):684–688
4. Gie GA, Linder L, Ling LS et al (1993) Contained morselized allograft in revision total hip arthroplasty surgical technique. Orthop Clin North Am 24:717–725
5. Halliday BR, English HW, Timperley AJ et al (2003) Femoral impaction grafting with cement in revision total hip replacement. Evolution of the technique and results. J Bone Joint Surg Br 85(6):809–817
6. Moreland JR, Moreno MA (2001) Cementless femoral revision arthroplasty of the hip: minimum 5 years follow up. Clin Orthop Relat Res Dec(393):194–201
7. Norwegian Arthroplasty Register annual report 2009
8. Paprosky WG, Greidanus NV, Antoniou J (1999) Minimum 10-year-results of extensively porous-coated stems in revision hip arthroplasty. Clin Orthop Relat Res Dec(369): 230–242
9. Reikerås O, Gunderson RB (2006) Excellent results with femoral revision surgery using an extensively hydroxyapatite-coated stem: 59 patients followed for 10–16 years. Acta Orthop 77(1):98–103
10. Seth S, Leopold M et al (1999) Current status of impaction allografting for revision of a femoral component. J Bone Joint Surg Am 81:1337–1345
11. Swedish Arthroplasty Register annual report 2008

5.2 Removing a Well-Fixed Corail® Stem: It's Not As Hard As You Think

Jean-Claude Cartillier and Jens Boldt

The full hydroxyapatite coating of the Corail® stem promotes effective stem osseointegration without compromising subsequent stem removal. The Corail® stem is implanted in a sheath of compacted cancellous bone and not against the cortical bone. Should the stem be explanted, it is possible to resect all newly formed bone bridges around the implant by using special instruments that combine flexible blades and Kirschner wires (K-wire). This chapter describes the indications for explantation and details the required technique. Since the remaining bone stock is preserved, a new Corail® stem can be inserted in conditions similar to those which occur in a primary implantation. Should this technique fail, more invasive surgical techniques are available such as a posterior longitudinal osteotomy or an extended trochanteric osteotomy.

Introduction

Removal of a well-fixed, uncemented femoral stem during revision hip arthroplasty remains a challenging procedure for all hip surgeons. In particular, the removal of a well-fixed Corail® stem is one of the often mentioned concerns for potential new users. Despite the fact that aseptic loosening of a Corail® stem is very unlikely, removal may be indicated due to:

1. Fracture of the neck of the femoral stem or damage to the stem taper, which is so severe that it prevents the insertion of a new femoral head or a salvage 'sleeve'.
2. Serious Biomechanical defects:

   – Major leg lengthening or shortening
   – Inappropriate offset
   – Inadequate anteversion angle

   These defects may present with dislocation, gait disturbance or symptomatic leg length discrepancy.

3. Infection: A stem which has loosened significantly due to infection will be easy to remove. Often, however, infection will require removal of a well-fixed stem to allow thorough debridement before reconstruction in one or two stages.

The removal of an uncemented stem is normally considered a highly challenging and risky procedure for any surgeon and has the potential to cause devastating damage to the femur. The Corail® stem is, however, often easier to remove than anticipated by the surgeon, especially if the surgeon has experience in removing other uncemented implants previously. This is due to the integrated design of the stem and the insertion technique. The compaction broaching technique results in a compacted layer of trabecular bone between the implant and the inner cortical surface of the femur. When extraction is required, it is this layer that is penetrated, which is relatively straightforward. By contrast, 'fit and fill' type designs of uncemented stem result in abutment of the implant against the inner cortical surface, thereby leaving no gap for the insertion of extraction instruments. The macrostructure of the Corail® stem surface also facilitates removal. The horizontal metaphyseal grooves, aligned in a reverse stair-stepped manner, facilitate the insertion of the flexible osteotome blades. The diaphyseal vertical grooves facilitate the axial insertion of the K-wires and allow the K-wires to converge in the underlying femoral canal.

Surgical Technique

The following recommended surgical technique does not require a special approach. Any approach that the surgeon feels comfortable with is possible, provided it gives sufficient access to the entire proximal metaphysis and stem. Specially designed narrow and flexible osteotomes, drill-mounted K-wires and a screw-in, slap hammer are part of the Corail® extraction set. Very occasionally, a lateral or posterior unicortical osteotomy with widening of the proximal femur may be helpful before hammering the stem out safely. Fortunately, an extended trochanteric osteotomy (Wagner) is almost never required, but if required is performed in a standard fashion, ensuring the osteotomy is long enough to allow access to the entire length of the stem.

Following adequate exposure of the proximal femur and once all scar tissue, capsule and preferably the femoral head have been removed, the surgeon must clear the interface of all remaining tissue and debris using the small and flexible osteotomes (Fig. 5.4). This process is continued until the depth at which solid osseointegration occurs is reached and the osteotomes start to bend. Instead of sacrificing further osteotomes

Fig. 5.4 The flexible
osteotomes being used to
develop the interface
proximally (Copyright
DePuyInternational
Limited)

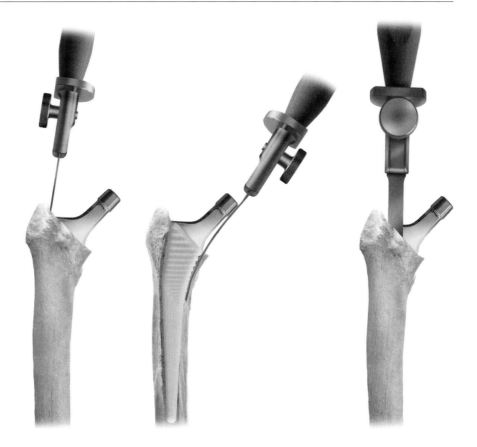

and potentially femoral bone, the surgeon should then
switch to using the drill mounted on 1.8 mm Kirschner
wires to further loosen the interface on all sides
(Fig. 5.5). As is often the case in femoral stem removal,
cancellous bone should be removed from the trochanteric bed area adjacent to the shoulder of the implant.
This will allow safe passage of the stem and prevent
fracture of the greater trochanter. Once the K-wires
cease to move forward easily the surgeon may possibly
switch between osteotomes and K-wires. It usually
takes two to three cycles to sufficiently loosen the bone
bridges at the tip of the stem.

At this point the specially designed Corail® slap-
hammer device is attached to the proximal screw hole
at the lateral shoulder of the prosthesis (Fig. 5.6). It is
essential to ensure that the thread of the slap-hammer
device is fully seated in the screw hole. We would recommend to initially hit the hammer distally and then
proximally. In our experience, this helps loosen the
remaining distal bone bridges at the tip of the stem
within the diaphysis. Following this, the surgeon
should now hit the hammer proximally with increasing
force. While hammering, it is very important to double
check that there is no angulation in order to prevent

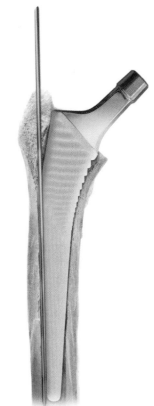

Fig. 5.5 A Kirschner wire
being used to develop the
distal interface (Copyright
DePuyInternational Limited)

Fig. 5.6 The screw-in slap hammer attached to the shoulder of the implant (Copyright DePuyInternational Limited)

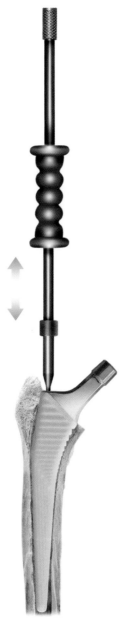

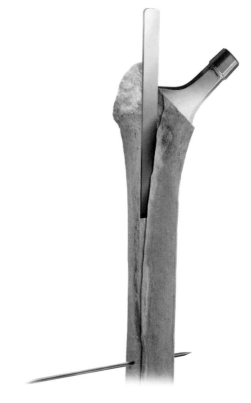

Fig. 5.7 A longitudinal split osteotomy (Copyright DePuy-International Limited)

non-axial stresses, since angulation may potentially fissure or crack the metaphysis. The surgical assistant must be instructed to closely monitor any movement of both, the stem and the femoral bone, in order to optimise and fine-tune both the forces and direction of the hammering actions. In about half of the cases the Corail® stem will come out easily. If that is not the case, the surgeon should simply pause and redo the

entire extracting procedure for about 10–20 min. Very often, repetitive hammering will eventually loosen the remaining bone bridges, setting the Corail® stem free. Standing firmly with a solid base is recommended when hammering due to the fact that sudden loosening and withdrawal of the stem could upset the surgeon's balance.

If, despite all efforts and correct surgical technique, the Corail® stem still does not loosen, the surgeon can apply the following technique to create a posterior longitudinal easing osteotomy (Fig. 5.7). Elevation of the posterior edge of the vastus lateralis muscle allows access to the linea aspera of the femur. A longitudinal cut is performed with a reciprocating saw from the posterior edge of the greater trochanter down to the anticipated depth of the Corail® stem −2 cm. Large, wide, and straight osteotomes are then introduced into the proximal end of the osteotomy to open up the femur slightly. At this point, the surgeon

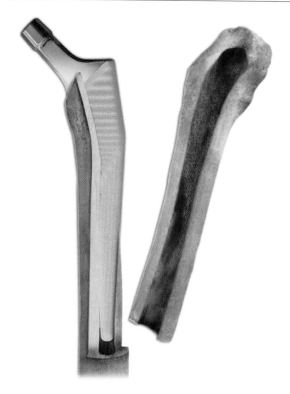

Fig. 5.8 An extended trochanteric osteotomy (ETO) (Copyright DePuyInternational Limited)

should simply repeat the hammering procedure as mentioned above and in virtually all cases this will lead to a successful removal of the Corail® stem without damage to the femoral bone stock. Prior to femoral preparation and insertion of the new stem, one or two cerclage cables are applied around the femur, distal to the lesser trochanter. The postoperative regime and rehabilitation is not jeopardised when using this technique. Only on very rare occasions is it necessary to resort to an extended trochanteric osteotomy (ETO) (Fig. 5.8) to remove a Corail® stem, but this can be achieved in the standard fashion, if necessary.

Collared or Collarless

Removal of the collared Corail® stem does not differ greatly in technique from that described above. This is due to the design of the collar, which protrudes from the stem medially and only slightly anteroposteriorly. This allows almost full access for osteotomes and Kirschner wires to the proximal bone-implant interface. When removing a collared stem, however, a small 5–10 mm horseshoe piece of bone may be removed underneath the medial collar from the medial calcar to facilitate access to the medial most aspect of the implant-bone interface.

Reconstruction

Following Corail® stem removal, an assessment should be made of the quality of the femoral bone stock. If the femur is adequately supportive and osteotomy has not been necessary, then a larger size Corail® stem can be used for the revision. If either the proximal metaphysis does not provide adequate support for a Corail® stem or a full, extended trochanteric osteotomy has been undertaken, then it is recommended to reconstruct the femur with a Corail® Revision Stem to achieve fixation in good quality bone or to bypass the distal extent of the osteotomy. If a longitudinal split osteotomy has been performed, it is not absolutely necessary to bypass the spilt provided adequate cerclage wiring has been undertaken.

Conclusion

There are several advantages when removing a well-fixed Corail® compared to other uncemented stems. Firstly, stem removal is rare with the Corail® stem due to its outstanding clinical performance and proven durability. Secondly, the special extraction instruments provide the surgeon with a tried and tested technique that is relatively straightforward. Thirdly, the surgical technique is minimally invasive and retains as much femoral bone stock as possible. Lastly, the procedure usually allows the surgeon to simply replace the stem with a larger Corail® primary or Corail® Revision stem, thereby maintaining the principles of 'conservative revision.'

5.3 Retaining a Well-Fixed Corail® in Revision: Building on Solid Foundations

Jean-Christophe Chatelet

Fully hydroxyapatite (HA) coated cementless femoral stems have shown excellent long-term survivorship, particularly with the 25-year follow-up of the Corail® stem. However, among the myriad of different cup designs, there has not yet been any one design that has shown similarly excellent results. Registry data clearly shows that cup failure is a more frequent problem than stem failure. We are therefore often faced with the surgical issue of a well-fixed femoral stem with a loose socket. In cemented stems, aseptic loosening secondary to polyethylene wear debris often progresses down the stem necessitating full revision. However, in this mode of failure with the Corail® stem, it is not uncommon to see proximal osteolysis and granulomas that do not extend past zones 1 and 7. This is due to the active osseointegration around the stem, which prevents the distal migration of polyethylene particles. This situation raises a number of issues:

> Can the acetabular cup be changed while leaving the Corail® stem in place, allowing simpler revision surgery?
> How can proximal femoral granulomas and cavitary lesions be managed when retaining the stem?
> If retaining the stem, how should a damaged Morse taper be managed?
> Will the osteolytic process induced by macrophage activation and osteoclastic bone resorption secondary to polyethylene wear debris continue after revision of the bearing surfaces?
> Surgical techniques to address these issues and the results of such surgery are discussed in this chapter.

Surgical Technique

Cup Revision and Stem Retention

Revision of the acetabular cup with retention of the stem is a relatively straightforward process. As the Corail® stem is modular it is possible to remove the femoral head, protect the Morse taper and proceed with

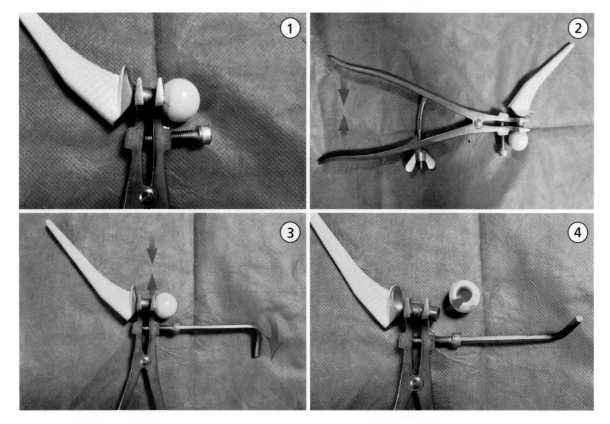

Fig. 5.9 The mechanical, screw action femoral head remover

Removal of the Femoral Head

The safest and most efficient method of femoral head removal is to use a mechanical extractor (Fig. 5.9). This applies a gradually increasing force to the junction eventually allowing the head to break free. The alternative is to use a mallet and head pusher. This technique may be acceptable for metallic heads, but is not recommended for ceramic heads due to the risk of fracture. The Morse taper can then be protected throughout the procedure by wrapping in a small swab and tying the swab in place with heavy suture thread.

Reusing a Damaged Morse Taper

The Morse taper must be carefully inspected after removal of the femoral head. If there is significant cup revision as normal. The protection of the Morse taper is of paramount importance, particularly if the surgeon wishes to use a ceramic head for the revision.

scratching or corrosion damage, then a metallic head must be used for the revision. If there is very little corrosion or no macroscopic damage, then we have frequently used a ceramic head on the retained stem. The classical recommendations are not to use a ceramic head on a retained Morse taper; however, we have not seen any ceramic head fractures in these cases. Newer technologies have allowed the manufacture of ceramic heads with metallic internal sleeves. These devices are recommended for use on retained stems, even if they are damaged, and their use will undoubtedly become more popular in the future (Fig. 5.10).

Dealing with Proximal Granulomas

Proximal osteolysis or granulomas around a distally well-fixed stem should be attended to at revision surgery. We recommend a technique of curettage of the areas, removal of membranous material and polyethylene wear debris followed by irrigation. The resulting cavities can then be filled with allograft and impacted.

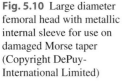

Fig. 5.10 Large diameter femoral head with metallic internal sleeve for use on damaged Morse taper (Copyright DePuy-International Limited)

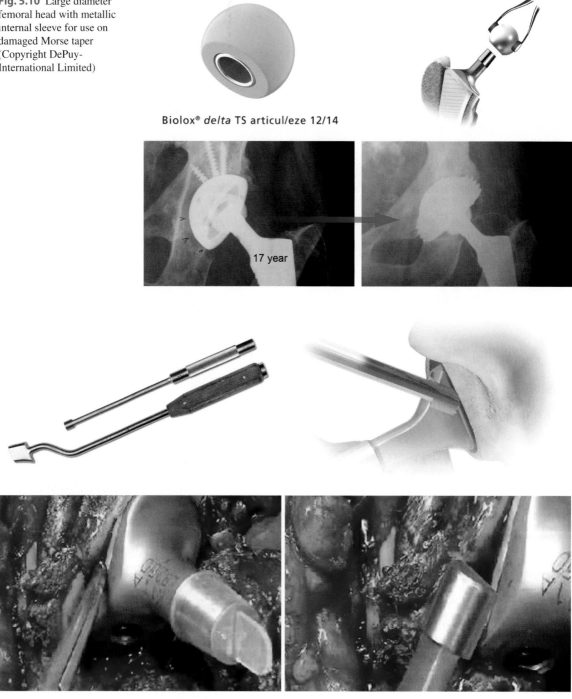

Biolox® *delta* TS articul/eze 12/14

17 year

Fig. 5.11 The bone impactor from the Corail® primary set – a useful instrument for bone impaction around a well-fixed Corail® stem

Femoral head allograft is normally used for this purpose. The femoral head is cleaned of all soft tissue and then milled in a commercially available bone mill. Prior to impaction, the bone is washed with normal saline. The bone impactor from the Corail® set is useful for the process of impaction (Fig. 5.11). This is a simple and fast technique, the results of which are discussed below.

Evidence for Retaining a Corail® Stem in Revision

Patient Series

Between 1993 and 2002, 228 revision hip arthro-plasties were performed in our centre. We retrospectively reviewed 115 cup revisions on a stable Corail® femoral stem. The remaining 113 cases underwent total hip prosthesis revision for cemented implant loosening and are not discussed here. Indications for cup revision surgery included cup loosening (98 cases) and severe polyethylene wear (17 cases).

The mean age of the patients was 71 years (range 40–89 years). In this study, 61 males and 54 females were included, and the mean time from primary surgery to revision was 11 years (range 7–15 years). The Corail® femoral implant was stable in all cases.

Femoral Issues

Of the 115 cup revisions, 97 stems were fully ingrown with no radiographic signs of loosening. Calcar rounding was seen in 28% of these cases. In the remaining 18 cases, there was granuloma formation and loosening around the proximal stem, assumed to be related to polyethylene wear. This subgroup was also younger and more active (mean age 63 years). Of these 18 cases, 11 were asymptomatic (Fig. 5.12). The stability of the Corail® stem was evaluated on preoperative radiographs and confirmed intraoperatively. The femoral head was removed by means of a mechanical extractor as described above and the Morse taper was thoroughly protected throughout the procedure. The quality of the titanium Morse taper was macroscopically evaluated. As discussed above the taper was deemed acceptable in 98 cases and in these cases an alumina ceramic head was used for the revision. In 17 cases there was marked damage or notching of the taper and a stainless steel head was used. The Morse taper was systematically cleaned and dried at the time of femoral head replacement.

The femoral granulomas (18 cases) were located in the following Gruen zones: Z1: 11, Z7: 1, Z8 and Z 14: 6 The mean diameter of granulomas was 38 mm on AP radiographs of the femur. Granuloma curettage with removal of polyethylene wear debris was performed as outlined above and the defects bone grafted using irradiated femoral head (Fig. 5.13).

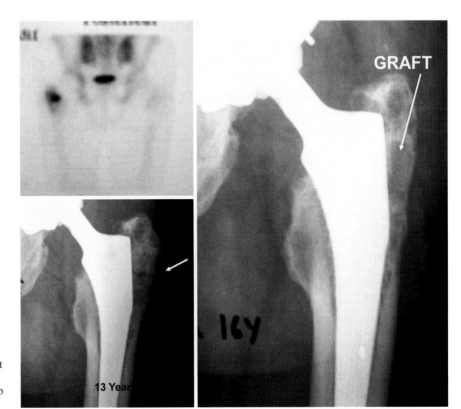

Fig. 5.12 Pain resulting from a crack in the greater trochanter induced by polyethylene wear debris (diagnosis confirmed by scintigraphy), curettage-graft of the lesion at 3-year follow-up (16-year follow-up for the Corail® stem)

Fig. 5.13 Proximal
osteolyses at 15-year
follow-up secondary to
severe polyethylene wear.
Grade 1 incorporation.
Curettage + graft and cup
revision at 7-year follow-up
(22-year follow-up for the
Corail® stem)

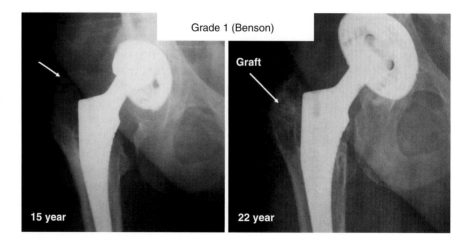

Acetabular Issues

Of the 115 cup revisions, the acetabular component
was loose in 98 cases. In the remaining 17 cases, there
was significant polyethylene wear, which was the reason for revision. All 115 sockets were revised with a
threaded Spirofit™ revision cup (Fig. 5.14). The cup is
HA coated and has equatorial spires to enhance initial
fixation. The bearing combinations were alumina on
poly in 83 cases, alumina on alumina in 15 cases and
metal on poly in 17 cases. The diameter of the revision
component was three sizes larger than that of the initial
cup to achieve intimate contact with the host bone. The
mean diameter was 58 mm. Bone grafts were used in
30 cases, but only to fill in cavitatory defects.

Results

Of the 115 cup revisions, 87 patients with radiographs were reviewed in 2009 at a mean follow-up of
9 years (range 7–11 years). Twenty three patients
had died demonstrating no prosthetic complication
and five were lost to follow-up. On the femoral side,
no femoral head fractures were observed and no separation of the alumina heads from the taper occurred.
Of the 18 cases of granuloma curettage and bone
grafting, all cases demonstrated cessation of the
osteolytic process and evidence of graft incorporation. Radiographic evaluation of the granulomas
was performed according to the Benson classification [1]:

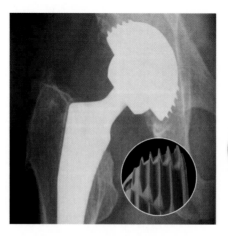

Fig. 5.14 The Spirofit™ cup
(Copyright DePuy-
International Limited)

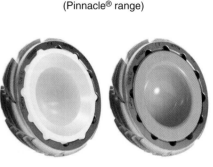

Spirofit™ acetabular cup
(Pinnacle® range)

Fig. 5.15 Proximal osteolysis at 15-year follow-up secondary to severe polyethylene wear. Grade 2 incorporation. Curettage + graft at 6-year follow-up and cup revision (21-year follow-up for the Corail® stem)

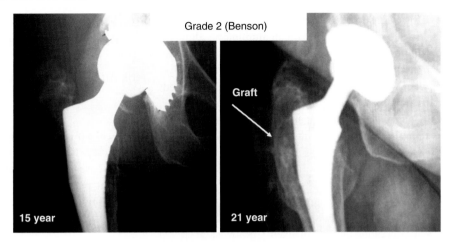

Grade 2 (Benson)

Graft

15 year

21 year

Grade 2 (4 cases) – disappearance of the border line, bone ingrowth and formation of trabecular (Fig. 5.15).

Grade 1 (14 cases) – graft incorporation with persisting border line.

Grade O (0 cases) – no radiographic change in the osteolysis and absence of trabecular bone.

At final follow-up, no stems had been revised; however, three cups had been re-revised, two for recurrent dislocation and one for early migration at 7 months induced by poor primary fixation of an undersized implant. The centre of rotation was d isplaced with a mean upward displacement of 3.2 mm secondary to the increase in diameter of the revision component compared to the primary.

Conclusions

The excellent long-term survival of the Corail® stem raises the problem of what to do when the acetabular cup is loose or worn and needs to be revised and the femoral stem is stable and ingrown. It has been shown in this chapter that retention of the Corail® stem in such a revision situation is a successful solution which lead to 100% stem survival at 9 years. In the presence of proximal osteolysis and granuloma formation around the stem, curettage and bone grafting has been shown to be a satisfactory approach both in terms of continuing stem survival (100% at 9 years) and reconstitution of the patient's bone stock. Furthermore, it would seem that this approach, combined with

revision of the bearing surface, halts the progression of the osteolytic process. Therefore, it is recommended that any stable Corail® stem should be left in situ, thus reducing the risks and potential complications inherent in stem revision. The concomitant problem of the potential damage to an existing Morse taper can be successfully addressed either by the use of a metallic head or a ceramic head with metallic sleeve. Undamaged tapers can be used with a standard ceramic head, but with caution.

The decision to proceed with revision for osteolysis should be made early in symptomatic patients, particularly in cases of impending fracture of the greater trochanter. Similarly, early revision should be undertaken prior to a total polyethylene liner failure. Therefore, these patients and the radiographic evolution of their osteolysis should be reviewed on a regular basis.

On the acetabular side, the use of threaded HA coated cups (Spirofit™) was a very effective solution in the management of acetabular revisions where the acetabular bone was of poor quality. The equatorial spires seem to be effective in revision surgery, since they offer better initial mechanical fixation than press-fit systems and provide good primary stability even in fragile or sclerotic bone. The fact that they are HA coated provides secondary fixation by means of bone consolidation, ingrowth and osseointegration.

On the acetabular side, curettage and bone grafting appeared sufficient to suppress osteoclastic activity. A similar result was obtained in other series in which curettage and bone grafting were combined with revision of the polyethylene liner [2–4].

However, in these cases, we recommend that the bearing couple is revised with an alumina-on-alumina or alumina-on-high density cross-linked polyethylene couple to prevent further generation of harmful polyethylene wear debris. The use of threaded HA coated cups has been successful and obviated the need for cemented fixation. The equatorial spires of the Spirofit™ system provided reliable intraoperative fixation in the living bone and promoted bone ingrowth in contact with HA coating.

Key Learning Points

> Preservation of a well-fixed Corail® stem is possible when revision surgery is performed for acetabular loosening or in the management of polyethylene wear-related granulomas.

> Curettage of granulomas combined with cancellous bone grafting provides long-term stem survival and reconstitution of bone stock.

> Change of the bearing couple helps reduce the amount of wear particles and decreases the risk of further osteolysis.

> On the acetabular side, threaded cup designs such as Spirofit™ seem to provide good fixation even if the bone is sclerotic or of poor quality.

References

1. Benson E, Christensen C, Monesmith E et al (2000) Particulate bone grafting of osteolytic femoral lesions around stable cementless stems. Clin Orthop Relat Res Dec(381): 58–67
2. Learmonth ID, Hussell JG, Grobler GP (1996) Unpredictable progression of osteolysis following cementless hip arthroplasty. Acta Orthop Scand 67:245–248
3. Maloney W, Jasty M, Harris WH (1990) Endosteal erosion in association with stable uncemented femoral components J Bone Joint Surg Am 72:1025–1034
4. Wanz Z, Dorr LD (1996) Natural history of femoral focal osteolysis with proximal ingrowth smooth stem implant. J Arthroplasty 11:718–725.

5.4 The Corail® Stem in Revision: Bigger Is Not Necessarily Better

Tarik Aït Si Selmi and Camdon Fary

The use of a primary fully hydroxyapatite (HA) coated, cementless stem in revision can be advocated in selected cases. This conservative approach has given consistent results in cases where the proximal bone loss was limited and where stable primary fixation was achievable.

Introduction

As a general rule, the use of a long stem in hip revision cases where the bone stock is compromised is a good solution in order to achieve adequate fixation for secondary integration to occur. However, long stems can be associated with complications such as femoral fracture, false route insertion, stress shielding and thigh pain. In some instances, the use of a standard primary stem can be considered in the revision situation when the available proximal bone stock allows adequate fixation. In the recent literature, there is a trend for experienced surgeons in high volume institutions to address revisions earlier in order to preserve bone stock and minimise complications [1]. Earlier intervention improves the outcome as a more conservative procedure can be used.

Indications

In aseptic loosening, good axial and rotational primary fixation can be consistently achieved with the Corail® stem. Appropriate indications include partial calcar erosion or limited proximal bone loss – for example isolated granuloma or contained metaphyseal bone defects (Paprosky grade I or II) as in Fig. 5.16a.

In well-fixed stems when revision is indicated for poor stem positioning (e.g. limb leg discrepancy, inappropriate off-set, dislocation due to inadequate anteversion, etc.) the use of a primary stem is the logical choice, if the femur is not damaged during the removal

Fig. 5.16 (**a**) Aseptic loosening with isolated distal granuloma. (**b**) Septic loosening after total hip arthroplasty (THA) removal (note the fractured greater trochanter)

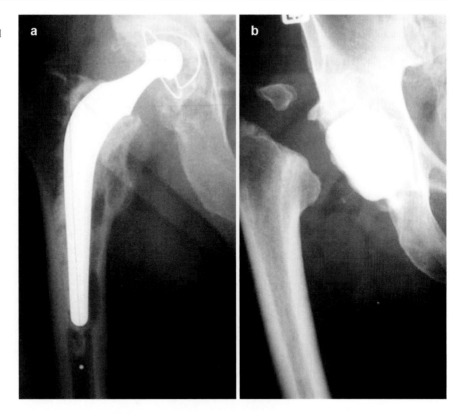

of the initial stem. Revision of a well-fixed femoral stem is also indicated when the taper is damaged or has an obsolete profile and when a metal sleeve is not available. Occasionally, the stem-neck junction of a well-fixed modular stem fails and requires revision.

In septic loosening, we believe that the smaller the implant the better, in order to limit as much as possible the effect of the implant as a foreign body and so to attempt to reduce the recurrence of the infection (Fig. 5.16b). The aim is to remove the necrotic bone, while retaining as much healthy bone as possible.

In proximal periprosthetic fractures with good bone quality, such as undetected intraoperative calcar cracks that extend distally as the patient's weight bears a standard primary cementless stem may be used for revision. This is provided that there is good fracture reduction and that the fracture is firmly fixed with appropriate cerclage wiring (Fig. 5.17a, b).

In acetabular loosening of very stiff or ankylosed total hip arthroplasty (THA), the removal of a well-fixed stem, with or without femoral osteotomy, is sometimes the safest and simplest way to reach the hip cavity and to obtain adequate exposure.

In some rare situations where the femoral canal is obstructed it may be impossible to use a long stem (Fig. 5.18a, b).

Technique

Templating is of crucial importance, especially in revision. The appropriate sized stem is selected and its final position is clearly identified using the lesser trochanter as a reference. The stem size is usually one size bigger than a primary stem, because of the lack of cancellous bone. When planning to use a primary stem in a revision situation one must be aware of the potential damage that can occur during the removal of a well-fixed stem and one must have a revision stem available as a backup.

The techniques of exposure and removal of the initial stem or components are not component-specific. In cemented stems, the entire cement mantle must be removed to optimise the bone-stem interface. If a window or a femoral osteotomy must be performed, or if a

Fig. 5.17 (**a**) A periprosthetic, displaced, oblique
fracture. (**b**) Femoral revision
with a Corail® stem. Three
wires have been used to
maintain the femoral
reduction prior to stem
insertion. The collar prevents
proximal migration of the
medial fragment

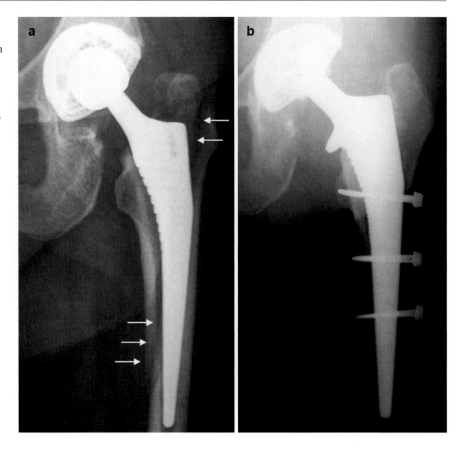

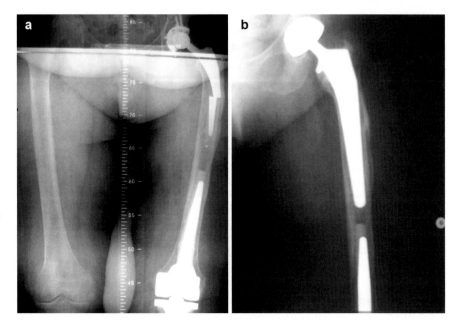

Fig. 5.18 (**a**) Loosened
fractured femoral stem above
a revision total knee
arthroplasty. The canal is
obstructed by the proximal
extension of the knee
prosthesis. (**b**) Revision with
the use of a standard Corail®
stem

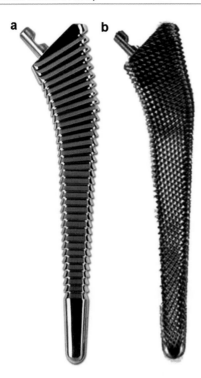

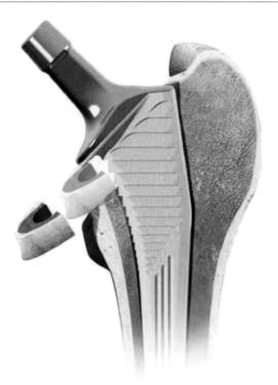

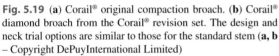

Fig. 5.19 (**a**) Corail® original compaction broach. (**b**) Corail® diamond broach from the Corail® revision set. The design and neck trial options are similar to those for the standard stem (**a, b** – Copyright DePuyInternational Limited)

Fig. 5.20 Insertion of a 'horseshoe' bone graft to restore a calcar defect. Once the graft has been put into place the final stem is inserted. The collar of the stem keeps the graft in position and applies a compressive load (Copyright DePuyInternational Limited)

canal perforation occurs, a longer stem must be used. In small proximal fractures or if a limited osteotomy is to be performed, a cerclage wire must be placed distal to the fracture or osteotomy prior to femoral broaching, to prevent further extension.

The standard Corail® femoral broaches are used as usual to compact any remaining cancellous bone, such as in the revision of a primary cementless stem (Fig. 5.19a). If a cemented stem has been removed or if the bone is sclerotic, the canal is prepared using the more aggressive 'diamond profile' broaches from the Corail® Revision set. These broaches have the same profile as the primary Corail® (Fig. 5.19b). In revision situations, fixation does not rely on the compacted bone, but rather on the intimate contact between the stem and cortical bone. These more aggressive broaches are used to create a superficial groove pattern on the inner cortical bone surface and to initiate bleeding from the sclerotic bone. Successive broaches are used in the usual manner to achieve axial and rotational stability.

A constant anteversion must be maintained during the process. It is important to only check rotational stability once axial stability has been achieved, as early rotation of the broach can destroy the vertical grooves created by the broaches and prevent the realisation of adequate stability. The appropriate position of the stem is checked from the lesser trochanter according to the preoperative planning. The broaches are used as a trial implant with the selected neck trial. When there is a small amount of calcar bone loss, a cortical bone graft may be used to restore the calcar height from the lesser trochanter (Fig. 5.20). When a bone graft is required, it is inserted with the final stem and fixed by impaction under the collar. Additional morsellised bone graft can be used to fill any gaps around the proximal part of the stem as required, but it is important to note that primary fixation must be achieved with the stem only.

Clinical Case Series

We reviewed 41 femoral revisions performed with a primary Corail® stem undertaken at our institution between 1989 and 2005. The mean age of the patients was 62 years (28–82). Indications for surgery were aseptic loosening (30 cases), deep sepsis (6 cases), femoral stem neck fracture (2 cases) and mechanical issues (3 cases). In 14 cases there was no bone loss as the femoral components were well fixed. In the cases with femoral loosening the bone loss was classified according to the Paprosky classification as type I in 12 cases, type II in 14 cases and type IIIA in 1 case. A collared implant was used were possible.

Results

Three cases had been lost to follow-up. The remaining 38 cases were followed up at a mean of 30.4 months (range 12–120). There had been no cases of repeat femoral revision. Two patients suffered from dislocation (4.8%), one patient from superficial infection (2.4%) and one patient underwent repeat acetabular revision due to loosening (2.4%). There were no cases of deep infection. All stems had osseointegrated and there was no evidence of stress shielding or subsidence. Harris Hip scores improved from 65/100 (9–100) preoperatively to 90/100 (50–100) at last follow-up. This was statistically significant ($p < 0.05$). There was no difference in functional score between groups based on extent of femoral bone loss.

Conclusion

The use of a standard Corail® stem for hip stem revision has previously been reported by Reikeras and Gunderson [3]. A primary Corail® stem was used in 18 femoral revisions out of 66 cases. All 18 cases were classified as Paprosky type I or II femoral defects. At a follow-up of 10–16 years no primary stems had been revised and there was no evidence of loosening or significant migration. Our case series [2] document clinical scores and overall results which are similar to other hip revision series in the literature. Bone integration was achieved in all cases and no failures were related to femoral loosening. We believe that a standard primary stem is a safe and reliable option in appropriate patients, provided that adequate primary fixation has been achieved using the recommended surgical technique. If primary fixation cannot be adequately achieved with a primary stem, a Corail® Revision Stem with its additional distal fixation is recommended.

Key Learning Points

> The use of a primary collared Corail® stem in revision can be recommended in Paprosky grade I and grade II cases as a conservative procedure.

> A precise surgical technique plus the use of revision broaches enable appropriate primary fixation to be achieved.

> In any case a revision stem must be available as a backup.

References

1. Ferney BJ, Blumenfeld TJ, Bargar WL (2007) Time to revision of primary THA is shorter for specialists than non specialists. Clin Orthop Relat Res 485:175–179
2. Pinaroli A, Lavoie F, Cartillier J-C et al (2009) Conservative femoral stem revision: avoiding therapeutic escalation J Arthroplasty 24(3):365–373
3. Reikeras O, Gunderson RB (2006) Excellent results with femoral revision surgery using an extensively hydroxyapatite-coated stem: 59 patients followed for 10–16 years. Acta Orthop 77(1):98–103

5.5 The Corail® Revision Stem (KAR™): When the Going Gets Tough

Tim Board and Alain Machenaud

This chapter details the development of the Corail® Revision Stem, the indications for use of the stem and the results in terms of the clinical and radiological outcome. The techniques required for removal of previous implants are discussed, as well as the specific techniques required for reconstruction of the femur with this stem system. An independent analysis of results is presented which shows a 97.3% survivorship at a maximum of 17 years for aseptic loosening in 161 Corail® Revision Stems. No evidence of radiological stress shielding was demonstrated and there was no clinical evidence of significant thigh pain. It is suggested that these results are as good, if not better, than those obtained with any other reconstruction system available.

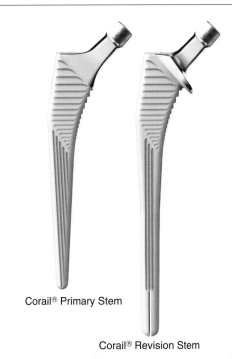

Corail® Primary Stem

Corail® Revision Stem

Fig. 5.21 The Corail® Revision Stem and the Corail® stem showing the increased length and distal slots in the revision stem (Copyright DePuyInternational Limited)

Development of the Corail® Revision Stem

This implant was developed in 1990 as an extension of the successful Corail® Hip range and was specifically designed for femoral revision cases. Originally, the stem was named the KAR™ stem, but in 2010 it was renamed the Corail® Revision Stem. The stem is indicated for use in revisions, where bone loss is such that supplementary fixation is required distal to the previous stem and where the use of a standard Corail® stem is not suitable. The stimulus for the development of this stem was the well-known problem of stress shielding of the femur that was seen with the traditional cylindrically shaped, long, porous coated stems (Wagner type) that relied on a distal press-fit for initial stability. These stems were bulky and manufactured from cobalt chrome alloy and hence were very stiff. Thigh pain was seen in as many as 31% of cases and concomitant stress shielding was frequently observed [4]. These drawbacks led to the development of a new prosthesis.

The Corail® Revision Stem (Fig. 5.21) shares the same morphologic characteristics as the Corail® collared stem and has the following features:

The endomedullary section has a Trapezoidal cross section and a bi-dimensional frontal and sagittal flare providing rotational stability and homogeneous metaphyseal load distribution. The macrostructure of the surface is made up of both horizontal grooves to minimise the potential for subsidence and vertical grooves, which further reinforce rotational stability and increase the bone-implant contact area by 15%.

The extramedullary section is available in two offset options: standard and high offset. Both stems are collared and have the same cervico-diaphyseal (CCD) angle of 135°. The high offset stem provides up to 7 mm of lateralisation depending on stem size.

As in the Corail® stem, the Corail® Revision Stem is manufactured from titanium alloy (Ti6Al4V) and the hydroxyapatite (HA) coating is plasma sprayed with a total thickness of 150 μm.

Each stem is 40 mm longer in the diaphyseal section than the equivalent Corail® counterpart.

The distal stem features two asymmetrical distal slots: the sagittal one is shorter than the coronal one. The sagittal slot increases the elasticity of the stem and helps the stem adapt to the varus femoral curves. The coronal slot has been designed to adapt to the

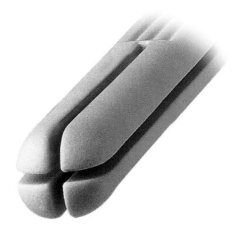

Fig. 5.22 Close-up image of the distal slots (in both planes) (Copyright DePuyInternational Limited)

anteroposterior femoral curve. The slots increase the stem flexibility and therefore increase the proximal loading of the femur to prevent stress shielding (Fig. 5.22).

The Corail® Revision Stem is available in sizes 10, 11, 12, 13, 14, 15, 16, 18 and 20.

The Articul/eze® Mini-Taper (AMT) and neck geometry exactly mirror the standard Corail® stem and give a range of motion of 148° when paired with a Pinnacle™ cup.

Indications for Use of the Corail® Revision Stem

Classification systems of femoral bone loss such as the Paprosky system can be useful as a guide to implant choice [5]. However, it must be emphasised that the final choice of implant must be based on the ability of that implant to achieve primary stability whilst minimising the risk of postoperative complications such as fracture. For the revision of type I deficiencies, where there has been minimal loss of metaphyseal bone and the diaphysis is intact, a standard Corail® stem can often be used. However, if there is uncertainty about the fixation achieved, a Corail® Revision Stem should be used. Consideration should be given to using a collared implant in all revision situations to act as a secondary preventer of subsidence during the ingrowth period. In type II deficiencies where there has been marked loss of metaphyseal cancellous bone, but the diaphyseal bone is intact, the Corail® Revision Stem can be used with great reliability. In type III femurs, where the metaphysis is severely damaged and offers little support, the Corail® Revision Stem can still be used if the diaphyseal bone offers adequate support (typically in type IIIA). In type III femurs, when the diaphysis is also damaged (i.e. type IIIB) it may still be

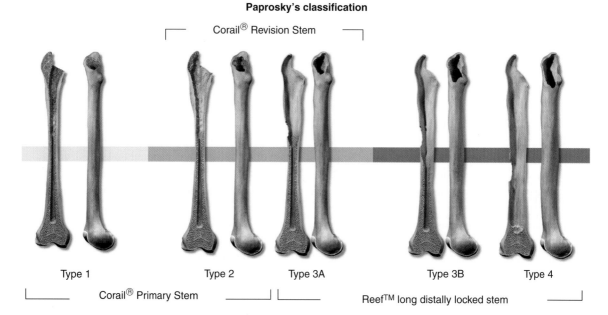

Fig. 5.23 General guide for implant choice in revision based on the Paprosky classification of bone loss (Copyright DePuyInternational Limited)

possible to achieve satisfactory stability with the Corail® Revision Stem, however, if implant stability is tenuous then consideration should be given to using the Reef® distally locked stem (Fig. 5.23).

Surgical Approach and Extraction of Implants

The most taxing part of revision hip surgery is often the safe exposure of the hip and the removal of previous implants and cement, if present. Avoidance of intra-operative complications such as femoral perforation or fracture, bone loss and nerve injury is of paramount importance. There are many surgical approaches to the hip that are appropriate for revision surgery; however, it is beyond the scope of this book to fully discuss these. The authors' preferred approaches are

the posterior approach (TB) and the anterolateral approach (AM). A list of tips and tricks for exposure and component removal are given in Table 5.1.

In most cases the old implant and cement can be removed from the top and this would be the first choice in maintaining the 'conservative revision' philosophy. Occasionally, however, it proves impossible to remove implants by this method and a femoral osteotomy is needed. The most common form is the extended trochanteric osteotomy (ETO). This is a well-recognised osteotomy that is undertaken by first making a sagittal saw cut in the posterior aspect of the femur to the tip of the previous stem. A drill and multihole guide is then used to perforate the anterior cortex opposite the posterior cut (Fig. 5.24). A drill is also used to connect the posterior cut to the anterior line distally. Osteotomes are then used from a posterior direction to complete the osteotomy and elevate the femoral flap with its

Table 5.1 A 'Box of Tricks' listing common problems in revision surgery and suggested solutions

Problem	Tip
Concern over sciatic nerve	Always attempt to identify nerve during posterior approach and pass nerve tape for later referencing. If nerve cannot be identified stick to orthopaedic principles of "get on bone and stay on bone" whilst entering joint posteriorly
Possible femoral perforation	If it is considered that a perforation may have occurred then femur in that area must be exposed to confirm
Definite femoral perforation/ crack	Cerclage wiring should ALWAYS be undertaken distal to a perforation or crack in the femur *If you think about – DO IT!*
Initial dissection (finding the fascia)	If fascial layer difficult to identify extend incision distally into virgin tissue to indentify fascia and then trace proximally
Dislocation of implants	When using a posterior approach ALWAYS release the Gluteus Maximus tendon from the femur and perform a full capsular release before attempting to dislocate the femur to reduce the chance of periprosthetic fracture
Difficult cement plug extraction	A 2 cm wide cortical fenestration can made on the anterior aspect of the femur. Its lower limit should be located 1.5 cm below the cement plug and its length should be identical to that of the cement plug. Chisels are used to release the visible part of the cement plug then a short screw is inserted for rotational and upward to downward mobilisation of the cement plug in order to bring it up in its entirety for removal through the prepared window. The window is closed and secured with cerclage wiring
Cement plug extraction with reamers	If using a reamer for cement plug extraction, using a cannulated femoral phantom inserted into the femur to guide the initial drill hole helps to maintain the correct alignment of the subsequent reamers
Standard cement extraction	Use of the Moreland™ osteotomes are recommended to remove the proximal, easily visible cement. An ultrasonic cement removing device can then be used to perforate through the cement plug distally to allow access for the "back scratching" Moreland instruments to remove the final cement
Removing an well fixed uncemented stem	If removal of the implant without osteotomy has not been accomplished a longitudinal split can be made in the posterior femur with an oscillating saw. An osteotome is introduced into the superior end of the cut to open the osteomty slightly. This will often allow the implant to be removed without the need to resort to a full ETO

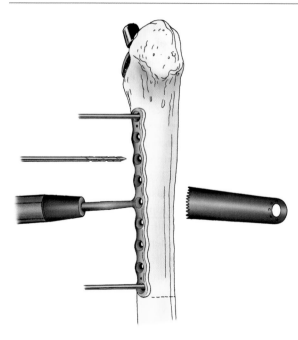

Fig. 5.24 Schematic showing drill template used to create the anterior osteotomy during an extended trochanteric osteotomy (Copyright DePuyInternational Limited)

aspect of the femur to cause the bone to bleed. This is an integral part of the technique as it promotes bony integration. Broaches of increasing size are used until the alignment, stability and predicted height of the broach is similar to that estimated from preoperative templating using either digital software systems or acetate templates. The most important factor is to achieve good axial and rotation stability of the broach. The broach is then removed and the trial prosthesis is inserted to the same level. The appropriate neck is selected (standard or high offset) and the hip reduced. If satisfactory stability and length are achieved, then the real implant may be inserted. As with the primary stem, it should be possible to insert the implant by hand until the last 3–4 cm. A mallet is then used to seat the implant to the desired height. Often the collar will not be supported by the calcar due to calcar loss. This has not been a problem in our experience and no cases of subsidence have been observed secondary to this. The ARTRO Group advocates the use of a cortical calcar 'horseshoe' graft to fill this defect, but this is not a prerequisite and primary stability should be achieved prior to insertion of such a graft.

attached vastus lateralis muscle anteriorly, exposing the contents of the proximal femur. The osteotomy is closed by means of cerclage wiring after removal of the implants. Closure can be either before or after insertion of the new stem, depending on stem choice.

Corail® Revision Stem Technique

The technique of insertion of the Corail® Revision Stem is similar to that of the Corail® stem in the primary situation, but with some important differences. Following removal of the previous implant and all cement and debris, the diaphysis is reamed with the hand reamers. All sizes of Corail® Revision Stem are 11 mm in diameter distally and therefore the canal must be reamed to a minimum 11 mm. It is often necessary to over-ream by 1 or 2 mm to ensure free passage of the trial. Broaches of increasing size are then used to open out the metaphysis. The broaches for the revision system are diamond tooth cutting broaches unlike those in the primary system, which are compaction broaches. The cutting broaches are designed to roughen the sclerotic cortical surface of the inner

Supplementary Bone Graft

Due to the rectangular cross section of the stem, there are often areas of non-contact with the stem proximally after final insertion. It is possible to fill these spaces by impacting cancellous bone graft from fresh frozen femoral head, or another source. It should be emphasised that adequate stability of the stem should be achieved before insertion of the graft, which only provides supplementary stability and is not a prerequisite.

Independent Analysis of the Outcome of the Corail® Revision Stem

The ARTRO Group began to implant the stem in 1990 and since then over 16,000 stems have been implanted worldwide (data obtained from DePuy). In 2008, one of the authors (TB) was invited to conduct an independent review of the series of Corail® Revision Stems implanted by the ARTRO Group. The review was undertaken between 2008 and 2009 and consisted of a case note review of all 161 cases and analysis of all available radiographs.

Patients

Between 1991 and 2007, 161 revisions were done by the ARTRO Group using the Corail® Revision Stem. The mean age at revision was 70 years (range 41–95). There were 74 men and 87 women. The reason for revision was aseptic loosening and osteolysis in 134 patients, periprosthetic fracture [12], implant fracture [8], infection [6] and polyethylene wear [1]. Of the femoral stems revised, 30 were uncemented and 131 were cemented. The revision procedure was the first revision in 139 patients, the second revision in 21 and the third revision in one patient. All stems were revised with the Corail® Revision Stem. Of the acetabular implants used 125 were uncemented, 2 were cemented, 5 were cages or support rings and 29 sockets were not revised or just underwent liner exchange. Ninety-one patients received a 28 mm femoral head, 68 had 32 mm heads and 2 patients had a 36 mm. Bone grafting of the metaphyseal area was performed in 120 cases and in 59 cases a horseshoe calcar graft was used. Intraoperatively, minor cracks occurred in the greater trochanter in 13 cases, calcar cracks in 10 cases, 2 of which were wired. Femoral fractures occurred in 20 patients, 11 of which required fixation.

Follow-Up

Forty-four patients died with stem in place before the final follow-up period. Follow-up analysis was either by clinic visit, postal questionnaire or telephone contact. Nine patients were lost to follow-up. At the last follow-up period, three stems had been revised for aseptic loosening and two for deep infection. This left a residual group of 103 stems. The mean follow-up period was 8 years (range 1–17.4 years). Kaplan-Meier survivorship analysis showed the survivorship for aseptic loosening to be 97.3% (95% confidence interval 53–100) at 17.4 years (Fig. 5.25).

The overall survivorship with revision for any reason as the endpoint was 94.7% (95% CI 34–100) at 17.4 years. The three cases that were revised for aseptic

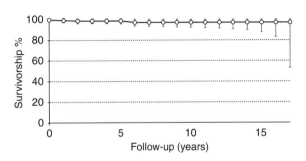

Fig. 5.25 Kaplan-Meier survival curve for aseptic loosening of the Corail® Revision Stem at 17.4 years

loosening merit further discussion. In two of these cases large volumes of ox bone graft were used to support the stem proximally and no evidence of ingrowth was seen. In one of these cases, the stem was probably undersized due to insufficient distal reaming and therefore had little proximal support and the combination of the ox bone graft not incorporating led to the failure of the stem. The third case again failed due to under sizing of the stem. The stem used in this case was a size 16, which was the largest stem available at the time (stem sizes up to 20 are currently available). The femur was described in the operation note as a 'drain pipe' femur and the surgeon was concerned about the stability of the fixation but the Reef® stem was not available at this time. The lessons to be learnt from these cases are:

1. The stem should be adequately sized with combined proximal and distal contact with the femur generating 3-point fixation.
2. Bone graft should not be relied upon for primary stability of the stem.

Radiographic Remodelling

Sixty eight cases had complete radiographic series and were analysed. Ninety six percent of cases showed proximal ingrowth and only one stem showed no distal ingrowth. Non-progressive radiolucent lines were observed in 10 stems, all in zones 1, 2, 7 and 8. No progressive radiolucent lines were observed. In order to analyse proximal remodelling and distal hypertrophy the cortical thicknesses and canal diameter were measured at two fixed levels as shown in Fig. 5.26.

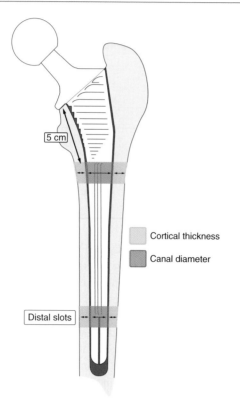

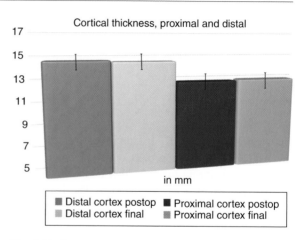

Fig. 5.26 The figure shows the technique for measuring cortical thickness and canal diameter at two fixed points along the stem (Copyright DePuyInternational Limited)

Fig. 5.27 Graph showing no significant change in proximal or distal cortical dimensions between initial postoperative and final follow-up radiographs

stems was 0.4 mm. Seven stems subsided more than 2 mm, all of which subsequently became ingrown. Remodelling of balloon defects adjacent to the stem was often seen (Fig. 5.28a, b). Significant resorption of the horseshoe calcar graft was seen in 52% of cases and partial resorption in a further 38%.

Functional Outcome

Statistical analysis of this data showed no evidence of distal cortical hypertrophy and no evidence of proximal stress shielding (Fig. 5.27). Mean subsidence of

The mean preoperative Harris Hip Score was 33.3 and the mean score at final follow-up was 81.8. No patients complained of significant thigh pain. In terms

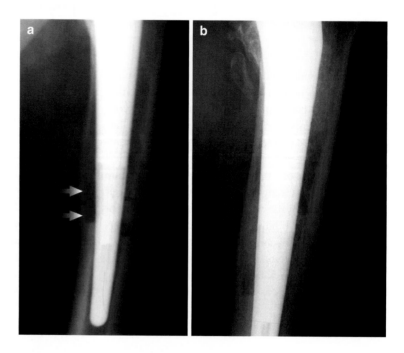

Fig. 5.28 (a) Immediate postoperative radiograph showing balloon defect medial to midpoint of stem. (b) Radiograph taken 4 years postoperatively showing filling in of the defect

of postoperative complications, dislocation occurred in 14 patients (8.7%), thrombosis in 5 (3%), femoral fracture was observed in 8 patients, only 2 of which required fixation. Sciatic nerve injury was observed in one patient.

Comparison with Other Studies

The independent analysis described above highlights the favourable results of the Corail® Revision Stem in comparison to the survivorship of other revision stems including cemented stems, cemented stems with impaction bone grafting and other uncemented stems [2–4]. The independent analysis also confirms the previously presented success of this stem as published in a report by the designing surgeons [7]. Indeed it could be argued that the results of the Corail® Revision Stem are better from a combined functional, bone preserving and survivorship point of view than any other stem currently available.

Reikerås and Gunderson [6] reported on 60 revisions performed with the Corail® (18 stems) or Corail® Revision Stem (42 stems) followed up for 10–16 years and showed a survivorship of 98.3% with revision for any reason as an endpoint. They also observed a very low incidence of distal cortical hypertrophy and proximal bone loss and surmised that this was due to the

very low net transfer of stress proximally to distally by the stem, therefore, allowing a somewhat physiological loading of the proximal femur. In agreement with the independent analysis detailed above, they also commented that no patient suffered from significant thigh pain.

Data from Wrightington Hospital, UK [1] showed no re-revisions in a consecutive series of 67 stems followed for a minimum of 12 months. The mean age was 67 years (range 36–83) and the indications for surgery were loosening or fracture. Four intraoperative calcar cracks and two canal perforations were observed, all occurring prior to stem insertion and treated with cerclage wiring. At follow-up there was one case of subsidence of 1 cm, which occurred following a fall resulting in a periprosthetic fracture. There were no dislocations, no infections and no cases of thigh pain. The functional outcome as measured by the Oxford Hip Score improved from 38 preoperatively to 24 at follow-up.

Conclusions

Multiple studies have demonstrated excellent medium-term results for the Corail® Revision Stem. Distal cortical hypertrophy and thigh pain do not occur with this stem. Proximal bone remodelling is therefore possible

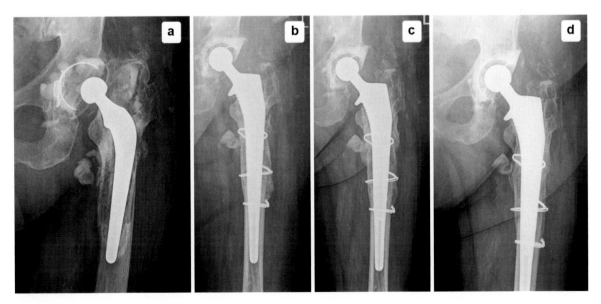

Fig. 5.29 (**a**) Preoperative radiograph showing severe proximal osteolysis and subsidence of a Charnley stem with periprosthetic fracture. (**b**) Postoperative radiograph of a Corail® Revision Stem with multiple cerclage wires. The socket has been revised with impaction bone grafting and a cemented socket. (**c**) Radiograph at 3 months postoperative showing remodelling of the proximal femur, especially adjacent to the lateral side of the proximal cerclage wire. (**d**) Same as (**c**), but at 18 months

as the stresses imparted on the proximal femur are relatively physiologic (Fig. 5.29a–d). The reasons for the success of this stem are thought to be twofold. Firstly, the stem is extensively HA coated which encourages bony ingrowth. Secondly, the stem is manufactured from titanium alloy and has crossed slots distally. These features allow the stem to be relatively flexible, thereby allowing semi-physiologic loading of the proximal femur. The flexibility of the stem also encourages stability in a wide range of situations. When the proximal bone is less supportive, more initial stress is taken distally until ingrowth occurs proximally. This allows greater proximal stress transfer. Where support is good proximally, then reliable bone ingrowth and early proximal stress transfer occur.

Key Learning Points

> The Corail® Revision Stem is suitable for a broad range of revision indications.

> Survivorship was 97.3% at 17.4 years.

> No evidence of distal hypertrophy or proximal resorption was observed.

> There were no cases of significant thigh pain.

> The revision procedure was simple to perform, fast and reliable.

References

1. Board TN, Gambhir AK, Hoad-Reddick A et al (2008) Uncemented Stems in Revision Hip Arthroplasty. Presented at the British Hip Society meeting, Norwich, 2008
2. Crawford SA, Siney PD, Wroblewski BM (2000) Revision of failed total hip arthroplasty with a proximal femoral modular cemented stem. J Bone Joint Surg Br 82(5):684–688
3. Halliday BR, English HW, Timperley AJ et al (2003) Femoral impaction grafting with cement in revision total hip replacement. Evolution of the technique and results. J Bone Joint Surg Br 85(6):809–817
4. Paprosky WG, Greidanus NV, Antoniou J (1999) Minimum 10-year-results of extensively porous-coated stems in revision hip arthroplasty. Clin Orthop Relat Res Dec(369):230–242
5. Paprosky WG, Burnett RS (2002) Assessment and classification of bone stock deficiency in revision total hip arthroplasty. Am J Orthop 31(8):459–464
6. Reikerås O, Gunderson RB (2006) Excellent results with femoral revision surgery using an extensively hydroxyapatite-coated stem: 59 patients followed for 10–16 years. Acta Orthop 77(1):98–103
7. Vidalain JP (1998) HA coated long stems in revision arthroplasty. Retrospective analysis of a continuous series of 109 KAR™ prostheses. Paper presented at the European Hip Society meeting. Beaune, 1998

5.6 The Reef® Stem: Anchorage in the Deep

Jean-Charles Rollier and Rémi Philippot

Revision hip arthroplasty in the reconstruction of major deficiencies of the metaphyseal-diaphyseal region remains challenging. The Reef® is a long, fully Hydroxyapatite (HA) coated, distally interlocked modular femoral stem specifically intended for use in the reconstruction of stages III and IV femoral defects according to the Paprosky classification. Stem interlocking ensures stable primary distal fixation. The full HA coating encourages osseointegration throughout the length of the stem, hence allowing stress distribution over a wide area and potential protection from proximal stress shielding. A thorough preoperative planning combined with a well-codified surgical procedure ensures satisfactory mid- and long-term results in this challenging surgery, as demonstrated in our clinical series of more than 100 patients.

Introduction

When managing severe femoral bone loss in revision total hip arthroplasty (THA), the surgeon usually faces two challenging problems: the first one is of mechanical origin and consists in achieving the long-term fixation of the femoral stem in thin or even absent metaphyseal cortices. The second and more recent challenge is of biological origin and consists in promoting bone regeneration in the metaphyseal region.

Several different techniques to address this problem have been suggested with largely disappointing clinical results. In particular: cemented implants [5, 13], reconstructing techniques using allografts [2, 9], uncemented implants with or without HA coating [12, 15, 17].

In this context, the ARTRO Group developed a femoral revision implant to complete the Corail® system, which is perfectly suited to situations where proper fixation of the proximal metaphyseal region of the implant is not possible and where distal diaphyseal fixation is essential. The implant is the Reef® stem, which has been used since 1995 by the whole ARTRO Group. The aim of the chapter is to report the experience of the group in treating these high-grade femoral revisions and to point out the key elements in this type of surgery.

History

In the management of moderate bone defects (grades I, II, III A according to Paprosky) use of the standard and long revision Corail® stems is a suitable treatment option. However, extensive defects (grades III B, III C and IV) require the use of a different implant design with distal interlocking, a greater choice of stem length and diameter and full HA coating to further improve osseointegration and enhance reconstruction of damaged regions. This is the Reef® concept.

Modularity

The modularity of this type of implant allows the surgeon to reconstruct the femur even when the level of bone destruction is somewhat greater than was apparent from preoperative imaging, a situation not uncommonly encountered in complex revisions. Modularity between stem and trochanteric component allows adjustment of anteversion and gives the opportunity to add an optional lateral trochanteric wing.

Distal Interlocking

Press-fit stabilisation of a conical stem is limited: the anatomical shape of lower femoral diaphysis makes it impossible. Distal interlocking is the only reliable option in this part of the femur. Vives [17] invented the concept of multiple screw distal locking in a smooth femoral stem, although he suggested that the implant should be removed and replaced with a shorter stem once reconstruction of the upper femur had been achieved. His procedure has rarely been used in practice, but the mechanical effectiveness of distal locking has been proven.

Full HA Coating

Like all implants from the Corail® range, full HA coating encourages secondary biological fixation through

Fig. 5.30 The modularity, distal interlocking Reef® system (Copyright DePuy-International Limited)

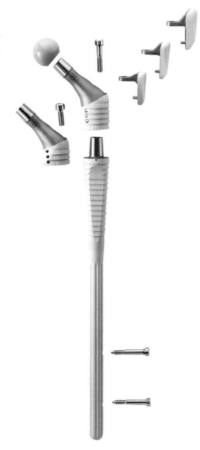

the osseointegration process where bone enables it. It promotes bone healing and reconstruction of the upper metaphysis under loading conditions.

The Reef® stem was created in 1995. It is a distally interlocked modular femoral reconstruction prosthesis with full HA coating. It is composed of the following parts (Fig. 5.30):

1. A monobloc metaphyseal-diaphyseal stem made of two parts:

    (a) A conical metaphyseal section featuring horizontal grooves.
    (b) A cylindrical diaphyseal section, bowed to adapt the anatomical femoral curve, and featuring vertical macrostructures. It is provided with 1–3 distal locking holes depending on the stem length. The stem is available in a comprehensive range of sizes: from 125 to 275 mm in length and from 10 to 20 mm in diameter.

2. A trochanteric component connected to the stem via a morse taper secured by means of a locking

screw, once the desired anteversion has been chosen. It features a series of medial cerclage cable holes for the fixation of the trochanteric osteotomy. It is available in two heights, 25 and 35 mm, with or without collar.

3. An optional trochanteric lateral wing is available in three different sizes and is used for stabilisation (and lateralisation) of the greater trochanter or of the femoral osteotomy itself.

Main Indications

The Reef® stem is indicated for the treatment of major femoral defects for which a primary Corail® stem or a revision KAR™ stem cannot provide adequate stabilisation.

Extensive loosening of types III and IV according to Paprosky are the main indications for distal locking fixation. If there is sepsis, a large femoral osteotomy may be performed to allow efficient curettage.

Periprosthetic fractures have an increasing incidence. The use of a Reef® implant is indicated in cases of an unstable femoral stem and periprosthetic fracture, either around the stem or distal to it (Vancouver types B2, B3 and C).

Femoral resection due to tumour treatment is a rare indication but the Reef® stem may act as a reconstruction prosthesis due to its distal stabilisation in the healthy part of the femur.

Preoperative Planning (Fig. 5.31)

Preoperative planning is an integral part of the surgical strategy and allows the following to be determined:

1. The level of the femoral osteotomy to achieve removal of the failed stem and, if necessary, the surrounding cement.
2. The level of the Reef® stem implantation. This is done by measuring the distance between the reference mark corresponding to the metaphyseal-diaphyseal junction of the stem, indicated on the template, and the lower border of the osteotomy.
3. The dimensions of the different components necessary for the reconstruction in terms of:

    (a) Diameter to achieve optimum filling of the healthy femoral diaphysis.

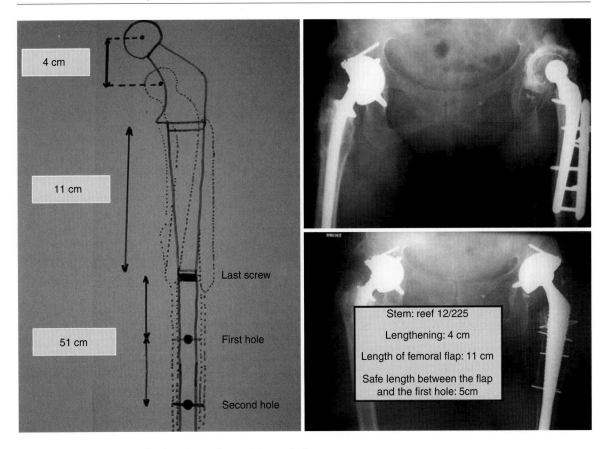

Fig. 5.31 Preoperative planning is an integral part of the surgical strategy

(b) Length to ensure reliable anchorage in the diaphyseal or lower diaphyseal-metaphyseal region knowing that the most proximal locking hole should be positioned at least 5 cm below the lower border of the osteotomy.

(c) Trochanteric component type, available in two different heights and various neck lengths, to restore the proper leg length.

4. The required number of locking screws, their length and position.

Surgical Technique

Surgical Approach

Regardless of the initial approach selected (posterior, lateral or anterior), the most effective surgical technique is an extensive Wagner transfemoral osteotomy (otherwise known as an extended trochanteric osteotomy) approach that includes the greater trochanter. This approach prevents further damage to an already weak femur by allowing straightforward removal of components and cement. Care should be taken to preserve vascularity and muscle insertions of the osteotomy flap. At the distal end, the external cortex is cut with a saw around the lateral hemicircumference and an osteotomy is made at the level determined during preoperative planning. Posterior osteotomy is performed on the linea aspera using the oscillating saw. The anterior border of the flap is prepared by drilling a series of holes guided by the osteoclasis drilling plate and passing through the quadratus femoris muscle. The drilling template should be positioned anteriorly directly opposite, and parallel to, the linea aspera. It is held in place with two drill sleeves to ensure the perforations are perfectly aligned. The anterior osteoclasis completes the osteotomy allowing the femur to open like a book.

Implant Removal

The failed implant, the surrounding cement, fibrous membrane and the debris may be removed rapidly and thoroughly without risk of a breach in the cortex and subsequent propogation of a fracture distally. The intramedullary cavity is cleared and curetted down to healthy bone and eventually reamed. The accurate assessment of defects can now be established. The examination should include the condition of the cortical walls, the actual loss of bone stock and any need for grafting.

Trial Stems

Once the distal diaphysis has been reamed, a trial stem of the same diameter or smaller by 1 mm is chosen. Two criteria must be determined:

1. The depth of insertion (the distance between the marker groove on the trial stem acting as a landmark for the metaphyseal-diaphyseal junction and the lower border of the osteotomy). The 'D' distance should be measured with a ruler.
2. The rotational and axial primary stability of the trial stem should be assessed prior to locking.

The trial stem is assembled on the stem inserter and introduced into the femoral canal to the depth estimated during templating. The anterior surface is marked 'ANT' to facilitate the orientation with respect to the femoral curvature. The junction between the cylindrical distal portion and flared metaphyseal part of the stem is shown on the trial stem by a marker groove. The trial stem should be stable within the femoral canal. With the trial stem in place, the stem inserter is then removed.

The chosen trial trochanteric component is attached. The anteversion of the trochanteric component is determined according to the stability and potential risk of impingement. Reference marks on the anterior and posterior faces of the trial stem help to find the version of the trochanteric component that best matches the patient's anatomy. When the trochanteric component is set to the required version, the locking screw may be tightened. A trial reduction is carried out once the trial head has been applied. Mobility and stability assessments are then performed. A trial trochanteric wing may be selected to enhance stabilisation of the greater trochanter or of the femoral osteotomy flap. At this stage, anteversion, height of the trochanteric component and neck length can be further adjusted.

Definitive Stem

Once the components to be used have been selected, the definitive stem is prepared for insertion.

(a) Targeting Device
The definitive stem, of the same length and diameter as the trial stem, is attached to the appropriate targeting device (right or left). A test is performed on the table to check the curvature and alignment of the locking holes with the final implant.

(b) Implantation of the Metaphyseal-Diaphyseal Stem
The stem may be inserted either directly attached to the targeting device or by using the stem inserter. It is impacted to the level which was determined during preoperative planning and which was confirmed with the trial stem. To ensure that the definitive stem is impacted to the same level as the trial implant, the distance between the proximal end of the vertical grooves of the metaphyseal-diaphyseal stem and the horizontal osteotomy should be measured again with a ruler.

(c) Distal Locking
The stem inserter is removed. The appropriate targeting device (right or left) is then inserted onto the taper and firmly locked into place. Drill bushes placed into the holes of the targeting device are designed to guide the trocar and drill bits used to prepare the femoral cortices for the locking screws. For enhanced precision, the proximal screw is inserted first. The most proximal locking hole should be located at least 5 cm from the lower border of the osteotomy. The trocar is passed through the 5 mm drill guide and lightly tapped to indent the cortex. It is then removed and replaced by the 5 mm drill bit, which is used to drill the lateral cortex only. The 3.5 mm drill guide is then passed through the 5 mm drill guide and the 3.5 mm drill bit used to drill the inner cortex.

The most appropriate screw length is determined by means of the screw length gauge. The screw is locked by means of the screwdriver, which is left in situ for additional bracing of the targeting device and to allow precision drilling of the distal screw holes. All screw holes should be used. When locking has been completed, the screw driver and targeting device is removed.

(d) Placement of the Trochanteric Component

The definitive trochanteric component, with or without collar, is then firmly impacted ensuring that the version is set to the value established during preoperative planning. It is highly recommended to use the specific impacter to ensure a reliable morse taper.

(e) Trochanteric Wing

Tightening of the upper screw allows the trochanteric component to be connected to the stem with the selected anteversion and also allows the definitive lateral wing to be attached, if necessary.

(f) Femoral Head Impaction

The selected prosthetic femoral head is impacted onto the morse taper in the standard fashion. A final reduction is then performed.

(g) Final Reconstruction

Reconstruction of the femoral shaft around the stem can be undertaken by putting the pieces of the cortical jigsaw together again, the lateral trochanteric osteotomy being the key element. Reattachment of the osteotomy flap is achieved by means of cerclage cables.

Postoperative Management

As a rule, weight bearing is dependent upon the healing rate of the femoral osteotomy. Patients are prevented from full weight bearing until there is radiographic evidence of osseointegration in the healthy part of the stem and of healing of the osteotomy and/or of the proximal femur defects up to the lower limit of the conical metaphyeal-trochanteric section. This is usually achieved after a mean period of 45–90 days. Partial protected weight bearing with crutches is then allowed.

Results of Our Clinical Study of 109 Patients

In order to assess the performance of the Reef® stem we conducted a prospective, continuous, multicentre study (four centres). Patients who received a Reef® stem between April 1999 and April 2005 were enrolled in the study. All patients had a femoral osteotomy and the preoperative planning and implantation technique were as described above.

Method

This was a prospective study during which patients were clinically and radiographically evaluated at 6 weeks, 3 months, 6 months and each year. All patients were assessed during the inclusion phase (preoperative) and at last follow-up, according to the Postel-Merle d'Aubigné and Harris scores. Radiographic examination was based on AP pelvic radiographs and AP and lateral hip and femur radiographs. These were updated at each review. During the inclusion phase, femoral loosening was noted and classified according to the Vivès classification modified by the SOFCOT in 1999. During the follow-up period, the bone-prosthesis interface was analysed according to the Gruen zones by studying radiolucencies, reactive lines, bone pedestals, osteolyses and reactions at the level of the calcar, in order to assess the quality of diaphyseal osseintegration and potential metaphyseal reconstruction. Heterotopic ossifications were classified according to Brooker. Femoral stem subsidence was evaluated and only subsidence over 5 mm were considered as significant. Radiographic follow-up was used to analyse femoral osteotomy healing and the occurrence of femoral stress shielding.

Clinical and Radiological Results

During the inclusion period, 109 patients of mean age at surgery 72.1 ± 12.5 years were enrolled. There were 66 females and 43 males. The mean follow-up period was 5 years (range 1–14). At last follow-up, 19 patients had died.

The indications for revision of the femoral component included aseptic loosening in 52 cases, periprosthetic fracture leading to loosening in 25 cases, revision of the femoral component for septic complication in 9 cases, revision of the fractured femoral component in 6 cases, femoral revision associated with correction of malunion in 16 cases and one case of stem revision for recurrent dislocation of a screwed Bousquet stem with difficult removal of the trochanteric component thus requiring a femoral osteotomy for extraction.

The preoperative femoral lesions in our series were graded preoperatively as follows: 16 stage 0, 15 stage I, 17 stage II, 42 stage III and 18 stage IV loosenings. They were re-graded intraoperatively and 6 stage II became stage III and 10 stage III became stage IV.

Revision of both stem and socket was undertaken in 35 cases and only involved the femoral side in 74 cases. The length of the femoral osteotomy performed during the surgical approach averaged 13.0 ± 4.6 cm. The clinical Harris Hip Score increased from 39 ± 12 to 83 ± 15 at last follow-up. The PMA score increased from 6.4 ± 3.4 to 14.7 ± 2.3 at last follow-up.

Intraoperative complications included: one case of sciatic nerve palsy which fully recovered within 1 year and three cases of femoral fracture demonstrating good healing at last follow-up.

Early or late postoperative complications included:

Four patients with repeated episodes of prosthetic instability

Six patients with recurrent sepsis, one of whom required stem removal

One non-displaced fracture of the femoral osteotomy secondary to a fall 6 months after surgery and managed with weight bearing

Three isolated revisions of the acetabular component

Two patients had their femoral stem unlocked after complaining of pain at the level of the screws which were removed (the implant was stable at last follow-up)

Two patients reported stem fracture managed with femoral implant replacement in the first case and plate osteosynthesis in the second case (both implants were stable at last follow-up).

The survival rate of the femoral implant at 8 years according to an actuarial method and using implant revision for aseptic loosening as the endpoint was 95.8% ± 0.03 (95% CI). This is shown in Fig. 5.32.

The radiographic outcome at last follow-up showed no significant subsidence and healing of the femoral osteotomy around the stem occurred in all cases except one. In this one case, fracture of the femoral osteotomy resulted in non-union. There were also three cases of greater trochanter non-union. At last follow-up there were non-progressive radiolucencies in Gruen zones 1, 2, 7 and 14 in 7 patients and 10 cases of severe calcar and proximal metaphysis atrophy. There was no evidence of stress shielding or equivalent, thus showing good secondary osseointegration of the implant (Fig. 5.33). There were no screw failures. Ossifications were graded as follows: 2 grade IV, 6 grade III, 9 grade II and 14 grade I.

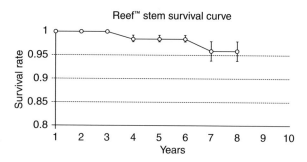

Fig. 5.32 Survival curve for the Reef® stem using implant revision for aseptic loosening as the endpoint. The survival rate at 8-years was 95.8%

Discussion

Our results confirm those of Vidalain [16], who demonstrated that the Reef® implant is a suitable option for the treatment of the most challenging femoral arthroplasty revision cases associated with severe metaphyseal-diaphyseal bone destruction (stages III and IV according to Paprosky). The suitability of the Reef® stem is due to its modularity, its distal interlocking and its full HA-coating.

Femoral Osteotomy

We systematically performed a transfemoral approach and our results demonstrated good healing of the osteotomy site, complete cement extraction and a reduced intraoperative complication rate (there were only three intraoperative fractures). Our results also confirmed those reported by Migaud [10] who underlined that femoral osteotomy could allow complete cement and granuloma extraction and could reduce the risk of intraoperative fractures. The use of a femoral osteotomy provided important advantages, not only since it provided good quality exposure during surgery, but also since it offered biological advantages by stimulating osteogenesis and metaphyseal reconstruction. It allowed precise positioning of stem locking and accurate adjustment of leg length.

Choice of Implant

We chose an interlocked implant since implant locking enhances rotational stability and avoids distal stem

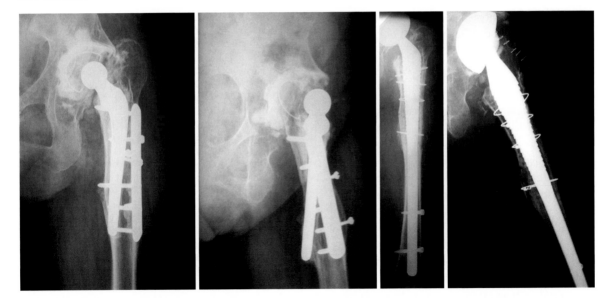

Fig. 5.33 The Reef® system demonstrates good long-term radiological results

migration. Unlike femoral revisions using diaphyseal press-fit fixation as in Wagner stems, no significant stem subsidence was reported at last follow-up. The 5-year survival rate of more than 98% confirms the results of Philippot et al. [11] and Kim et al. [6] at a minimum of 5 years using a coated interlocked stem. According to the work of Mahomed et al [7], interlocking enhances rotational stability by 320% and axial stability by 230%. Interlocking therefore appears to be a good option to prevent rotational micromovement, which according to Harris et al. [3] and Chandler et al. [1] promotes femoral loosening.

Radiographs revealed lytic lesions in the metaphysis, but these were rare and non-progressive. Radiographs also revealed good osseointegration, which proved that HA coating is effective and reliable in revision surgery as well as in primary surgery. HA coating improved distal fixation by encouraging secondary proximal fixation of the implant. These results confirm those obtained by the Wrightington team, which reported worse results using cemented revision stems and better results using HA coated stems [14]. This result they attributed to the poor quality of the biological interface between cement and the sclerotic bone and to the fact that in revision surgery sclerotic bone of poor quality is usually encountered.

Implant modularity provided many benefits. It allowed the implant construction to be varied intraoperatively in order to adapt the implant to the bone deficiencies, often underestimated at the preoperative planning stage. It permitted intraoperative adjustment of femoral leg length and anteversion. It facilitated exposure in cases of acetabular revision, a benefit which is not provided by anatomic stems [4]. It also permitted optimum filling of the femoral metaphysis and thus long-term biological fixation [8].

Conclusions

The use of the Reef® stem with diaphyseal interlocking in femoral revision surgery involving extensive damage (grades III and IV according to the Paprosky classification system) provided good rotational and axial stability, a prerequisite for secondary fixation using HA coating. Distal interlocking is an outstanding technique for the reconstruction of proximal femoral mechanical deficiencies and for the treatment of femoral fractures around a loose stem. In our continuous series of 109 patients the Reef® stem with distal interlocking gave reliable and reproducible results. Patients recovered a painless hip with a functional range of motion under weight bearing. Metaphyseal bone stock was improved by means of a femoral osteotomy without the need for bone grafting. Full HA coating of the

femoral stem contributed to the good results. There
was a low rate of complications and only 2 cases of
stem loosening. The survival rate at 8 years with
implant revision for aseptic loosening as the endpoint
was 95.8%.

> **Key Learning Points**
>
> ❯ In cases of major femoral deficiency involving
> extensive bone defects, stabilisation of a coni-
> cal femoral implant in the metaphyseal or dia-
> physeal region is difficult and requires instead
> the use of a longer, distally interlocked femo-
> ral stem.
> ❯ Full HA coating allows effective (but tempo-
> rary) distal screw fixation to be replaced by
> secondary osseointegration.
> ❯ In stages III and IV according to Paprosky, use
> of a modular implant such as the Reef® pros-
> thesis helps resolve intraoperative technical
> difficulties.
> ❯ In our series of more than 100 patients with a
> mean follow-up of 5 years (range 1–14), the
> long-term survival was good and the compli-
> cation rate was low. These good results dem-
> onstrate the valuable contribution made by
> this type of implant to the treatment of major
> femoral deficiencies.

References

1. Chandler HP, Ayres DK, Tan RC (1995) Revision total hip replacement using the S-ROM femoral component. Clin Orthop Relat Res 130:319–322
2. Gie GA, Linder L, Ling RS et al (1993) Impacted cancellous allografts and cement for revision total hip arthroplasty. J Bone Joint Surg Br 73:14–21
3. Harris WH, Mulroy RD, Malone WJ et al (1991) Intraoperative measurement of rotational stability of femoral components of total hip arthroplasty. Clin Orthop Relat Res May; (266):119–121
4. Hozack WJ, Mesa JJ, Rothman RH (1996) Head-neck modularity for total hip arthroplasty; Is it necessary? J Arthroplasty 11:397–399
5. Kempf JF, Hhuten D, Giraud P et al (1989) Résultats des rescellements fémoraux. Rev Chir Orthop 75(1):48–52
6. Kim YK, Kim HJ, Song WS et al (2004) Experience with the BICONTACT revision stems with distal interlocking. J Arthroplasty 19:27–34
7. Mahomed N, Schaztker J, Hearn T (1993) Biomechanical analysis of a distally interlocked press-fit femoral total hip arthroplasty. J Arthroplasty 8:129–132
8. Massin P, Geais L, Astoin E et al (2000) The anatomic basis for the concept of lateralized femoral stem: a frontal plane radiographic study of the proximal femur. J Arthroplasty 15:93–101
9. Migaud H, Jardin C, Fontaine C et al (1997) Reconstruction fémorale par des allogreffes spongieuses impactées et protégées par un treillis métallique au cours de révisions de prothèses totales de hanche. Dix neuf cas au recul moyen de 83 mois. Rev Chir Orthop 83:360–367
10. Migaud H, Gueguen G, Duhamel A (2000) Reprise fémorale dans les arthroplasties de la hanche. Avantages et inconvénients des abords osseux extensifs Rev Chir Orthop 86(I):69–72
11. Philippot R, Delangle F, Verdot FX et al (2009) Femoral deficiency reconstruction using a hydroxyapatite-coated locked modular stem. A series of 43 total hip revisions. Orthop Traumatol Surg Res 95(2):119–26
12. Raman R, Kamath RP, Parikh A et al (2005) Revision of cemented hip arthroplasty using a hydroxyapatite-ceramic-coated femoral component. J Bone Joint Surg Br 87:1061–1067
13. Rubasch HE, Harris WH (1988) Revision of nonseptic loose, cemented femoral components using modern cementing techniques. J Arthroplasty 3:241–248
14. Subramanian S, Argawal M, Board T et al (2010) Distally locked, fully hydroxyapatite coated modular long stems in salvage revision hip arthroplasty: a report of early experience Eur J Orthop Surg Traumatol 20:17–21
15. Trikha SP, Siongh S, Rayhnam OW et al (2005) Hydroxyapatite-ceramic-coated-femoral stems in revision hip surgery. J Bone Joint Surg Br 87:1055–1060
16. Vidalain JP (2001) Advantages of a modular interlcked ha coated stem in revisions with major bone deficiencies. J Bone Joint Surg Br 83(II):112
17. Vives P, Plaquet JL, Leclair A et al (1992) Revision of interlocking rod for loosening of THP. Concept – preliminary results Acta Orthop Belg 58(1):28–35
18. Wagner H (1989) Revisions prothese für das Hüftgelenk. Ortopäde 75(I):25–60

Approaches

6

David Beverland

Contents

J.-P. Vidalain et al. (eds.), *The CORAIL® Hip System*,
DOI: 10.1007/978-3-642-18396-6_6, © Springer-Verlag Berlin Heidelberg 2011

6.1 Introduction and General Considerations

Charles Clark

This section focuses on the surgical approaches through which the Corail® hip system can be implanted. Implant design features, which make the Corail® hip amenable to a variety of approaches, will also be presented. Various surgical approaches are presented and the technical details of the approaches as well as the associated indications, advantages, and disadvantages are explained. The surgical approach chosen for a patient should allow sufficient exposure for accurate implant placement, while minimizing soft tissue trauma.

Introduction

The Corail® hip system includes a very versatile femoral stem which can be efficiently and effectively implanted via common surgical approaches to the hip ranging from anterior to posterior. I have personally implanted Corail® femoral components extensively via both anterior and posterior approaches. The implant has unique design features that make it amenable to a variety of surgical approaches which will be described in this section. The techniques described include the anterior approach both with and without the use of a traction table, the anterolateral approach, the lateral approach, the posterior approach, and the double incision approach.

Foremost among the design features which facilitate the versatile use of the Corail® hip system are the tapered stem and the hydroxyapatite coating. The lateral shoulder on the stem makes this implant particularly amenable to implantation via the anterior approach. Mobilization of the femur is one of the technically demanding components of an anterior approach and the design of both the shoulder of the stem and the stem and broach facilitates broach and stem placement.

An important aspect of stem design is having multiple options available to meet the demands of various patient anatomies. The Corail® stem offers both

collared and collarless versions, standard and high offset necks, as well as a coxa vara stem.

Patient Selection

Patient selection is an important consideration when considering the use of a specific approach. I believe it is important for a surgeon to have at least two approaches for a hip arthroplasty, which he or she uses regularly, since unique patient anatomies may make one approach advantageous over another. For example, a patient with a neurological disorder is often at high risk for dislocation, in which case the surgeon may prefer an anterior approach. Another patient with a particular body habitus such as a very wide pelvis or substantial truncal obesity may be better suited for a posterior or lateral approach. Various anatomic considerations which are important factors in deciding the approach to the hip joint will be described in the individual approach sections. In general, however, a patient with a narrower pelvis may be an ideal candidate for an anterior approach, whereas a morbidly obese patient with a large panniculus may be better approached posteriorly.

Approaches

The surgeon needs to appreciate the technical aspects of a particular approach including the extent to which a particular approach is capable of accommodating anatomical differences. The advantages and disadvantages of each approach should be carefully considered by the surgeon before embarking on implanting a total hip arthroplasty in a particular patient. Regardless of the approach, however, the Corail® hip system is versatile enough to be well suited for any approach, which the surgeon may choose and because of its various options, is well suited for the majority of proximal femoral anatomies.

Specific approaches are associated with specific anatomic considerations. Knowledge of internervous planes, local vascular anatomy, and the extensile ability of an approach is important. Regardless of the approach selected, the exposure of the acetabulum and proximal femur must be adequate to allow for accurate implant placement, which is a prerequisite for the long-term success of the arthroplasty.

6.1.1 Anterior Approach with Orthopedic Table: Supine Position

Joel M. Matta and Danielle Berberian

Introduction

The first hip arthroplasty performed through this approach was by Robert Judet in 1947 and the surgery was facilitated by operating on the Judet Table with the patient in the supine position. The reasons for Judet's choice of this approach for hip arthroplasty were the following:

1. The hip is an anterior joint, closer to the skin surface anteriorly than posteriorly.
2. The approach follows the anatomic interval between the zones of enervation of the superior and inferior gluteal nerves laterally and the femoral nerve medially.
3. The approach exposes the hip without detachment of muscle from the bone.

A little over a decade later in the 1960s Charnley started implanting the first consistently successful total hip replacement. The initial emphasis regarding total hip arthroplasty was to find a workable prosthesis with satisfactory longevity. Charnley was the first to do this. Other surgeons adopted the Charnley® prosthesis and thereby adopted the Charnley transtrochanteric approach. It is worthy of note that both Charnley and Judet developed their techniques around the supine position to have better control of cup position and leg length.

Sarmiento felt that the soft tissue dissection was too extensive and the trochanteric osteotomy problematic with Charnley's approach, and therefore began using a posterior approach total hip arthroplasty. This had a worldwide influence. The posterior approach compromised the abductors less, however it was necessary to adopt the lateral position.

Over the past 20 years the most common approaches for total hip arthroplasty have been posterior (most popular) and lateral transgluteal (Harding). The main criticism of the lateral approach is postoperative limp due to partial abductor detachment. The main criticism of the posterior approach is dislocation. The anterior approach, by contrast, preserves the posterior structures important for preventing dislocations, and the lack of disturbance of the minimus and medius help facilitate the recovery of a normal gait.

In 1996, the Judet-Tasserit table was out of production and no longer available for purchase. As a result, Dr. Joel Matta decided to bring his ideas for the design of a new table to the manufacturer Mizuho-OSI and enlisted their support for both a table and for teaching. The result of the collaboration was the PROfx™ table and the HANA™ table. The new tables operate inside the wound, with the femoral lift hook's ability to raise and lower the femur as well as maintaining the traditional external positioning function [3–5].

Advantages of Anterior Approach with the Orthopedic Table

While there are numerous advantages of the anterior approach for total hip replacement, the main benefit is that it is not necessary to detach or split any muscle from the pelvis or the femur and the "hip deltoid" is not disturbed. The result is that there is an immediate stability of the hip that obviates the need for dislocation precautions as well as permitting a more rapid recovery. Another advantage of the technique is the ability to apply the use of fluoroscopy for immediate information and increased accuracy regarding acetabular position and femoral length and offset [1]. Also, this technique facilitates bilateral hip replacement [2].

Brief Summary of Technique

The patient is placed supine on either the HANA™ or PROfx™ table with their feet in boots that are attached to the table's leg spars (Fig. 6.1). The normal incision starts 2–3 cm posterior and 1–2 cm distal to the anterior superior iliac spine and extends in a distal and slightly posterior direction to a point 1–2 cm anterior to the greater trochanter. The joint is reached through an interval between the sartorius and the tensor facsia latae. In the process, the anterior capsule may be either excised or preferably opened as flaps, and repaired as part of the closure.

The hip is dislocated anteriorly and the femur is externally rotated 90° and the capsule freed from the medial neck. The hip is relocated, the femoral neck cut,

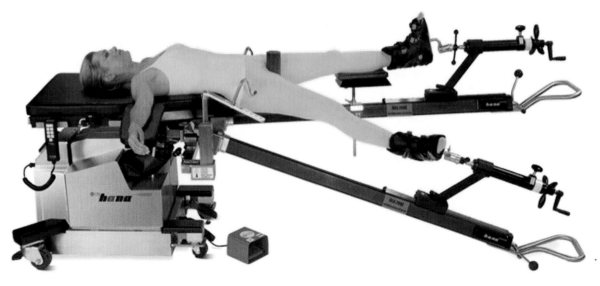

Fig. 6.1 Patient supine on the HANA™ table

and the femoral head removed. Reaming begins under direct vision and later a check is done with the fluoroscope to control the depth of reaming and adequate circumference. Following acetabular insertion under fluoroscopy (Fig. 6.2), the gross traction control on the leg spar is released and the femur internally rotated to neutral. The vastus ridge is palpated and the femoral hook placed just distal to this and around the posterior

femur. The femur is now externally rotated 90° and the hip hyperextended and adducted (Fig. 6.1).

The tip of the first Corail® broach enters the neck near the posterior medial cortex (Fig. 6.3). When broaching is complete, a trial head is put on and the femur hook jack is lowered and the hook removed. The leg is flexed and the hip is relocated by using manual traction and internal rotation. Images of both hips are

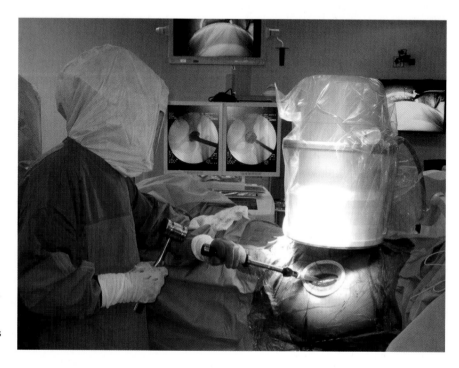

Fig. 6.2 Fluoroscopic control of acetabular position during insertion; a goal of 20–25° of anteversion and an inclination angle of 40–45° is ideal

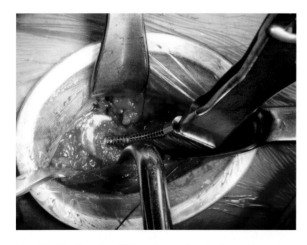

Fig. 6.3 The first Corail® broach entering the femoral canal

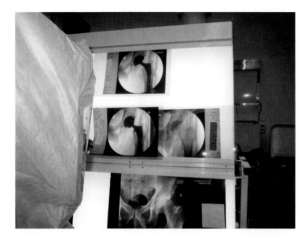

Fig. 6.4 X-ray images of the final components are taken and viewed. The surgeon can make the final check of leg length and offset at this point and make any adjustments necessary prior to closing

taken with the fluoroscope and printed to determine accurate leg length and offset. The two transparencies can be viewed on the x-ray viewing box by overlying them. After the decision is made for the femoral prosthesis, the trial components are taken out (utilizing the same steps previously mentioned with respect to the femoral hook and leg spar positioning) and the final femoral stem prosthesis and head are implanted. Another transparency is printed with the fluoroscope confirming leg length and offset, and serves as the immediate postoperative x-ray (Fig. 6.4).

Clinical Results

From November 1996 to December 2009 JMM performed a consecutive, unselected series of 2,126 primary total hip arthroplasties using the anterior approach. Body mass index ranged from 15 to 69 with a median of 26. Operative duration had a median time of 1.2 h and the median blood loss was 300 cc.

One hundred and seventy cemented femoral components were implanted including 41 cemented femoral resurfacing components. One thousand nine hundred and fifty-six femoral components were inserted without cement including 1,542 Corail® stems. Revisions were performed for loosening or fracture in 10 cemented femoral components including two resurfacings. Revision of uncemented femoral components for loosening was performed for 2 of 371 Alloclassic® stems and 1 of 1,542 Corail® stems. Two Alloclassic® stems and one Corail® were revised for early fracture around the stem [6].

The collared Corail® was the preferred implant and comprised the large majority of the Corail® cases.

References

1. Anterior Total Hip Arthroplasty Collaborative (ATHAC) Investigators (2009) Outcomes following the single-incision anterior approach to total hip arthroplasty: a multicenter observational study. Orthop Clin North Am 40(3):329–342
2. Mast NH, Munoz M, Matta JM (2009) Simultaneous bilateral supine anterior approach total hip arthroplasty: evaluation of early complications and short-term rehabilitation. Orthop Clin North Am 40(3):351–356
3. Matta JM et al (1994) Single incision anterior approach for THA on an orthopaedic table. Clin Orthop Relat Res 298:89–96
4. Matta JM, Ferguson TA (2008) THR after acetabular fracture. Orthopaedics 28:959
5. Yerasimides JG, Matta JM (2005) Primary total hip arthroplasty with a minimally invasive anterior approach. Semin Arthroplasty16(3):186–190
6. http://www.hipandpelvis.com

6.1.2 *Direct Anterior Without Traction Table: Supine Position*

Hans-Erik Henkus and Tom Hogervorst

Patient Selection

The anterior supine intermuscular approach without traction table can be used in patients with osteoarthritis, avascular necrosis, rheumatoid arthritis, a subcapital femoral fracture, and revision surgery for inlay, cup, and stem when no extended trochanteric osteotomy is needed.

Contraindication

The surgery can be performed in almost every patient. Care should be taken with the very obese, although the least fat is found in front of the hip. An overhanging paniculus can obstruct the broaching of the femoral canal, but can be held proximally with tape. The approach is not recommended for short muscular male patients especially in combination with a short femoral neck or a low CCD angle.

Positioning and Incision Placement

Patient positioning is on a radiolucent table that can extend at the level of the anterior superior iliac spines (ASIS). Draping is done so that both limbs can move freely. The interval between the tensor fascia lata laterally and the sartorius muscle medially can be palpated following a line between the ASIS and the lateral side of the patella.

The incision starts 2–3 cm distal to the ASIS and runs over the midline of the tensor fascia latae muscle belly to 2–3 cm distal to the tip of the greater trochanter. This avoids damage to the lateral femoral cutaneous nerve that follows a variable course within the fascia of the sartorius muscle.

Superficial Dissection

The incision is deepened through the subcutaneous fat in line with the skin incision. The fascia over the tensor muscle is opened in its midline. The fascia on the medial side is lifted and the intermuscular interval between the sartorius and the tensor is entered using a finger. The capsule on the lateral side of the hip and the anterior part of the greater trochanter can now be palpated. A Homan retractor is positioned outside the capsule on the lateral aspect of the neck thus retracting the tensor muscle. During the whole procedure care should be taken to protect the tensor muscle from tearing.

The lateral femoral circumflex vessels cross the intermuscular interval just distal to the inter-trochanteric line. These vessels must be clamped or cauterized: "If you can't find these vessels, they will find you!" The rectus femoris muscle follows the lateral acetabular rim and can be elevated from the anteromedial part of the capsule using a Cobb's elevator. A second Homan can now be placed extracapsularly on the medial side thus retracting the rectus femoris muscle medially and exposing the whole anterior part of the capsule.

Deep Dissection

The capsule can be incised in an inverted T or H shape or excised according to the surgeon's individual preference. The intertrochanteric line forms the inferior border and can be palpated at the origin of the vastus lateralis muscle. Homan retractors can now be placed within the capsule on both sides of the neck. The intertrochanteric line, which can also be seen on the AP x-ray can be used as a reference for the osteotomy of the femoral neck. The femoral head is removed with a corkscrew. When removal of the head is difficult it can be facilitated taking a slice of bone of the femoral neck first. The preparation of the cup is similar to any other approach. With the supine position an image intensifier can be used to check the position of the cup (Fig. 6.5).

For the femur, the critical step is to release the capsule at the posterosuperior neck junction. This can be accomplished by pulling the femur forward while using electrocautery to release the capsule. Care should be taken not to release the piriformis tendon. The piriformis can be seen medial to the neck-trochanter junction when the leg is in (90°) of external rotation. The femur is pulled forward with a bone hook allowing us to judge the effect of release as we cut. The proximal femur can then be presented into the wound by putting the leg in a "lazy figure of 4" position, extending the operating table by 20–30° and elevating the femur using a double bend Homan positioned behind the

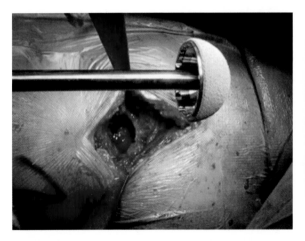

Fig. 6.5 The view of the acetabulum is excellent with the anterior approach. You can use the anatomic landmarks like the transverse ligament, as well as determine the position of the cup relative to the operating table and floor (Rights belong to Hans-Erik Hankus, Tom Hogervorst)

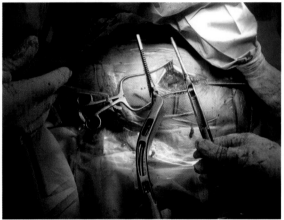

Fig. 6.7 The Corail® system has excellent offset handles for patients where the ASIS tends to obstruct a straight entrance to the femoral canal (Rights belong to Hans-Erik Hankus, Tom Hogervorst)

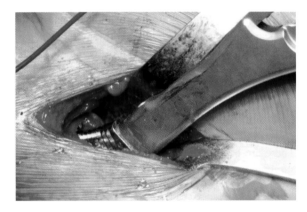

Fig. 6.6 The proximal femur is presented within the wound by extending the operating table by 20°–30°and elevating the femur using a double bend Hohmann positioned behind the greater trochanter (Rights belong to Hans-Erik Hankus, Tom Hogervorst)

greater trochanter (Fig. 6.6). Inadequate release of the posterior capsule can hamper the exposure of the proximal femur by preventing its anterior translation relative to the ilium. Broaching the femur is similar to any other approach. With the anterior approach the stem can easily be malpositioned in varus. Care should be taken to broach posterolaterally. The Corail® system has excellent offset handles for patients where the ilium tends to obstruct a straight entrance to the femoral shaft (Fig. 6.7).

Test reduction is easy and the supine position gives you optimal control of stability and leg length.

Deep Repair and Closure

Capsular closure can be performed if desired. The fascia lata is closed with a running suture, followed by subcutaneous and skin sutures. A wound drain can be used if so desired.

Advantages

The anterior intermuscular approach is a safe, reproducible approach using a true internervous plane without any muscle interference. We believe the supine position has several advantages over the lateral decubitus position. The pelvis is in a constant stable position. The view of the acetabulum is excellent affording us to use both anatomic landmarks, like the transverse ligament as well as determine the position of the cup relative to the operating table and floor. Fluoroscopy can be used in difficult cases. Leg length and implant stability can be assessed much more easily without a traction table.

No special tools are needed except for a double-bent Homan retractor and a bone hook to pull the femur forward during release of the posterior joint capsule.

Disadvantages

The lateral femoral cutaneous nerve is at risk during the procedure. It can be damaged directly if the incision is made too medially or indirectly by overstretching.

A painful neuralgia has been described in the literature. When the femur is inadequately exposed a varus malposition of the stem or fracture may occur. There is clearly a learning curve and this should be addressed by mastering the approach in cadavers first and by visiting appropriate learning centers.

6.1.3 Direct Anterior Without Traction Table: Lateral Position

Markus C. Michel

Patient Selection

The Direct Anterior Approach (DAA), or MicroHip™, can be used in a wide range of indications including in the obese and in all age groups. It is not implant dependent, so it can be used for cementless and cemented implants, but uncemented implants with a low shoulder profile, such as the Corail®, are the most suitable for this approach. When the surgeon first starts to use this approach, patient selection is extremely important. It is key to build up your initial experience with easy cases such as females with a normal body mass index (BMI) and a standard anatomy. It is recommended that you gradually stretch the range of indications toward the heavy muscular male with a short femoral neck and a varus hip. This is certainly the most demanding type of patient.

Contraindications

There are no specific contraindications as long as the surgeon operates within his/her comfort zone.

Positioning and Incision Placement

The patient is positioned in a lateral decubitus position, where the posterior foot part of the table has been removed. A strong support in the back of the patient is needed in order to prevent the pelvis from moving. It is critical to have good access to the femur. The surgeon stands in front of the patient as shown in Fig. 6.8. Specific landmarks are used for the incision. We draw a line from the middle of the anterior border of the greater trochanter to the anterior iliac crest. The distal 6–8 cm of this line is used for the incision (Fig. 6.9).

Superficial Dissection

The subcutaneous tissue is dissected down to the level of the fascia. We then access the border of the Ilio-Tibial

Fig. 6.8 Placement of the patient (Copyright DePuy International Limited)

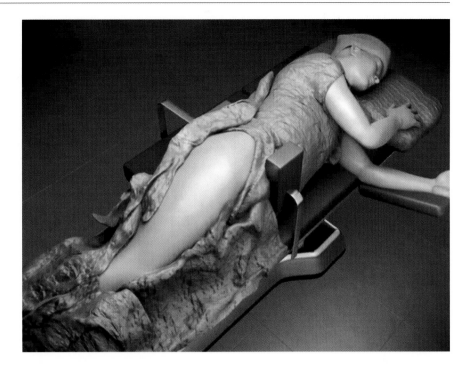

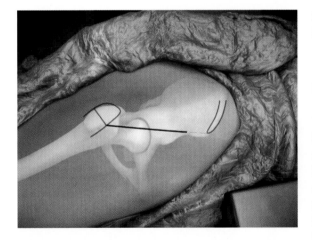

Fig. 6.9 Landmarks (Copyright DePuy International Limited)

Band (ITB), where the incision is placed 2–3 mm in the ITB following the longitudinal fibers. This is for two reasons. Firstly the border of the ITB is easier to suture when closing than the sometimes fine fascia of the tensor muscle. Secondly, the superficial lateral nerve of the thigh can be avoided by proceeding with blunt dissection of the tensor muscle from underneath the fascia.

The lateral cutaneous nerve might be close, but it always runs on the superficial side of the fascia. The first blunt retractor is set on the lateral side of the femoral neck in order to move all the musculature to the lateral side and give access to the femoral neck.

Deep Dissection

The anterior neck is covered with a thin double layer of fascia containing the yellow fat pad in the middle. The reflected rectus tendon runs medially. A longitudinal incision of the superficial layer is followed by a blunt dissection of the yellow fat pat moving it medially together with the reflected rectus tendon and holding it in place with a second blunt retractor. The capsule is incised in a T-shaped manner lateral to the insertion of the reflected rectus tendon. It is better to dissect the capsule from the intertrochanteric line in an inside out technique to avoid the main branches of the circumflex artery (Fig. 6.10). The ascending branch, which runs along the deeper surface of the tensor muscle, needs to be coagulated or ligated. The blunt retractors are placed around the femoral neck and the osteotomy is performed prior to dislocation of the femoral head. Then, for dislocation, a corkscrew is inserted into the lateral femoral neck. It is used to flip the femoral neck toward you. Now the corkscrew is repositioned into the longitudinal axis of the femoral neck and can be used to twist the head several times until it is completely loose.

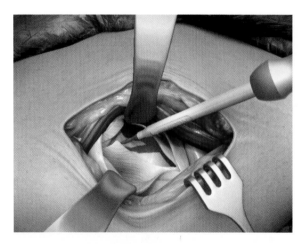

Fig. 6.10 Capsular incision (Copyright DePuy International Limited)

After removing the head you will have a great 360° view of the acetabulum, which can be further enhanced by adding a third double bent Hohmann retractor at the lateral insertion of the transverse acetabular ligament (TAL), so as to distalize the femur. Identify the TAL, which is an important local landmark for controlling version of the cup. When implanting the cup also be aware that in the lateral decubitus position the pelvis tends to adduct and that combined with the impact of version on radiographic inclination means the surgeon should aim

for an operative inclination of about 35° in order to achieve a 45° angle on the postoperative AP radiograph.

For preparation of the femur, a blunt retractor is placed over the tip of the greater trochanter before the leg is dropped behind the table (Fig. 6.11. With this retractor the tensor muscle can be flipped over the greater trochanter at the same time as the trochanter is moved with the tip of the retractor medially in order to prevent the femur from impinging against the lateral acetabular rim. In standard hips no special release is needed. If the hip is very stiff, we first perform a release of the posterior capsule, second a release of the piriformis tendon, and third a partial release of the tensor muscle from the anterior iliac crest.

Before broaching, make sure that you have a good overview of the femur in order to have the correct entry point for the implant. The most common error is to start broaching too medial, in which case the broach will be in varus. This increases both the risk of under sizing and of cracking the calcar.

Deep Repair and Closure

After implantation, all you have to do is close the capsule with a few stitches and then a running suture to the fascia, and finishing with skin closure.

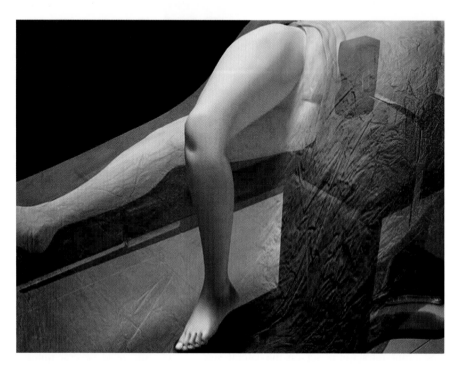

Fig. 6.11 Position for access to the femur (Copyright DePuy International Limited)

Advantages

The main advantages are avoidance of the hip deltoid in an internerveous plane, so the rehabilitation is extremely fast and the outcome has been shown to be superior to a standard Harding approach even after 5 years. In the lateral decubitus position hardly any release is needed, blood loss is minimized and no specific tools like an extension table are involved. Therefore, not only does the surgeon have an excellent view of the acetabulum and femur, he/she also has full control over the procedure.

Disadvantages

It is a completely different procedure from any standard approach and therefore needs special training and education in order to protect both surgeons and patients from unnecessary risks. For further information go to: www.do-surgery.com or www.ozm.com.

6.1.4 Anterolateral with Traction Table: Supine Position

Alain Machenaud

Introduction

Derived from the Watson-Jones approach, the GK MacKee anterolateral approach provides easy access to the joint cavity without causing significant muscle damage, which makes it very attractive in terms of postoperative stability and early recovery. The use of a traction table has acknowledged drawbacks with respect to patient positioning and evaluation of the lower limb (LL) length. However, its benefits include the need for fewer assistants thus decreasing the overall cost of the procedure and the risk of infection and also the facilitation of computer-assisted navigation (CAS).

The surgical approach described here is that of GK MacKee. It is a modified Watson-Jones approach to which Professor G. de Mourgues added the use of the traction table. It has been widely and continuously used since 1974 without restriction with respect to patient selection and is therefore considered suitable for all primary total hip arthroplasties (THAs), irrespective of patient morphotype, age or etiology.

Patient Positioning

The patient is placed supine on a traction table, which is inclined 30° toward the nonoperated side. Apart from the surgeon, only two assistants are necessary: one scrub nurse who is in charge of the instrument trays and one unsterile assistant who looks after the traction table and the handling of the lower limb. The patient is prepped and draped to allow access to a rectangular area which includes the iliac crest and the upper one-third of the femur, thus obviating the need for prepping the genital region and the rest of the lower limb (LL) (Fig. 6.12).

Incision

The skin incision commences 1.5 cm posterior to the anterior superior iliac spine (ASIS) and is extended

Fig. 6.12 Positioning of the patient

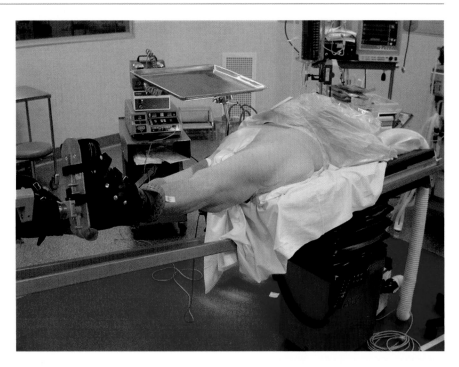

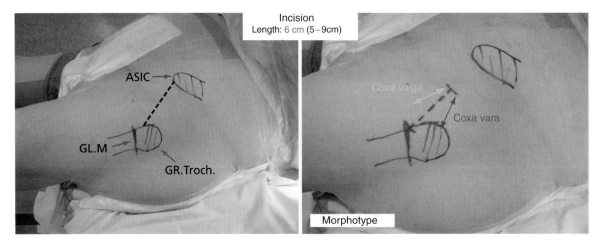

Fig. 6.13 Skin incision

over the anterior aspect of the tip of the greater trochanter. The mean length of the skin incision is 12 cm going up to a maximum of 15 cm in obese patients. In mini-invasive surgery (MIS) the mean length of the skin incision is 6.5 cm (range 5–9.5 cm). Such measurements are suitable for a standard hip. In coxa-valga deformity of the hip, the skin incision should be placed 1.5 cm anteriorly whereas in coxa-vara, it should be 1.5 cm posteriorly. With MIS, the incision must be

properly centred according to the patient's hip morphology (Fig. 6.13).

The Intermuscular Plane

The intermuscular plane can be easily identified. It corresponds to the interval between the "red and the white" the tensor fascia lata anteriorly and the gluteus

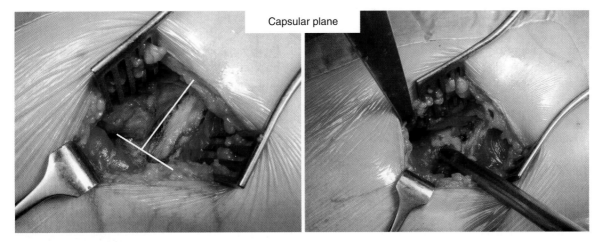

Capsular plane

Fig. 6.14 Joint-capsule incision

medius posteriorly. These two muscles can be easily separated using a self-retaining retractor placed into the lower part of the incision thus clearly exposing the dissected window between these two muscles. Muscle splitting should stop once the tendon of the rectus femoris muscle is visualized to avoid damage to the inferior branch of the superior gluteal nerve. This now provides direct access to the capsule.

Capsuloligamentous Plane

An inverse T-shaped capsular incision is made with the vertical incision being made along the neck axis, ending at the rectus femoris muscle tendon and the transverse incision running along the anterior intertrochanteric line as far as the upper and lower borders of the neck, which are then easily exposed using two Hohmann retractors (Fig. 6.14).

Hip Joint Procedure

1. The unsterile assistant places the lower limb in external rotation, while the lesser trochanter is palpated, acting as a landmark for initial femoral neck resection. The femoral neck is initially resected slightly above the pre-plannned level, prior to hip dislocation. This conservative resection level ends at the junction of the upper border of the femoral neck and the base of the tip of the greater trochanter. The femoral head is then removed with some simple maneuvering, which includes manual traction to the lower limb via the traction table.

With the head removed there is excellent exposure of the acetabulum with good visualization of common anatomical landmarks such as the anterior and posterior horns, the acetabular roof, and the transverse acetabular ligament (TAL).

2. The definitive neck cut and femoral preparation requires that the lower limb be placed in extension, adduction, and external rotation. The unsterile assistant is in charge of these manipulations once the lower limb has been released from the traction table. A Hohmann retractor is then placed posterior to the greater trochanter and is used to elevate the femoral neck. In the case of a stiff hip, a slight release of the gluteus minimus and/or the piriform fossa will improve the exposure. After direct visualization of the lesser trochanter, definitive neck resection may be performed at the level defined during preoperative planning.

3. Femoral preparation starts by inserting a canal finder to determine the axis of the femoral canal. If it cannot be easily inserted, repositioning of the leg will help achieve proper orientation for the canal finder and subsequent femoral broaches. Cancellous bone compaction and broaching are thus facilitated. The use of a Hohmann retractor at the level of the greater trochanter ensures that broach insertion is sufficiently lateral.

4. Stem insertion should be performed by taking into account the key elements elsewhere described (Sect. 3.3.1).

Wound Closure

The capsule is repaired and the split muscles are approximated using either continuous or interrupted sutures.

Advantages

There are some theoretical advantages related to the anterior approach:

1. Early mobilization (thus resulting in a shorter hospital stay and rehabilitation period).
2. Low rate of hip dislocations (early and late), even in the absence of anti-dislocation prophylactic measures (Sect. 3.4). The use of MIS also contributes to reducing this rate.
3. Very good visualization of the acetabulum.

There also some theoretical advantages that are related to the use of a traction table:

1. Reduced infection risk, no lower limb manipulations and limited skin preparation.
2. Reduced overall cost of the surgery due to the smaller surgical team.
3. Easy use of x-ray to detect any malorientation or assess leg length.
4. Reliable computer-assisted navigation; both iliac crests can be easily instrumented and good pelvic stabilization is obtained using the traction table.

Disadvantages

1. Longer operative time – patient's positioning on the traction table usually requires 10–15 min. However, skin preparation and placement of surgical drapes are quicker than in other surgical approaches.
2. Direct visual control (by comparison) of leg length equality is not possible.
3. Longer learning curve compared with posterior approaches due to the absence of complete lower limb visualization.

Key Learning Points

> Access to the joint capsule does not require muscle resection, thereby making functional recovery faster and reducing the dislocation rate.
> Can be easily converted into a minimally invasive approach without any specific change of technique or instrumentation, but requiring a longer learning curve.
> The required surgical team consists of fewer people, thereby reducing both the cost and the risk of infection.
> Due to the supine position, access to the contralateral ASIS is easy and pelvic stabilization using the traction table is good.
> Can be easily and reliably used with computer-assisted navigation (CAS)

6.1.5 *Direct Lateral: Supine Position*

Rüdiger von Eisenhart-Rothe and Jens Boldt

Introduction

In 1954 McFarland and Osborne introduced a direct lateral approach without trochanteric osteotomy, the latter having been described by Charnley. While this approach was described with the patient placed on his side, Kevin Hardinge performed the same approach with the patient supine on the operating table. This, he felt, was associated with two advantages; firstly, better component orientation and secondly, improved control of leg length. The Hardinge approach has been often modified since its introduction in 1982 and remains one of the most popular hip joint approaches worldwide.

The Hardinge Approach

The patient is placed in the supine position with the greater trochanter hanging slightly over the lateral edge of the table. The skin incision can either be made parallel to the femur or at an angle of about 20° relative to the femur directed posteriorly at its proximal end with the tip of the greater trochanter at its midpoint (Fig. 6.15). Incision length varies from 6 to 12 cm depending on the state of the soft tissues and the gender of the patient. The fascia lata is divided in line with the skin incision between the gluteus maximus and tensor fascia

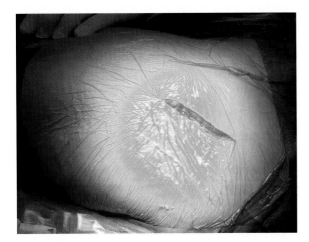

Fig. 6.15 Skin incision for lateral modified Hardinge approach

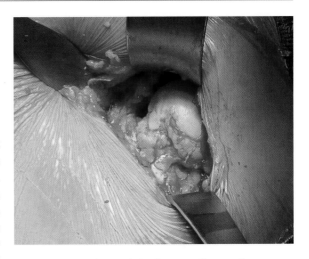

Fig. 6.16 Split being made in gluteus medius muscle

lata muscles. Then the tensor fascia lata is retracted anteriorly and the gluteus maximus posteriorly.

The anterior and posterior dimensions of the gluteus medius are identified and blunt dissection is used to separate the muscle fibers between the anterior 30% and the posterior 70% of the muscle (Fig. 6.16). This dissection is limited to 3 cm proximal to the insertion on the greater trochanter to avoid injury to the inferior branch of the superior gluteal nerve.

Distally, the incision passes down to the bone through the vastus lateralis near the anterior surface of the femur. It is important to maintain functional continuity through the thick tendinous periosteum covering the greater trochanter. Then the gluteus medius is reflected anteriorly in continuity with the vastus lateralis. The periarticular soft tissue, particularly the reflected head of the rectus muscle is retracted from the anterior joint capsule and a curved Hohmann retractor can be placed over the anterior wall of the acetabulum. Occasionally, cutting the reflected head of the rectus femoris is necessary depending on how tight the hip is. The capsule is now opened by a T-incision and may be resected. The tendinous insertion of the anterior portion of the gluteus minimus can be detached during external rotation of the leg. Dislocation of the femoral head can be achieved at this point by full adduction and external rotation of the leg (Fig. 6.17).

It should be noted that the posterior part of the gluteus medius with its thick tendon is left undisturbed.

One blunt retractor is placed behind the greater trochanter and a second one above the lesser trochanter for better exposure for the monoplanar osteotomy

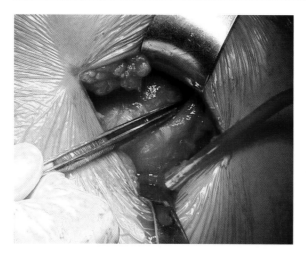

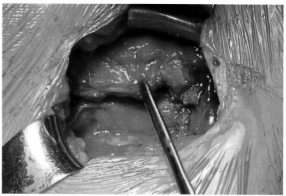

Fig. 6.19 Reconstruction of the undamaged vasto-gluteal muscular complex

Fig. 6.17 Dislocation and preparation for neck resection

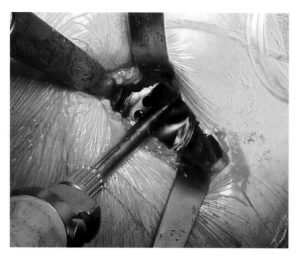

Fig. 6.18 Placement of the cup under full 360° vision

which is performed with an oscillating saw at a 90° angle to the femoral neck axis running from the piriform fossa laterally to the medial calcar 1 cm above the lesser trochanter medially. The head is then removed and the labrum and capsule are excised as required for better exposure of the acetabulum. Finally, three retractors are placed in a three-point (Mercedes) star fashion around the acetabulum. The acetabulum is then reamed and the cup implanted (Fig. 6.18).

Preparation

For the preparation of the stem, the contralateral leg is lowered and the operated leg placed in external rotation

and adduction and with the knee flexed. A Hohmann retractor is positioned at the lesser trochanter and an additional Hohmann retractor is placed medial to the level of neck resection at the transition to the greater trochanter to protect the laterocranial muscular tissue during stem preparation. If necessary, further correction of the femoral neck resection is now possible.

Preparation of the femoral canal can then be done exactly as described in Sect. 3.3.1. Preparation of the lateral aspect of the proximal femoral neck can be minimized and gluteal muscle integrity remains untouched with the Corail® stem.

After relocation of the hip joint, a stability and motion check is performed with special attention being given to adduction with external rotation and full flexion with internal rotation. Possible impingement between implant and bone as well as between bone and bone should be ruled out. A fluoroscopic check should be done to verify correct positioning of the components. The closure is made in layers. The tendinous part of the gluteus minimus is repaired. The anterior part of the gluteus medius and vastus lateralis falls back into place as a flap and the tendinous part of the gluteus medius is sutured which brings tendon to tendon (Fig. 6.19).

Advantages

The advantages of this approach are the excellent exposure even in very muscular, obese patients or in cases of challenging hip joint pathology. Furthermore, postoperative complications are significantly lower when comparing the lateral to the posterior approach, particularly the dislocation rate [2].

Disadvantages

The often cited downside of the lateral approach is the potential damage to the superior gluteal nerve and the consequent Trendelenburg limp. However, in our own practice, with experience of over 1,000 procedures, this problem is uncommon (<1%). One must also consider that about 10–15% of patients will have some gluteal weakness irrespective of the approach [3]. Also Jolles and Bogoch found no significant difference between the posterior and lateral approach regarding postoperative Trendelenburg gait [1]. Another cited issue is an increased risk of heterotopic ossification (HO). However, this is observed more often when using the lateral Liverpool approach, where a slither of bone is taken with the gluteal flap to allow better reattachment [4]. Increased HO has not been an issue in our own series, provided the patient is treated with NSAIDs for 10 days postoperatively.

References

1. Jolles BM, Bogoch ER (2004) Surgical approach for total hip arthroplasty: direct lateral or posterior? J Rheumatol 31(9):1790–1796
2. Kwon MS et al (2006) Does surgical approach affect total hip arthroplasty dislocation rates? Clin Orthop Relat Res 447:34–38
3. Pai VS (1996) Significance of the Trendelenburg test in total hip arthroplasty. Influence of lateral approaches. J Arthroplasty 11:174–179
4. Pai VS (1997) A comparison of three lateral approaches in primary total hip replacement. Int Orthop 21(6):393–398

6.1.6 *Direct Lateral: Lateral Position*

Emilio Romanini and Attilio Santucci

Patient Selection

The approach can be used for virtually every primary hip arthroplasty.

Contraindications

MIS approaches, including the direct lateral in lateral decubitus, should be avoided in complex primary cases and for very stiff hips, which require more extensile exposures.

Positioning

The patient is positioned in lateral decubitus on a standard operating table and firmly held in place with conventional hip props. Care is taken such that the props do not impede the anterior translation of the femur and knee nor prevent adduction. Prepping is done in the standard fashion.

Incision

The greater trochanter (GT) is the main skin landmark. A longitudinal incision is made parallel to the long axis of the femur. The incision is centered at the mid portion of the greater trochanter 2 cm above the tip and is extended 5–8 cm distally. According to some authors, the incision can be angled at 30–45° (proximal to distal, posterior to anterior) to facilitate an even smaller incision.

Superficial Dissection

The subcutaneous tissue is sectioned in line with the skin incision, and it is carefully dissected from the iliotibial band to create a mobile window. The iliotibial band is usually incised slightly longer than the skin (less than 2 cm proximally and distally) and then retracted with a Charnley retractor with moderate tension. The fascia can be easily closed at the completion of the procedure because of the mobility of the overlying tissues. The trochanteric bursa is incised to identify the gluteus medius and vastus lateralis fibers.

Deep Dissection

A hockey stick incision is made at the anterior third of the gluteus medius fibers starting approximately 2 cm proximal and anterior to the tip of the GT. This incision is carried out anterior to the GT to leave behind a posterior tendinous cuff for later suturing. Two resorbable #2 sutures are used to identify and displace the tendons anteriorly and to ease final anatomical closure. The gluteus minimus is then identified under direct vision, is incised and marked with a suture, and its original insertion is also marked to check for length at closure.

Both the gluteus minimus and the anterior detached portion of the gluteus medius are elevated to expose the superior aspect of the hip capsule and then both are placed underneath the Charnley retractor.

With adequate exposure of the anterior capsule, an anterior capsulectomy is performed, exposing the neck, femoral head, and acetabular rim. The hip can be easily dislocated with external rotation, flexion, and adduction. The femoral neck cut can then be performed as indicated by matching preoperative planning with intraoperative direct visualization with the leg externally rotated.

After the femoral head is resected, the Charnley retractor can be removed if mobilization of the leg is obstructed. Standard or curved dedicated Hohmann retractors are placed anteriorly, posteriorly, and superiorly to achieve adequate visualization of the acetabulum, externally rotating the leg as needed. The acetabular labrum and capsular tissues, which obscure acetabular exposure, are removed before reaming, which is done in the standard fashion.

To perform femoral preparation, the leg is flexed and externally rotated into the pre-prepared anterior leg bag. Then the proximal femur is pushed out of the incision using a curved, blunt Hohmann retractor around the GT, a Hohmann retractor on the medial side of the cut above the lesser trochanter and a femoral elevator. The femoral elevator is pushed from the posterior aspect upward to deliver the femur from the wound. This allows for maximal femoral elevation and exposure. It is often useful to further externally rotate the leg while it is in the anterior leg bag to facilitate femoral broaching and stem placement. Straight access to the femoral canal is possible at this step and femoral preparation is performed in the standard fashion.

Careful soft tissue repair is key to the success of this approach. Soft tissue repair includes the re-approximation of the divided gluteus minimus to its original insertion or to the insertion of the gluteus medius and anatomical repair of the anterior muscle flap to the posterior tendinous cuff, using the same #2 resorbable suture already in place.

The fascia lata, subcutaneous tissues, and skin are closed in the usual fashion.

Advantages

  Safe and reliable procedure
  Clear visualization (surgeon and assistant), which is also advantageous for teaching purposes
  Straightforward implant positioning
  Low dislocation rate
  Very rare nerve/vascular complications

Disadvantages

  Partial damage to the abductor with potential weakness (limp)
  Potentially higher incidence of heterotopic ossification

6.1.7 *Posterior: Lateral Position*

Scott Brumby

Introduction

The posterior approach is the universal incision for hip arthroplasty surgeons. It provides excellent access and vision for all primary and revision hip surgery. If needed, the approach can be extended and modified for management of unexpected intraoperative adverse events and for more complex revision surgery.

According to Gibson (1950) [1], the first description of the approach was by von Langenbeck in 1874, modified by Kocher in 1887–1909, and later was translated into English by Stiles in 1911. In addition, many surgeons have modified the classic approach based on their teaching, experience and needs depending on the complexity of the surgery being performed.

Historically, dislocation has been cited as a major limitation of the approach. In the past, it was common to release the gluteus maximus insertion from the femur, the psoas tendon from the lesser trochanter and to perform a complete anterior capsulotomy in order to gain greater exposure. This massive soft tissue release was often further compromised by excision rather than repair of the posterior capsule. In more recent years, the deep dissection has been minimized and a strong repair of the external rotators and posterior capsule has been highlighted and improved. It is now accepted that dislocation is probably not related to surgical approach but rather to multiple other factors such as cup positioning, hip biomechanics, head diameter, and impingement.

There has been a gradual change making the approach less invasive; more recently, this has been promoted as the "mini posterior approach." Not only is the skin incision shorter today, but more importantly the deep dissection is more muscle preserving and repair of the posterior structures is more secure. The literature does not suggest that smaller incisions offer any clinically relevant advantage. Good visualization, minimal muscle trauma, and correct component position are far more important.

Positioning

The posterior approach is performed with the patient in the lateral decubitus position on a standard operating table. Positioning clamps that hold the pelvis firmly are required. Posteriorly, the clamp is placed centrally over the lumbar-sacral junction and anteriorly either on the symphysis pubis or on either the upper most or both anterior superior iliac spines. The pelvis should not move with movement of the lower limb. The surgeon should supervise patient positioning to ensure that it is optimal and to reduce the incidence of pressure-related injury or neuropraxia.

The patient is then prepped and draped to isolate the posterolateral hip.

An assistant holds the foot at the end of the bed and elevates the lower limb. The prepped area includes the lateral hip and buttock to a level superior to the iliac crest, the groin, and entire lower limb to the ankle. Drapes are then placed above and below the hip joint. The leg is free, draped within a sterile stockinet. An impervious hip extremity drape is then placed over the leg. The groin is isolated with a sterile ioband dressing; the lateral hip is covered with a large sterile ioband dressing. The pelvic anatomical landmarks should be palpable through the drapes. The lateral proximal half of the thigh is accessible. The free draped lower limb should allow the hip to be flexed to 90° and easily rotated to allow access to the hip joint and testing of joint stability.

Incision

Correct placement helps minimize wound edge tension and allows good visualization. A straight incision is made with the leg flexed at 45° and centered over the posterior aspect of the greater trochanter (GT). The length of the incision will vary according to the body habitus and complexity of the surgery. I routinely use a 15 cm incision one-third inferior and anterior to the greater trochanter and two-third posterior and superior.

Superficial Dissection

The skin and subcutaneous fat are incised down to the fascia lata and gluteus maximus fascia. Small blood vessels are encountered and cauterized. The gluteus maximus muscle can either be identified along the anterior border and reflected posteriorly (Gibson) or split in the line of its fibers over the posterior border of the greater trochanter, I choose the latter. Care should

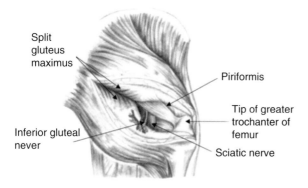

Split
gluteus
maximus

Piriformis

Tip of greater
trochanter of
femur

Inferior gluteal
never

Sciatic nerve

Fig. 6.20 dissection and location of the inferior gluteal nerve (With permission from Ling and Kumar [2])

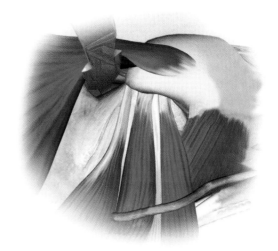

Fig. 6.21 Posterior hip anatomy showing single prong retractor placed to protect gluteals muscles and visualize the tendons of piriformis and the deep external rotators

be taken not to extend the split in the gluteus maximus too posteriorly or proximally. The inferior gluteal nerve and vessels enter the deep surface of the gluteus maximus approximately 5 cm superior to the GT [2]. The nerve is accompanied by several vessels which may bleed in the proximal deep surface if the split is extended too far. If the nerve is injured, the functional weakness is often minimal; however, a cosmetic wasting of the muscle may occur. The trochanteric bursa may be removed if prominent or reflected posteriorly (Fig. 6.20).

The surgeon should now have a clear view of the posterior border of the greater trochanter and gluteus medius. When the latter is retracted superiorly the piriformis and the other external rotators can visualized. The sciatic nerve lies deep and posterior to the external rotators, and will be protected if the muscles are released off the bone and then reflected back. However, the nerve is never far away and is particularly vulnerable in protrusio when it is pulled forward. It can be injured by a poorly placed retractor or dissection toward the sciatic notch. Anatomical variants do occur and the nerve should be formally identified in more complex cases.

Deep Dissection

Piriformis identification is the key to release of the remaining external rotators, namely, the obturator internus with the superior and inferior gemelli, the obturator externus and the quadratus femoris as well as the underlying capsule. A single prong retractor is placed between the piriformis and the gluteus minimus onto the ilium just above the superior border of the acetabulum. The piriformis and deep rotators are released from the GT as close as possible to their insertion so as to maximize their length for subsequent repair. The release continues inferiorly at least to the upper edge of quadratus femoris. The capsule is also released in the same manner (Fig. 6.21).

There are many variations to this deep release. Some surgeons choose to take the external rotators and capsule in two separate layers. Others have tried to preserve the piriformis muscle insertion to the femur.

I then use four separate 2-vicryl stay sutures with one each into the piriformis tendon, superior capsule, inferior capsule, and conjoint tendon of the obturator internus and the gemelli. The posterior capsule and external rotators are then reflected posteriorly to allow access to the acetabulum and also protect the sciatic nerve.

To dislocate the femoral head from the acetabulum, the capsule must be reflected posteriorly and the posterior aspect of the head must be clearly visible. The hip is internally rotated, slightly flexed and adducted. The neck cut can then be made with the leg vertically upright and in line with the longitudinal axis of the body.

To expose the acetabulum, I place the limb back on the other limb and slightly flexed and adducted. I place a single prong retractor anteriorly on the ilium to

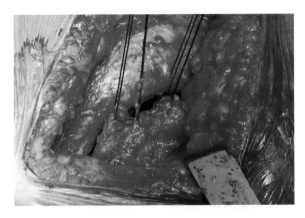

Fig. 6.22 Posterior capsule and external rotators repair: sutures are placed in capsule and deep rotators and then pulled through and tied over bone to reconstruct posterior soft tissues

translate the femur anteriorly, a Norfolk-Norwich self-retainer between abductors and posterior capsule, and external rotators and a double prong inferior retractor to identify the transverse acetabular ligament.

To expose the proximal femur to prepare the canal, the leg is internally rotated, flexed, and adducted. A long handle femoral elevator is very useful. The gluteal muscles are protected and the proximal femur and calcar must be clearly seen.

Posterior Capsular Repair Through Bone

A strong anatomical repair of the posterior capsule and deep rotators is essential. I make two drill holes in the proximal posterior aspect of the greater trochanter to allow repair of the capsule and deep rotators. The sutures are passed and then tied allowing a solid posterior repair (Fig. 6.22).

Summary

As Gibson wrote 60 years ago, the posterior approach is *facile princeps*; easily the first, an obvious leader. Nothing has changed today.

The main reasons for early revision of total hip arthroplasty (THA) are infection, dislocation, poor cup fixation, and femoral shaft fracture. The posterior approach allows excellent vision to assess these factors and manage any adverse event through the same incision. The acetabulum is clearly seen to allow accurate reaming and positioning of the cup and assessment of impingement. Various methods can be used to check leg length, offset, and stability with direct vision of the articulation. Cup fixation can be assessed and tested and screw placement if needed can be performed safely. The proximal femur and calcar are well visualized without excessive dissection to allow an accurate femoral neck cut, collar contact if required, and assessment of the calcar for undisplaced intraoperative fractures.

The posterior approach should be used and understood by all young arthroplasty surgeons before consideration of other approaches. More extensile approaches and osteotomies for revision surgery have been described but are beyond the scope of this chapter. The posterior approach however allows the surgeon to create a more extensile exposure if needed without changing patient position, or compromising the initial dissection.

> ### Key Points
>
> › The posterior approach is the universal incision for hip arthroplasty.
> › Good vision and care of soft tissues is more important than skin incision length.
> › The inferior gluteal nerve enters the deep surface of gluteus maximus 5 cm superior to the GT.
> › The Piriformis tendon is the key landmark to the posterior hip.
> › A strong anatomic repair of the posterior capsule and external rotators is essential.

References

1. Gibson A (1950) Posterior exposure of the hip joint. J Bone Joint Surg Br 32-B:183–186
2. Ling ZX and Kumar VP (2006) The course of the inferior gluteal nerve in the posterior approach to the hip. J Bone Joint Surg Br 88-B:1580–1583

6.1.8 Direct Two Incisions: Lateral Position

Robert Kipping

Patient Selection

This technique can be applied to the full spectrum of degenerative hip disease in all age groups irrespective of bone morphology. Obesity is not a contraindication.

Contraindications

On the femoral side: severe bone defects of the proximal femur, which require bony reconstruction via a transfemoral approach.

On the acetabular side: severely dysplastic hip joint with a pseudoarthrosis requiring reconstruction of the acetabular socket as described by Harris and other authors [1].

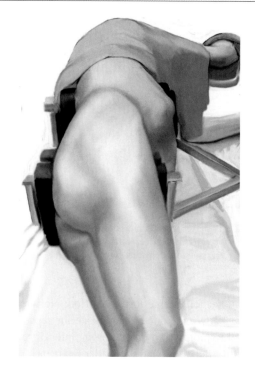

Fig. 6.23 Patient fixation in the lateral position (From Kipping [6] © Urban & Vogel)

Positioning and Incision Placement

The patient is securely fixed in the lateral decubitus position (Fig. 6.23). Once draped, the leg is placed in a slightly abducted position on a so called "Mayo-table," which is adjustable in height (Figs. 6.24 and 6.25).

The anterior incision is made in the palpable gap between the tensor fascia lata and the sartorius muscle in the region that would equate to the distal quarter of the Smith-Petersen approach [3, 4]. The posterior incision is made in line with the fibers of the gluteus maximus, midway between the posterior aspect of the greater trochanter and the ischial tuberosity. This is known as the Mini-Hardinge approach [5]. The length of each incision does not exceed 6–8 cm (Fig. 6.26).

Superficial Dissection

Anteriorly, the plane between the two muscles (tensor fascia lata and the sartorius) is developed manually until the femoral neck with the overlying capsule is palpable.

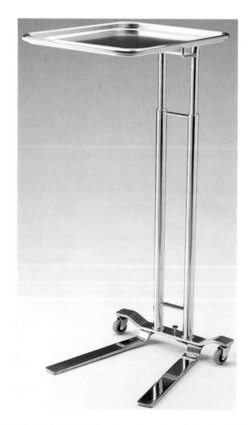

Fig. 6.24 "MAYO-table" undraped to place the leg in the lateral position (From Kipping [6] © Urban & Vogel)

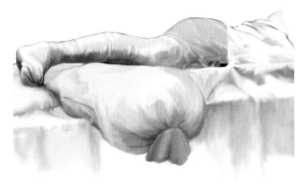

Fig. 6.25 Patient draped on the MAYO-table in the lateral position (From Kipping [6] © Urban & Vogel)

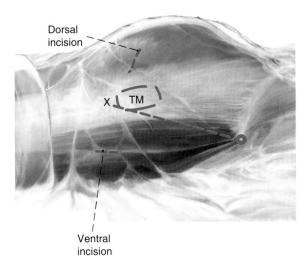

Fig. 6.26 Landmarks and incision lines frontal view (From Kipping [6] © Urban & Vogel)

Posteriorly, the fibers of gluteus maximus are separated manually until the external rotators are visible.

Deep Dissection

Anteriorly, a cobra retractor is placed around the femoral neck and Deaver retractors are placed medially and distally to expose the anteromedial aspect of the capsule. Then, the reflected head of the rectus femoris is dissected off the capsule and the latter is then opened. Osteophytes may be removed from the acetabular rim.

The surgeon then returns to the posterior window. A cobra retractor is placed between the glutei and the external rotators. The latter, apart from the piriformis, are cut together with the capsule. This creates a flap which exposes the posterior aspect of the femoral head.

The joint is then dislocated and the femur is internally rotated through 90°, flexed to 45°, and placed in an adducted position to enable the neck to be cut. The head is removed and the femoral canal broached easily under direct vision. The fit of a trial stem is then verified and left in place.

The leg is placed again on the "Mayo-table" and the surgeon moves back to the anterior window to ream and position the cup again under direct vision.

The trial stem is removed and replaced with the definitive stem. After positioning the final prosthesis, the stem is replaced into the socket.

Deep Repair and Closure

After copious wound lavage a deep drain is brought out anteriorly. A subcutaneous posterior drain may be used. Repair of the external rotators is not necessary. The subcutaneous tissue is closed in both wounds and skin closure may be performed with a resorbable suture.

Advantages

This double incision approach allows excellent visualization of the acetabulum and of the femoral canal via a direct approach without the requirement for navigation or fluoroscopy. Damage to the whole abductor group including the very sensitive fascia lata and the piriformis muscle can be avoided. No excessive force is necessary to expose the femur as compared to the anterolateral approach. Superior gluteal nerve palsy, which can sometimes occur when using a single anterolateral incision, is not observed.

Depending on the implant used, patients may commence full weight bearing in the first few days after surgery. Dislocation of the joint is observed less frequently than with other approaches [2–4]. Revision surgery, if needed, is easily performed by extending the minimally invasive incisions.

Disadvantages

The learning curve, even for experienced surgeons, is long. The first 20–30 operations should be supervised by a teacher who is familiar with the procedure. Precise lateral positioning of the patient is crucial, if optimal cup orientation is to be achieved.

References

1. Bauer R, Kerschbaumer F, Poisel S et al (1979) The transgluteal approach to the hip joint. Arch Orthop Trauma Surg 95:47–49
2. Berger RA (2003) Total hip arthroplasty using the minimally invasive two-incision approach. Clin Orthop Relat Res 417:232–241
3. Irving JF (2004) Direct two-incision total hip replacement without fluoroscopy. Orthop Clin North Am 35:173–181
4. Kipping R (2006) Der 2-Inzisionen-Zugang zur Implantation einer Hüfttotalendeprothese. Orthop Prax 42:598–603
5. Rittmeister M, Peters A (2005) Künstlicher Hüftgelenksersatz über eine posterior Mini-Inzision – Ergebnisse in 76 aufeinander folgenden Fällen. Z Orthop 143:403–411
6. Kipping R (2009) The standard implantation of a total hip prosthesis via two incisions. Oper Orthop Traumatol 21(3):335–348

Bearings

7

David Beverland

Content

J.-P. Vidalain et al. (eds.), *The CORAIL® Hip System*,
DOI: 10.1007/978-3-642-18396-6_7, © Springer-Verlag Berlin Heidelberg 2011

7.1 Tribological Aspects: To Wear or Not to Wear

John Fisher, Eileen Ingham, Louise Jennings, Zhongmin Jin, Joanne Tipper, and Sophie Williams

High demand, young and active patients need high performance bearings. Conventional polyethylene bearings have led to wear, osteolysis and failure in high demand patients. Alternative bearings, including: cross-linked polyethylene, metal on metal, ceramic on ceramic and ceramic on metal should be considered for high demand patients. The wear and tribological performance of these different bearing materials are described under normal walking conditions and under adverse conditions of rim loading, which can occur with incorrectly positioned components or abnormal anatomy. Bearing solutions are described that are predicted to give greater than 25 years lifetime in high demand patients.

Introduction

Wear with the associated risk of osteolysis is the major factor controlling the long-term survivorship of total hip replacements. In this chapter, the wear with associated osteolysis produced by historical metal on polyethylene bearings in the hip is compared to that produced by the new material combinations now available for high performance bearings. Relevant research from a single centre is reported and summarised.

Polyethylene Wear and Osteolysis: The Need for High Performance Bearings

Wear with the associated wear debris-induced osteolysis is the major cause of long-term failure in historical polyethylene bearings [14, 31, 32]. The failure pathways involve generation of polyethylene wear particles in the articulation [14] and adverse reactions to the wear particles in the periprosthetic tissues leading to macrophage activation, osteolysis and loosening [31, 32]. The wear of conventional polyethylene is determined by a number of independent variables including: oxidative stability,

counterface roughness, cross shear and the surface area being worn [19]. Polyethylene wear particles range in size from 10 to 100 μm [51, 54, 57], with the most biologically active being submicron in size [17, 26, 27, 43].

Historical polyethylene sterilised with gamma irradiation in the presence of air, was found to be susceptible to oxidative degradation, which led to an increased wear rate [15] and the generation of smaller and more reactive particles [5]. Since the late 1990s polyethylene has been sterilised by irradiation in an inert atmosphere or by alternative means, which has led to improved stability and resistance to oxidative degradation [31].

The wear of polyethylene is dependent on the surface roughness of the counterface [5], with an increased counterface roughness or discrete scratches or damage, substantially increasing the polyethylene wear rate [3, 4, 16, 54]. The use of a ceramic femoral head articulating against a polyethylene acetabular cup provides a smoother and more damage resistant counterface, which results in lower polyethylene wear rates [21, 44, 55].

The nature of the wear tracks, complexity of motion and resulting degree of cross shear also have a marked effect on wear. Linear tracks with low cross shear produce low wear [42], while multidirectional motions and higher levels of cross shear, as found in hip replacements, produce increased wear [2, 42]. Most recently, a fundamental quantitative relationship between cross shear and wear has been defined [37], which has now been used as an input to improved computational wear models [1, 24, 37–39].

The wear rate of 28 mm conventional polyethylene acetabular cups has been shown to be between 25 and 40 mm^3/million cycles [2, 3, 55, 58] depending on the material and quality of the femoral head. This agrees with retrieval studies [54] of conventional polyethylene bearings in the hip. In normal demand patients with conventional polyethylene who walk one million steps a year, it can take between 12 and 20 years to reach the threshold for osteolysis of 500 mm^3. However, for more active patients with up to two million steps per year or for hip prostheses with larger femoral heads articulating on conventional polyethylene, wear debris-induced osteolysis can occur in less than 10 years. This experience with conventional polyethylene and the concerns of failure due to wear debris-induced osteolysis, has resulted in the development of a range of new high performance bearings [31, 32] for higher demand patients and these are described in the following sections.

Cross-linked Polyethylene

Cross-linking of polyethylene was introduced in the late 1990s in order to reduce wear and to reduce oxidative degradation. There are a number of methods of cross-linking. Irradiation cross-linking in an inert atmosphere acts to reduce oxidative degradation, but does not eliminate it. Irradiation cross-linking in an inert atmosphere, followed by remelting, recombines the free radicals in the polymer, resulting in a much more stable material. Cross-linking is increased as irradiation dose is increased, with typical cross-linking levels of between 5 and 10 MRad being used in hip replacements. This level of cross-linking produces a two- to fivefold reduction in wear compared to conventional polyethylene [10, 20, 22, 23] with wear rates between 5 and 10 mm^3/million cycles; the lowest wear rate being with the 10 MRad material. Some companies and laboratories have reported a zero wear rate with cross-linked polyethylene in hip joint simulators. Scrutiny, however, indicates that the methods used either have reduced loading conditions or non-physiological, high levels of serum proteins that artificially reduce polyethylene wear. Physiologically relevant simulations have shown wear rates of 5–10 mm^3/million cycles, which is a 50–80% reduction compared to conventional polyethylene. This level of reduction in wear has also been reported in clinical studies. High levels of cross-linking also lead to a reduction in mechanical properties and in particular in the toughness of the polyethylene. This may result in an increased risk of rim fracture. It is recognised that rim loading of the acetabular insert by the head, due to microseparation, an incorrectly positioned cup or impingement occurs in many patients [19]. While conventional polyethylene cups with a thick cross-sectional wall can withstand this type of rim loading [58], highly cross-linked polyethylene inserts may not possess sufficient toughness. Medium levels of cross-linking of polyethylene of 5–7 MRad are recommended in hip replacements.

While there is substantially less volume of wear debris produced by cross-linked polyethylene, it has been shown that the wear particles are smaller and more reactive, so the extension of the osteolysis free lifetime may not be as great as indicated by the reduction in volumetric wear [33]. A ceramic head articulating on medium cross-linked polyethylene will provide an excellent tribological solution for many patients; however, it is questionable whether the reduction in wear and risk of osteolysis is adequate for the young high demand patient expecting 'fifty active years after fifty.' Alternative hard on hard bearings need to be considered.

Metal on Metal Bearings

Metal on metal bearings manufactured from cobalt chrome alloys have lower wear rates than polyethylene bearings, due to the hardness of the metallic alloy. The wear rates under normal walking conditions have been reported to be between 0.1 and 1 mm^3/million cycles [12, 13], depending on the lubrication conditions. Metal on metal bearings operate under the mixed lubrication condition [36] and are sensitive to the loading regime and protein concentration of the lubricant. High serum concentration and low swing phase load have been shown to reduce friction and metal wear rates [6, 60] by improving the mixed lubrication regime. Wear has been shown to be higher during the initial bedding in phase of wear, after which the surfaces become more conforming, the lubrication is enhanced and wear is reduced [12, 13, 30, 40]. Bearings with a larger radial clearance have higher initial bedding in wear [40], but after initial bedding in, the conformity of the worn bearings with different clearances converge and the steady state wear rates are similar. Larger diameter heads have reduced initial wear due to greater conformity [30, 40]. Although a larger head theoretically gives better lubrication [36] for head sizes above 40 mm, no significant reduction in long-term wear has been found [40].

There has been much debate regarding the metallurgy of metal on metal bearings. It has been clearly shown that high carbon cobalt chrome alloys should be used in preference to low carbon alloys, which give high wear [13, 53]. There is, however, no significant difference in the wear between as-cast and wrought bearings and between as-cast and as-cast and heat treated bearings, assuming high carbon content alloys are used [34, 48]. There is a long history of success of metal on metal bearings and when they wear at low levels they can last for very long periods of time [9]. In well-functioning metal on metal bearings, the mechanical and corrosive wear mechanisms, the wear particles and the metal ion release is reduced due to effective protein boundary layers on the surface of the cup and head [50, 62, 63]. The wear rates quoted above for standard walking conditions of 0.1–1 mm³/million cycles are equivalent to combined metal ion levels in the patient of 1–10 parts per billion. At these low levels of wear and ion release, adverse reactions to the particles or ions have not been documented. Wear particles from cobalt chrome metal on metal bearings are in the nanometre size range (10–100 μm) and readily distributed around the body. At high concentrations, the wear particles have been shown to be cytotoxic to cells in vitro, and at sub-cytotoxic concentrations they have been shown to be genotoxic [7, 8, 25, 49]. However, for well-functioning prostheses, metal ion and particle concentrations are low and do not cause adverse reactions. The exception to this is in the low percentage of patients who are immunologically sensitive to metal ions, for whom metal on metal bearings are contraindicated.

Metal ion levels of 10–100 parts per billion, however, have been reported in some patients, which is consistent with a much higher wear rate. Elevation of wear has been simulated in the laboratory by steeply inclined cups, which leads to rim loading, and by microseparation (offset deficiency) and rim loading [41, 61]. In these cases, wear rates of up to 10 mm³/million cycles have been recorded, and this is consistent with the increase in clinical ion levels. Offset deficiency, joint laxity and microseparation have been shown to generate the highest wear rates. Clinically, steep cup angles and cups with a low profile or coverage of the head have been associated with elevated metal ion levels. There is evidence emerging that microseparation and accelerated rim wear can produce a greater number of larger particles, which are more likely to be retained around the joint (rather than disseminated around the body as with small particles) and therefore cause adverse local reactions and masses or pseudo-tumours in periprosthetic tissues Metal on metal bearings require good surgical technique and do not tolerate variations in cup position or head position and offset, without introducing rim loading and substantial increases in wear. Under these conditions increased wear can cause elevated ion levels and local adverse reactions in periprosthetic tissues. Total hip replacements, which have fuller cup coverage of the head provide a more robust solution and better tolerate variations in surgical position, resulting in less variation in clinical wear rates. Clinically, it is the high wear bearings associated with rim wear that cause early failure.

Ceramic on Ceramic

The alumina ceramic on ceramic bearing is the hardest and lowest wearing of the bearing surfaces, with wear rates under standard walking conditions of 0.01–0.1 mm³/million cycles [46]. Unlike metal on metal, an increase in cup angle up to 60° has not been shown to increase wear. Clinically, low wear has also been recorded [47]. However, retrieved components have shown stripe wear on the head and wear on the rim of the cup [45, 47]. While this type of wear is not generated by steeply inclined cups, we have shown that it is produced by microseparation of the head and cup (by as little as 0.5 mm) and this can increase the wear rates in alumina ceramic bearings up to 1 mm³/million cycles. The rate of stripe wear has been validated against retrievals. This level of wear is still much less than with cross-linked polyethylene. Under standard conditions without rim wear, the ceramic wear particles produced are nanometre in size, but with rim wear, larger particles up to 1 μ in size have also been demonstrated [28, 56].). This bimodal distribution of wear particle size has been found in simulators under microseparation and from retrieved tissues [28, 56]. Biocompatibility studies of alumina ceramic wear particles have shown that they are far less cytotoxic compared to metal on metal particles [25] and that they have a lower potential to induce inflammation compared to polyethylene wear particles [29]. In the last 5 years alumina ceramic matrix composite bearings have become available (Biolox® Delta, CeramTec). This material has a higher toughness, a reduced risk of fracture and a reduced wear compared to alumina ceramic (Biolox® Forte, CeramTec). The wear of the composite is less than 0.5 mm³/million cycles under microseparation and rim wear conditions [52] The alumina ceramic matrix composite bearing couple is the lowest wearing combination under standard and under rim wear conditions. There remain concerns, however, about fracture of the acetabular insert in a limited number of patients and potential for chipping of the insert, either during insertion in the cup or following rim loading.

Ceramic on Metal

The hard on hard bearings, metal on metal and ceramic on ceramic are 'like on like' bearings, an approach rarely adopted in tribological science. Such bearing combinations results in stripe wear on the head when rim loading occurs. The concept of a ceramic on metal bearing was introduced to produce a hard on hard bearing couple with different materials and differential hardness [11, 58]. The harder ceramic head articulating on the lower hardness metal insert avoids stripe wear of the head during microseparation and rim loading. The ceramic head acts to reduce the corrosive wear found in metal on metal bearings, while the metal insert eliminates the risk of insert fracture or chipping in ceramic on ceramic bearings. The metal insert can be designed with a lower thickness than a ceramic insert which means that in the ceramic on metal bearing, a 36 mm head and insert can be used with a 50 mm acetabular shell, as compared to a 52 mm shell with a ceramic insert. The volumetric wear rates of ceramic on metal bearings have been shown to be equivalent to ceramic on ceramic bearings under both standard and microseparation rim loading conditions, that is 0.01–0.1 mm³/million cycles under standard conditions and approximately 1 mm³/million cycles under microseparation conditions. This is between two and ten times less than metal on metal bearings [11, 58]. Clinical studies [35, 58] have shown a reduction in metal ion levels compared to metal on metal bearings. The ceramic on metal bearing is now available worldwide as part of the Pinnacle™ (DePuy) bearing series.

Discussion

A range of different bearing options is now available for high demand patients. A ceramic or metal femoral head on cross-linked polyethylene represents the bearing of choice for many patients. For very high demand patients with potentially 'fifty active years after fifty,' the performance of alternative hard on hard bearings, which produce much lower wear than cross-linked polyethylene [18], is needed. This review has emphasised the importance of rim loading and microseparation in predicting clinical wear and the need to evaluate all bearing combinations under these conditions. It reinforces the importance of good surgical technique in both cup position and in terms of restoration of the offset.

Acknowledgements Support for research has been received from EPSRC, The Wellcome Trust – Centre of excellence in medical engineering WT 088908/z/09/z. ARC, NIHR, LMBRU, FCRF.

Industry support has been received from, DePuy, CeramTec, Mathys, JRI, BITECIC, Tissue Regenix, Corin.

References

1. Barbour PSM, Barton DC, Fisher J (1995) The influence of contact stress on the wear of UHMWPE for total replacement hip prostheses. Wear 181:250–257
2. Barbour PSM, Stone MH, Fisher J (1999) A hip joint simulator study using simplified loading and motion cycles generating physiological wear paths and rates. Proc Instn Mech Eng H 214:455–467
3. Barbour PSM, Stone MH, Fisher J (2000) A hip joint simulator study using new and physiologically scratched femoral heads with ultra-high molecular weight polyethylene acetabular cups. Proc Instn Mech Eng H 214:569–576
4. Besong AA, Hailey JL, Ingham E et al (1997) A study of the combined effects of shelf ageing following irradiation in air and counterface roughness on the wear of UHMWPE. Biomed Mater Eng 7:59–65
5. Besong AA, Tipper JL, Ingham E et al (1998) Quantitative comparison of wear debris from UHMWPE that has and has not been sterilised by gamma irradiation. J Bone Joint Surg Br 80:340–344
6. Brockett C, Williams S, Jin ZM et al (2007) Friction of total hip replacements with different bearings and loading conditions. J Biomed Mater Res B Appl Biomater 13:508–515
7. Brown C, Fisher J, Ingham E (2006) Biological effects of clinically relevant wear particles from metal-on-metal hip prostheses. Proc Instn Mech Eng H 220:355–369
8. Brown C, Williams S, Tipper JL et al (2007) Characterisation of wear particles produced by metal on metal and ceramic on metal hip prostheses under standard and microseparation simulation. J MaterSci Mater Med 18:819–827
9. Clarke MT, Darrah C, Stewart T et al (2005) Long-term clinical, radiological and histopathological follow-up of a well-fixed McKee-Farrar metal-on-metal total hip arthroplasty. J Arthroplasty 20:542–546
10. Endo M, Tipper JL, Barton DC et al (2002) Comparison of wear, wear debris and functional biological activity of moderately crosslinked and non-crosslinked polyethylenes in hip prostheses. Proc Instn Mech Eng H 216:111–122
11. Firkins PJ, Tipper JL, Ingham E et al (2001) A novel low wearing differential hardness, ceramic-on-metal hip joint prostheses. J Biomech 34:1291–1298
12. Firkins PJ, Tipper JL, Ingham E et al (2001) Influence of simulator kinematics on the wear of metal-on-metal hip prostheses. Proc Instn Mech Eng H 215:119–121

13. Firkins PJ, Tipper JL, Saadatzadeh MR et al (2001) Quantitative analysis of wear and wear debris from metal-on-metal hip prostheses tested in a physiological hip joint simulator. Biomed Mater Eng 11:143–157

14. Fisher J, Dowson D (1991) Tribology of artificial joints. Proc Instn Mech Eng H 205H:73–79

15. Fisher J, Chan KL, Hailey JL et al (1995) Preliminary study of the effect of ageing following irradiation on the wear of ultrahigh-molecular-weight polyethylene. J Arthroplasty 10:689–692

16. Fisher J, Firkins P, Reeves EA et al (1995) The influence of scratches to metallic counterfaces on the wear of ultra-high molecular weight polyethylene. Proc Instn Mech Eng H 209:263–264

17. Fisher J, Bell J, Barbour PSM et al (2001) A novel method for the prediction of functional biological activity of polyethylene wear debris. Proc Instn Mech Eng H 215:127–132

18. Fisher J, Jin Z, Tipper J et al (2006) Tribology of alternative bearings. Clin Orthop Relat Res 453:25–34

19. Fisher J, Jennings LM, Galvin AL et al (2010) 2009 Knee Society Presidential Guest Lecture: polyethylene wear in total knees. Clin Orthop Relat Res 468:12–18

20. Galvin AL, Tipper JL, Ingham E et al (2005) Nanometre size wear debris generated from crosslinked and non-crosslinked ultra high molecular weight polyethylene in artificial joints. Wear 259:977–983

21. Galvin AL, Williams S, Hatto P et al (2005) Comparison of wear of ultra high molecular weight polyethylene acetabular cups against alumina ceramic and chromium nitride coated femoral heads. Wear 259:972–976

22. Galvin AL, Kang L, Tipper JL et al (2006) Wear of cross-linked polyethylene under different tribological conditions. J Mater Sci Mater Med 17:235–243

23. Galvin AL, Tipper JL, Jennings LM et al (2007) Wear and biological activity of highly crosslinked polyethylene in the hip under low serum protein concentrations. Proc Instn Mech Eng H 221:1–10

24. Galvin AL, Kang L, Udofia I et al (2009) Effect of conformity and contact stress on wear in fixed-bearing total knee prostheses. J Biomech 42:1898–1902

25. Germain MA, Hatton A, Williams S et al (2003) Comparison of the cytotoxicity of clinically relevant cobalt-chromium and alumina ceramic wear particles *in vitro*. Biomaterials 24:469–479

26. Green TR, Fisher J, Stone MH et al (1998) Polyethylene particles of a 'critical size' are necessary for the induction of cytokines by macrophages *in vitro*. Biomaterials 19: 2297–2302

27. Green TR, Fisher J, Matthews JB et al (2000) Effect of size and dose on bone resorption activity of macrophages by *in vitro* clinically relevant ultra high molecular weight polyethylene particles. J Biomed Mater Res Appl Biomater 53:490–497

28. Hatton A, Nevelos JE, Nevelos AA et al (2002) Alumina-alumina artificial hip joints. Part I: a histological analysis and characterisation of wear debris by laser capture micro-dissection of tissues retrieved at revision. Biomaterials 23(16):3429–3440

29. Hatton A, Nevelos JE, Matthew JB et al (2003) Effects of clinically relevant alumina ceramic wear particles on TNF-α production by human peripheral blood mononuclear phago-cytes. Biomaterials 24:1193–1204

30. Hu XQ, Isaac GH, Fisher J (2004) Changes in contact area during the bedding-in of different sizes of metal on metal hip prostheses. Biomed Mater Eng 14:145–149

31. Ingham E, Fisher J (2000) Biological reactions to wear debris in total joint replacement. Proc Instn Mech Eng H 214:21–37

32. Ingham E, Fisher J (2005) The role of macrophages in osteolysis of total joint replacement. Biomaterials 26:1271–1286

33. Ingram JH, Stone M, Fisher J et al (2004) The influence of molecular weight, crosslinking and counterface roughness on TNF-alpha production by macrophages in response to ultra high molecular weight polyethylene particles. Biomaterials 25:3511–3522

34. Isaac GH, Thompson J, Williams S et al (2006) Metal-on-metal bearings surfaces: materials, manufacture, design, optimization, and alternatives. Proc Instn Mech Eng H 220:119–133

35. Isaac GH, Brockett C, Breckon A et al (2009) Ceramic-on-metal bearings in total hip replacement: whole blood metal ion levels and analysis of retrieved components. J Bone Joint Surg Br 91:1134–1141

36. Jin ZM, Dowson D, Fisher J (1997) Analysis of fluid film lubrication in artificial hip joint replacements with surfaces of high elastic modulus. Proc Instn Mech Eng H 211: 247–256

37. Kang L, Galvin AL, Brown TD et al (2008) Quantification of the effect of cross-shear on the wear of conventional and highly cross-linked UHMWPE. J Biomech 41:340–346

38. Kang L, Galvin AL, Brown TD et al (2008) Wear simulation of ultra-high molecular weight polyethylene hip implants by incorporating the effects of cross-shear and contact pressure. Proc Inst Mech Eng H 222:1049–1064

39. Kang L, Galvin AL, Fisher J et al (2009) Enhanced computational prediction of polyethylene wear in hip joints by incorporating cross-shear and contact pressure in additional to and sliding distance: effect of head diameter. J Biomech 42:912–918

40. Leslie I, Williams S, Brown C et al (2008) Effect of bearing size on the long-term wear, wear debris, and ion levels of large diameter metal-on-metal hip replacements-an in vitro study. J Biomed Mater Res B Appl Biomater 87: 163–172

41. Leslie IJ, Williams S, Isaac G et al (2009) High cup angle and microseparation increase the wear of hip surface replacements. Clin Orthop Relat Res 467:2259–2265

42. Marrs H, Barton DC, Jones RA et al (1999) Comparative wear under four different tribological conditions of acetylene enhanced crosslinked ultra high molecular weight polyethylene. J Mater Sci Mater Med 10:333–342

43. Matthews JB, Besong AA, Green TR et al (2000) Evaluation of the response of primary human peripheral blood mononuclear phagocyted to challenge with *in vitro* generated clinically relevant UHMWPE particles of known size and dose. J Biomed Mater Res Appl Biomater 52:296–307

44. Minakawa H, Stone MH, Wroblewski BM et al (1998) Quantification of third-body damage and its effect on UHMWPE wear with different types of femoral head. J Bone Joint Surg Br 80:894–899

45. Nevelos J, Ingham E, Doyle C et al (2000) Microseparation of the centers of alumina-alumna artificial hip joints during simulator testing produces clinically relevant wear and patterns. J Arthroplasty 15:793–795

46. Nevelos JE, Ingham E, Doyle C et al (2001) The influence of acetabular cup angle on the wear of "Biolox® Forte" alumina ceramic bearing couples in a hip joint simulator. J Mater Sci Mater Med 12:141–144

47. Nevelos JE, Prudhommeaux F, Hamadouche M et al (2001) Comparative analysis of two different types of alumina-alumina hip prosthesis retrieved for aseptic loosening. J Bone Joint Surg Br 83:598–603

48. Nevelos J, Shelton JC, Fisher J (2004) Metallurgical considerations in the wear of metal-on-metal hip bearings. Hip Int 14:1–10

49. Papageorgiou I, Brown C, Schins R et al (2007) The effect of nano- and micron-sized particles of cobalt-chromium alloy on human fibroblasts in vitro. Biomaterials 28:2946–2958

50. Pourzal R, Theissmann R, Williams S et al (2009) Subsurface changes of a MoM hip implant below different contact zones. J Mech Behav Biomed Mater 2:186–191

51. Richards L, Brown C, Stone MH et al (2008) Identification of nanometre-sized ultra-high molecular weight polyethylene wear particles in samples retrieved in vivo. J Bone Joint Surg Br 90:1106–1113

52. Stewart TD, Tipper JL, Insley G et al (2003) Long-term wear of ceramic matrix composite materials for hip prostheses under severe swing phase microseparation. J Biomed Mater Res B Appl Biomater 66:567–573

53. Tipper JL, Firkins PJ, Ingham E et al (1999) Quantitative analysis of the wear and wear debris from low and high carbon content cobalt chrome alloys used in metal on metal total hip replacements. J Mater Sci Mater Med 10:355–362

54. Tipper JL, Ingham E, Hailey JL et al (2000) Quantitative analysis of polyethylene wear debris, wear rate and head damage in retrieved Charnley® hip prostheses. J Mater Sci Mater Med 11:117–124

55. Tipper JL, Firkins PJ, Besong AA et al (2001) Characterisation of wear debris from UHMWPE on zirconia ceramic, metal-on-metal and alumina ceramic-on-ceramic hip prostheses generated in a physiological anatomical hip joint simulator. Wear 250:120–128

56. Tipper JL, Hatton A, Nevelos JE et al (2002) Alumina-alumina artificial hip joints. Part II: characterisation of the wear debris from in vitro hip joints simulations. Biomaterials 23:3441–3448

57. Tipper JL, Galvin AL, Williams S et al (2006) Isolation and characterization of UHMWPE wear particles down to ten nanometers in size from in vitro hip and knee joint simulators. J Biomed Mater Res A 78:473–480

58. Williams S, Butterfield M, Stewart T et al (2003) Wear and deformation of ceramic-on-polyethylene total hip replacements with joint laxity and swing phase microseparation. Proc Instn Mech Eng H 217:147–153

59. Williams S, Schepers A, Isaac G et al (2007) The 2007 Otto Aufranc Award. Ceramic-on-metal hip arthroplasties. A comparative in vitro and in vivo study. Clin Orthop Relat Res 465:23–32

60. Williams S, Jalai-Vahid D, Brockett CL et al (2006) Effect of swing phase load on metal-on-metal hip lubrication, friction and wear. J Biomech 39:2274–2281

61. Williams S, Leslie I, Isaac G et al (2008) Tribology and wear of metal-on-metal hip prostheses: influence of cup angle and head position. J Bone Joint Surg Am 90:111–117

62. Yan Y, Neville A, Dowson D et al (2008) Tribo-corrosion analysis of wear and metal ion release interactions from metal-on-metal and ceramic-on-metal contacts for the application in artificial hip prostheses. Proc Instn Mech Eng J 222:483–492

63. Yan Y, Neville A, Dowson D et al (2009) The influence of swing phase load on the electrochemical response, friction and ion release of metal on metal bearings. Proc Inst Mech Eng J 223:303–309

Cups

David Beverland

8

Contents

J.-P. Vidalain et al. (eds.), *The CORAIL® Hip System*,
DOI: 10.1007/978-3-642-18396-6_8, © Springer-Verlag Berlin Heidelberg 2011

8.1 Positioning the Acetabular Cup Using TAL: A Reliable Landmark

David Beverland and Pooler Archbold

In total hip arthroplasty (THA) excessive retroversion is associated with posterior instability, anterior impingement, and resultant groin pain. Excessive anteversion can lead to anterior instability and posterior impingement. The transverse acetabular ligament (TAL) straddles the inferior limit of the bony acetabulum. It is a strong load-bearing structure and in the normal hip, in association with the labrum, provides part of the load-bearing surface for the femoral head. It is our hypothesis that the TAL, in combination with the labrum, defines the normal version of the acetabulum. In Belfast, we found that using the TAL helped reduce our primary dislocation rate from 3.7% to 1%. In 50% of cases TAL is covered by either soft tissue or bone, but with care and a good exposure it can be found in well over 99% of cases. It has a number of advantages:

It is independent of patient positioning
It allows an individualised version for each patient
It is easy to teach and consistently present
It is valuable in MIS surgery

If the acetabular cup is cradled by and lies just deep to the TAL, we feel this helps to restore the acetabular joint centre. However, the TAL does not help with inclination. We recommend a maximum of 35° of operative inclination when using the posterior approach.

Introduction

Ensuring the placement of the acetabular component in an optimal position during THA is a complex problem. Correct cup orientation is critical to achieving stability, maximising range of motion and limiting wear. An intricate interplay exists between the cup position, cup orientation and the soft tissue balance of the hip. As proximal femoral and acetabular anatomy vary, a universally applicable set target for ideal cup orientation is hard to justify.

Instead a need has existed to develop and establish a reproducible and easy to use method that controls cup positioning to a patient-specific location. At our institution it has been our hypothesis that the transverse acetabular ligament (TAL) can be used to do this. Although still excised by some surgeons the TAL has been used by the senior author (DB) as the sole control of acetabular cup version in >5,500 consecutive THAs. Archbold et al. [1] in a published series of 1,000 consecutive hips, in which they used this technique to control cup version, had an acceptably low dislocation rate of 0.6%. This was using a 28 mm head with a standard posterolateral approach in combination with repair of the posterior capsule. Many factors contribute to dislocation, but correct placement of the cup is critical. This chapter examines the evidence for TAL-based cup placement and provides a detailed overview of this quick and simple to use technique, which is independent of patient position.

One of the most widely referenced papers on acetabular component orientation was published in 1978 by Lewinnek et al. [5]. With respect to version it recommended a "safe range" of 15° of anteversion (±10°). This was based on the x-ray analysis of 9 dislocations out of 300 total hip arthroplasties (THAs) done by five different surgeons. Six of the nine patients that dislocated had had a previous operation. Of the nine patients that dislocated three had an anterior dislocation and each had an anteversion of 25° or more, which was significantly different compared to those that did not dislocate where the average was 15.6°. The five posterior dislocations had an average anteversion of 19.2° which was not different. The "safe range" quoted in this paper should be viewed with caution because of the small numbers involved and the diversity of the group. Also x-rays were only available for analysis in 113 of the 291 hips that did not dislocate. Perhaps the most important conclusion of the paper was 'Acetabular component orientation is not the only factor (causing dislocation) as demonstrated by the fact that the most experienced surgeon in this study had only one dislocation out of 190 cases. He did not place a significantly greater number of acetabular cups within the safe range than did the other surgeons.' In reality, all experienced surgeons use subtle internal landmarks that are often difficult to explain and hard to reproduce. Furthermore, this more experienced surgeon was the only one to repair the posterior capsule.

In contrast to the version we have more proven boundaries when it comes to a safe range for abduction (inclination) angles for the cup. It is widely acknowledged that radiographic abduction angles above 50° are to be avoided. Patil et al. [8] demonstrated increased polyethylene wear with abduction angles >45°. De Haan et al. [3] found increased metal ion levels in large metal-on-metal articulations with inclinations >55°. Clearly, abduction angles are easier to measure than anteversion on the traditional anteroposterior x-ray and this could, in part, explain the greater emphasis and focus on abduction. Although we personally consider that anteversion and abduction of the cup are of equal importance, we think the crucial difference between them is the fact that the natural variation in version is much greater than for inclination. As a consequence, an excessive anteversion in one patient could be inadequate in another. This does not apply to inclination where the normal variation is smaller.

From our institution Archbold et al. [2] reported on 25 consecutive patients, who were being investigated for labral tears with an MRI arthrogram of the hip. The use of contrast allowed us to visualise the transverse acetabular ligament (TAL) and labrum and we were then able to look at the orientation of the plane created by these structures. This plane was determined manually by selecting points on the TAL and labrum. The best fit plane through these points was determined and its orientation expressed with respect to a constructed pelvic coordinate system. Perhaps, not surprisingly, we found very similar answers to the quoted literature in that the average operative anteversion of the TAL-labrum plane was 23.0° and the average abduction was 45.6°. However, the range for anteversion was >30° (5.3–36.1°) whereas the range for inclination was <12° (38.4–50.3°).

Based on these results, if firstly during surgery we aimed for and successfully achieved 20° of anteversion for every patient and secondly if we accept the philosophy that anteversion should be patient-specific, then for some patients the angle will either be too anteverted or too retroverted by 15°. The other problem is actually being able to correctly position the cup at 20° anteversion. There are surgeon factors and patient factors that make this difficult. Firstly from the surgeon's perspective, as can be appreciated from Fig. 8.1, we are generally not good at judging 20° and secondly, with respect to patient factors, positioning on the operating table is the main issue. This is particularly true with the lateral decubitus position where it is difficult to ensure correct patient position at the start of surgery compounded by the potential for the patient to move during surgery.

With respect to cup version, the ideal solution would be a patient-specific landmark that was easy

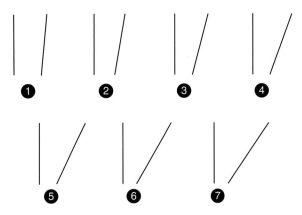

Fig. 8.1 Demonstrating the difficulty in judging which two lines are at 20° to each other. 7 = 35°, 6 = 30°, 5 = 25°, 4 = 20°, 3 = 15°, 2 = 10°, 1 = 5°

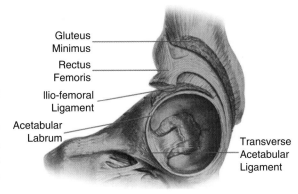

Fig. 8.2 Anatomical dissection illustrating that the TAL and labrum form a recognisable plane. Also emphasising the importance of good exposure during surgery if using the TAL (Adapted from Grant's *Atlas of Anatomy*)

to find, easy to use effectively and was independent of patient position on the table. We feel that the TAL, in combination with the labrum, provides at least one viable solution. Figure 8.2 shows an anatomical dissection that clearly illustrates that the TAL and labrum form a natural plane, but if you are going to use TAL for version you must see it as clearly as this. The key to using TAL is good exposure.

Surgical Technique

We use the posterior approach with the patient in the lateral decubitus position. The hip is dislocated and

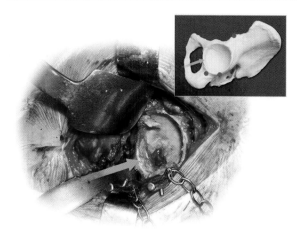

Fig. 8.3 Acetabular exposure during surgery showing the various retractors with a green arrow pointing to the TAL

the femoral head resected. A calliper is then used to measure femoral head diameter. If, for example femoral head diameter was 48 mm, then we feel that the acetabular cup size should be a maximum of 4 mm bigger or 52 mm.

Acetabular exposure is as shown in Fig. 8.3. The first Charnley pin goes into the ischium followed by a second Charnley pin into the posterior wall of the acetabulum, being careful that it does not go into the acetabulum. The anterior retractor goes anteriorly and superiorly so as not to go over the anterior wall. Placing this retractor over the anterior wall can damage the anterior wall and will also increase the risk of neurovascular injury because of the proximity of these structures. The exposure is then completed by placing an inferior teardrop retractor beneath the TAL.

As reported by Archbold et al. [1] we have created a classification of TAL based on 1,000 consecutive cases as shown in the table below.

So, in half the cases (49%), the TAL is immediately visible on exposing the acetabulum. But this means in the other half the surgeon has to make an effort to find and expose it. Approximately one-third (35.1%) are Grade II, which means the TAL is covered by soft tissue. In this situation, the soft tissue can be easily cleared by a combination of blunt and sharp dissection. The remainder (15.6%) are grade III and in this grade the TAL is covered by osteophyte. This can be removed to expose the TAL by using a small diameter reamer which is directed in a caudal direction. This needs to be done slowly and carefully so as to avoid damage to the TAL. The surgeon has to alternate between reaming and looking until the fibers of the TAL start to appear. There is also the rare (0.3%) grade IV TAL which cannot be found. In this situation we feel that the surgeon has inadvertently destroyed it. The greatest risk of damage to the TAL occurs when it is covered by osteophytes (grade III).

Having exposed the acetabulum and TAL, attention can then focus on the labrum. In almost 95% of cases the posterior labrum is present and relatively undamaged as reported by Archbold et al. [1]. The posterior labrum can usually be retained as it does not obstruct preparation of the acetabulum. Its inner surface can be shaved with the scalpel leaving the distal free margin which in continuity with the TAL provides an aid to alignment. In contrast, the anterior and superior parts of the labrum, if still present, are frequently torn and need to be excised as they do impede and obstruct acetabular preparation. Also any remains of the Ligamentum Teres are removed from the floor of the acetabulum but it is our practice to leave the fat pad intact and not to remove it.

Having exposed the acetabulum, an acetabular reamer which is the same size as the original femoral head is then used as a 'cup sizer.' It is our hypothesis that in the *normal* acetabulum the TAL and labrum form a plane that comes just beyond the equator of the acetabulum unlike the bony acetabulum which is less than a hemisphere. If the hemispherical 'cup sizer' (reamer) is positioned so as to be cradled by the TAL and orientated so as to sit parallel to and just deep to the line formed by the TAL and the remaining posterior labrum, this we feel is the ideal location for the

Grading of TAL – I to IV based on 1,000 consecutive cases.			
I	Normal TAL	49%	Easily visible on exposure of the acetabulum
II	Covered by soft tissue	35.1%	Cleared by blunt and sharp dissection
III	Covered by osteophytes	15.6%	Cleared using an acetabular reamer
IV	No TAL identified	0.3%	

cup. In this position, there should be no anterior overhang, joint centre in terms of offset and height should be restored and version should be correct. Our aim is to put the definitive cup in the same location. The only difference is that we reduce the abduction angle.

In contrast to this technique, much traditional teaching has been to ream the acetabulum down to true floor, but if this is done the cup will sit too deep relative to TAL and the joint centre will have been medialised, which results in a decreased acetabular offset. This is usually also associated with the cup sitting higher than the original joint centre and thus offset and height are both incorrect with respect to restoration of joint centre.

As discussed above, the key thing about the cup sizer is that it is the same diameter as the original femoral head. There are situations where, when the surgeon introduces the cup sizer (acetabular reamer) into the acetabulum, the face of the reamer will sit proud of the TAL and posterior labral plane. This, we feel, represents a degree of acetabular dysplasia and in these situations there will usually have been a low centre edge angle on the preoperative x-ray. In this situation, the acetabulum has to be deepened in order to achieve adequate bony cover for the acetabular component. In so doing the cup will be inevitably medialised and the acetabular offset and usually the height will be decreased compared to the pre arthritic state of that hip. In such cases, correct joint tension can be restored by compensating for the lost acetabular offset by increasing the offset and height of the femoral component.

Initial reaming begins with a reamer that is smaller than the original head size except in cases of protusio when a reamer equal to or even bigger than original head diameter is used so as to avoid any further deepening of the acetabulum. When reaming, the reamer is kept parallel to the TAL except for the final reamer, which is moved eccentrically just before it is removed. This is because normally the teeth on acetabular reamers do not come as far as the equator and therefore unless the reamer handle is moved eccentrically the reamed acetabular cavity will not be hemispherical. For the system that we use, the acetabulum should be reamed size for size or a maximum of 1 mm smaller. At the completion of reaming, bleeding sub-chondral bone should be visible and the fat pad should still be intact. Even when the acetabulum has been deepened because of mild dysplasia reaming will not have gone

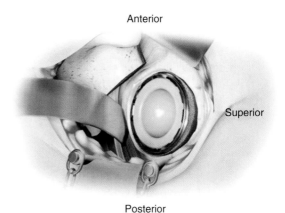

Fig. 8.4 Acetabular cup in place showing the exposed external surface of the cup both superiorly and posteriorly, but with no anterior overhang (Copyright DePuyInternational Limited)

as far as the true floor. Clearly, in the presence of significant dysplasia, the acetabulum may have to be reamed down to the true floor – this is uncommon in our practice.

When it comes to cup insertion, the cup will initially obscure the TAL. This can be counteracted by initially reducing the abduction angle (in lateral decubitus the surgeon lowers his/her hand). This then brings the TAL into view and the cup can be orientated so as to be parallel to the TAL. The surgeon can then lift his/her hand to the chosen abduction angle and then impact the cup. As discussed below, our recommendation is to aim for a maximum of 35° of operative inclination. Once the cup is in place the liner can then be inserted. It is critical that when the cup is inserted there is no anterior overhang. If the acetabular component is inserted parallel and just deep to the TAL, then there should be no anterior overhang and the cup should be flush with the psoas valley. In most cases, when using a cementless component, there will be exposed cup superiorly and posteriorly as shown in Fig. 8.4.

A summary of cup position is shown in Fig. 8.5. As can be seen from the figure we feel that by staying parallel to the TAL we can control version. In addition, by not reaming too deep to the TAL we can maintain acetabular offset. If the cup is deep to the TAL, then when using a cementless cup an offset liner can be used to compensate. Also by making sure the cup is cradled by the TAL we can ensure that the cup is not left too high.

Clearly, for the concept to be effective, the surgeon has to ensure that the cup is parallel to the TAL. As we

Cup too anteverted   Cup too retroverted

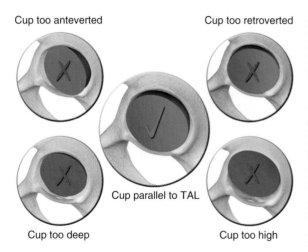

Cup parallel to TAL

Cup too deep   Cup too high

inclination. This is operative inclination as defined by Murray [6]. In lateral decubitus, this means that the cup introducer is held at 35° relative to the floor. This is based on work done in our institution by Hill et al. [4]. This work demonstrated that when using the lateral decubitus position, if the surgeon achieves 35° of operative inclination during surgery, this will, on average, translate to (35 + 13) 48° of radiographic inclination on the postoperative x-ray. Part of this 13° difference is predictably explained by the impact of operative anteversion, which increases radiographic inclination. This factor accounted for 6° of the difference, but the other 7° we feel is caused by adduction of the pelvis as a result of patient positioning as illustrated in Fig. 8.7.

Fig. 8.5 Central diagram is the ideal position with the cup parallel to the TAL and just deep to it. *Top left* is too anteverted. *Top right* is too retroverted. *Bottom left* is too deep and *bottom right* too high (From Archbold et al. [1]. Reproduced and adapted with permission and copyright © of the British Editorial Society of Bone and Joint Surgery)

Conclusion

The TAL is consistently present, patient-specific, independent of patient position on the operating table, easy to use and easy to teach. Previous work published from our institution by Ogonda et al. [7] has shown that it is also of value in MIS of the hip using the posterior approach. Most specifically, we feel that it helps to control version and restore joint centre, but not abduction angle. When using the posterior approach, we recommend that the surgeon aim for a maximum of 35° of operative inclination.

have already seen in Fig. 8.1, it is not easy to judge 20°, but how good are we at knowing when two lines are parallel? As can be confirmed in Fig. 8.6, the human eye is able to discern when two lines are out of parallel by only one degree.

The TAL does not assist with cup inclination, and when using the lateral decubitus position and the posterior approach we aim for a maximum of 35° of inclination.

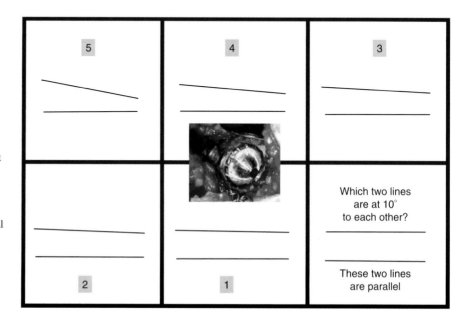

Fig. 8.6 Demonstrating that in contrast to the difficulty we have in judging 20° the human eye is very good at judging whether or not two lines are parallel. The central operative photograph shows the face of the cup lying parallel to the TAL. With respect to the diagrams −5 = 10°, 4 = 5°, 3 = 3°, 2 = 2°, 1 = 1°

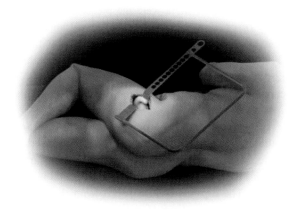

Fig. 8.7 Patient lying in lateral decubitus demonstrating the adducted position of the hip that we feel causes a secondary adduction of the pelvis (Copyright DePuyInternational Limited)

References

1. Archbold HAP, Mockford B, Molloy D et al (2006) The transverse acetabular ligament, an aid to acetabular component placement during total hip arthroplasty J Bone Joint Surg Br 88(7):883–886
2. Archbold H, Slomczykowski M, Crone M et al (2008) The relationship of the orientation of the transverse acetabular ligament and acetabular labrum to the suggested safe zones of cup positioning in total hip arthroplasty. Hip Int 18(1): 1–6
3. De Haan R, Pattyn C, Gill H et al (2008) Correlation between inclination of the acetabular component and metal ion levels in metal-on-metal hip resurfacing replacement. J Bone Joint Surg Br 90:1291–1297
4. Hill J, Gibson D, Pagoti R et al (2010) Photographical measurement of acetabular cup inclination in total hip arthroplasty using the posterior approach. J Bone Joint Surg Br 92:1209–1214
5. Lewinnek GE, Lewis JL, Tarr R et al (1978) Dislocations after total hip-replacement arthroplasties. J Bone Joint Surg Am 60:217–220
6. Murray DW (1993) The definition and measurement of acetabular orientation. J Bone Joint Surg Br 75: 228–232
7. Ogonda L et al (2005) A minimal-incision technique in total hip arthroplasty does not improve early postoperative outcomes. A prospective, randomized controlled trial. J Bone Joint Surg Am 87(4):701–710
8. Patil S, Bergula A, Chen P et al (2003)Polyethylene wear and acetabular component orientation. J Bone Joint Surg Am 85:56–63

8.2 Restoration of Acetabular Offset: Respecting the Hip Centre

Michel Bonnin and Michel-Henri Fessy

Conventional acetabular preparation consists of reaming down to the true floor. This technique medialises the centre of rotation of the hip (CRH) and can reduce the acetabular offset by up to 8.5 mm. In theory, this medialisation must be compensated for by increasing the offset of the femoral stem if the global offset is to be preserved. In contrast, an anatomical technique attempts to restore CRH relative to the acetabulum.

The purpose of the study was (1) to analyse the displacement of the CRH after simulated implantation of a total hip arthroplasty (THA), (2) to compare two acetabular positioning techniques, one conventional and one anatomical and (3) to analyse the consequences of anatomical placement in terms of acetabular offset, positioning and risk of cup overhang and protrusion. Our hypothesis is that the 'anatomical' technique makes it possible to achieve a better restoration of hip kinematics.

Introduction

During THA, global offset must be preserved in order to achieve proper function of the abductor muscles and to ensure that the hip is stable. Preoperatively, global offset depends on three factors; the anatomy of the proximal femur (femoral offset), the anatomy of the floor of the acetabulum (acetabular offset), and finally alteration of this anatomy as a result of the degenerative process (acquired change in offset) (Fig. 8.8).

There has been considerable focus on femoral offset both in terms of research and by the implant companies, and as a result femoral offset can be restored using prosthetic stems with a wide variety of head neck combinations (Sect. 4.2.6). There has been much less interest and fewer published studies on acetabular offset. *Conventional* acetabular preparation consists of reaming down to the true floor in order to optimise the bone anchorage and to limit the risks of prosthetic overhang, which can cause significant groin pain due to iliopsoas impingement. This technique medialises

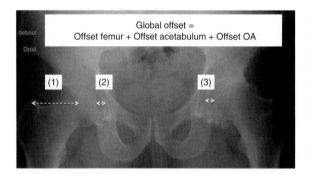

Fig. 8.8 Global offset of the hip depends on (1) the architecture of the upper end of the femur (femoral offset), (2) the anatomy of the floor of the acetabulum (acetabular offset) and finally (3) alteration of this anatomy as a result of the degenerative process (acquired change in offset)

the CRH and reduces the acetabular offset. In theory, this medialisation must be compensated for by the offset of the femoral stem, if the global offset is to be preserved.

Some authors would rather preserve the acetabular offset by maintaining a space between the true floor of the acetabulum and the acetabular cup [1, 7, 13]. To do this, they ream the acetabular cavity conservatively by stopping at the subchondral bone. This more *anatomical* technique makes it possible to limit the displacement of the CRH but can reduce the bone-cup contact surface and increase the risk of prosthetic overhang.

The purpose of the study was (1) to analyse the displacement of the CRH after simulated implantation of a THA, (2) to compare two acetabular positioning techniques, one conventional and one anatomical and (3) to analyse the consequences of anatomical placement in terms of acetabular offset, positioning and risk of cup overhang and protrusion.

Our hypothesis is that the 'anatomical' technique makes it possible to achieve a better restoration of hip kinematics.

Equipment and Methods

Fifty CT-scans of normal hips were selected from our large data bank of combined hip and knee scans that have been routinely performed in our centre prior to total knee arthroplasty since 2004 [3]. All patients signed an informed consent form and the Institutional Review Board (IRB) approved this retrospective

study. Exclusion criteria were the presence of a THA history of previous hip trauma or surgery and/or the presence of osteoarthritis. This provided us with the CT scans of 50 patients who had a total knee arthroplasty between 2008 and 2009. Their mean age was 73 years ± 8 (51–88), with 28 women (72 years ± 8) and 22 men (74 years ± 7).

All the scans had been performed using the same protocol with a multibar scanner (Siemens Sensation, Munich, Germany). The patients were placed in supine position, with extended knees, their feet set in neutral rotation. The hip had been scanned from the antero-inferior iliac spine down to the lesser trochanter, the knee from 5 cm above the upper rim of the patella down to the anterior tibial tuberosity. The study was carried out using the OsiriX® software, dedicated to the analysis of DICOM images (open-source software; http://homepage.mac.com/rossetantoine/osirix).

Femoral anteversion was measured after superimposition of the transverse section cut passing through the posterior femoral condyles and the femoral neck. Acetabular anteversion was determined on the transverse or horizontal cross section running through the middle of the femoral head. The femoral neck-shaft angle was determined from the appropriate CT coronal section.

In the transverse plane, the measurements were made on the section going through the level of the true floor of the acetabulum and cutting through the femoral head at the level of the fossa of the ligamentum teres. The centre of the femoral head (CF) was also referenced. The CRH was then determined after simulated implantation of the acetabular implant using each of the two techniques; firstly (a) with the acetabular cup in contact with the true floor of the acetabulum ("conventional" technique) and secondly (b) preserving acetabular offset, by positioning the cup at the level of the subchondral bone ("anatomical" technique). The theoretical diameter of the acetabular cup with these two techniques was also measured (Fig. 8.9). The CF–CRH distance was measured with respect to global distance, but also in terms of all three axes; mediolateral, longitudinal and anteroposterior.

For each of the two techniques, the global acetabular protrusion was defined as the distance measured between the centre of the simulated acetabular cup and the line linking the anterior and posterior walls of the acetabulum. In order to simulate surgical implantation, the cup was positioned in such a way that its anterior

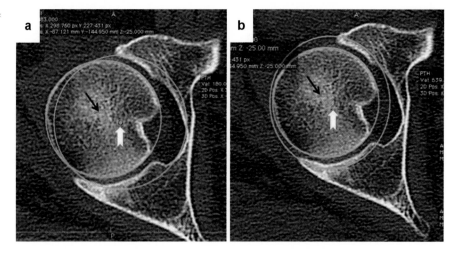

Fig. 8.9 (**a**) The centre of the femoral head (*black arrow*) and the centre of the simulated cup position as per the conventional technique (*white arrow*) are marked. The resultant CRH is displaced medially and posteriorly relative to the centre of the native femoral head by a significant amount. (**b**) The simulated cup is positioned as per the anatomical technique. The CRH (*white arrow*) is much closer to the centre of the femoral head

rim remained just deep to the anterior wall of the acetabulum. In this position, the posterior overhang of the cup relative to the posterior wall of the acetabulum was measured together with the cup anteversion. Thus we looked at both protrusion and posterior overhang.

Measurements of acetabular cup placement were then made in both the transverse and coronal planes. The CF of the femoral head was identified and then the CRH was determined using each of the two techniques, and finally the size of the cup was determined in the transverse plane. The CF–CRH distances were measured as a global distance and then along each of the three axes; longitudinal, mediolateral and anteroposterior.

Results

Prior to any intervention, femoral anteversion was $11.9° ± 10.5$ ($-8.9°$ to $37°$), the femoral neck-shaft angle was $132° ± 3.9$ ($124°–145°$) and the acetabular anteversion was $23.8° ± 6.8$ ($11–35°$). These values exhibited no significant differences between men and women. The femoral head diameter was 42.6 mm $± 2.5$ ($44–53$ mm) in women and 49.6 mm $± 2.7$ ($43–55$) in men ($p < 0.0001$).

After simulated cup implantation the global shift of the CRH was 1.04 mm $± 1.5$ ($0–4.4$) with the anatomical technique and 4.3 mm $± 1.8$ ($0–8.7$) with the conventional technique ($p < 0.0001$). Among the three components of the global shift, pure medialisation was 1.2 mm $± 1$ ($-1.5–3.7$) with the anatomical technique

and 4.0 mm $± 1.9$ (-1.5 to 8.5) with the conventional technique ($p < 0.0001$). Medialisation was greater than 5 mm in 46% of the cases with the conventional technique, but in no case when using the anatomical technique (Fig. 8.10). Posterior shift was $0.22 ± 0.6$ (-1.3 to 2) with the anatomical technique and $0.99 ± 0.9$ ($0–3.5$) with the conventional technique ($p < 0.0001$). Superior shift was 2.7 mm $± 1.5$ ($0–5.7$) with the anatomical technique and $3.9 ± 1.6$ ($0.4–7.7$) with the conventional technique ($p < 0.0001$). Differences between men and women were significant except for the posterior shift (Table 8.1).

No relationship was identified between the medialisation of the CRH and the neck-shaft angle (either with the conventional technique $r = 0.05$ or with the anatomical technique $r = 0.04$), nor with the femoral anteversion angle (with the conventional technique $r = 0.23$ or with the anatomical technique $r = 0.28$). Medialisation did correlate with the upward shift ($r = 0.44$ and $p = 0.01$) and with the posterior shift ($r = 0.4$ and $p = 0.01$). There was a significant relationship between the diameter of the femoral head and the CRH medialisation with the anatomical technique ($r = 0.477$ and $p = 0.001$) and the conventional technique ($r = 0.482$ and $p < 0.001$).

The diameter of the simulated cup was 52.4 mm $± 4$ ($44–63$) with the anatomical technique and 51.2 mm $± 4.2$ ($44–60$ mm) with the conventional technique ($p < 0.0001$). The protrusion of the centre of the cup relative to the anterior and posterior walls of the acetabulum was 1.6 mm $± 3.2$ (-8.4 to 5.1 mm) with the anatomical technique and -1.7 mm $± 2$ (-8.4 to 0.7 mm) with the conventional technique ($p < 0.0001$).

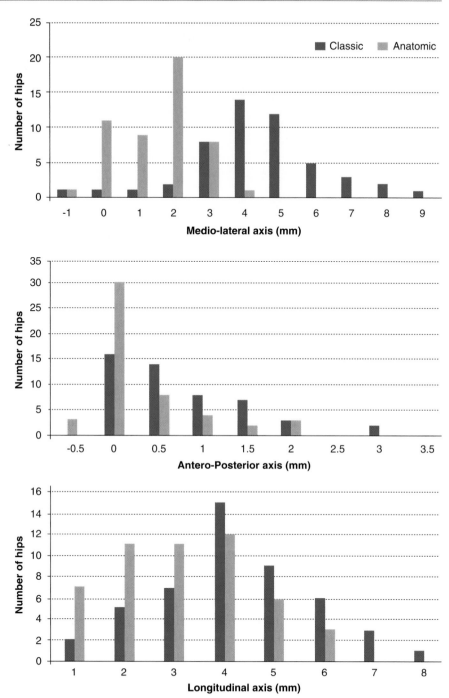

Fig. 8.10 Distribution of the displacement of the centre of rotation of the hip along the three axes (medial along the mediolateral axis, posteriorly along the anteroposterior axis and superiorly along the longitudinal axis) when comparing the two techniques of cup placement

The technique used had a net influence on the positioning of the cup and on the protrusion. Each cup was aligned such that its anterior rim sat just deep to the anterior wall of the bony acetabulum so as to avoid any impingement with the tendon of the iliopsoas. Using this method of placement the anteversion of the cup was $31.5° \pm (10–41.7°)$ with the anatomical technique and $23.1° \pm (9–35°)$ with the conventional technique ($p < 0.0001$) and the posterior overhang was 5.7 mm± (0–14.9 mm) with the anatomical technique and 0.62 mm± (0–3.6 mm) with the conventional technique ($p < 0.0001$).

Table 8.1 Results of the global series and in the men/women subgroups

	Techniques	Series mean ± SD (min-max)		<0.0001 Females mean ± SD (min-max)		Males mean ± SD(min-max)		P-value
Cup diameter	Classic	51.2 ± 4.25	(44 – 60)	48.2 ± 2.2	(44 – 54)	55 ± 2.9	(47 – 60)	<0.0001
	Anatomic	52.4 ± 4.4	(44 – 63)	49.2 ± 1.9	(44 – 54)	56.5 ± 3.3	(47 – 63)	<0.0001
	P-value			<0.0001*				
Translation of the Hip centre								
Medial	Classic	4.0 ± 1.9	(– 1.5 – 8.5)	3.7 ± 1.7	(– 1.5 – 5.4)	5.07 ± 1.5	(-1.5 – 8.5)	<0.0001
	Anatomic	1.2 ± 1.0	(– 1.5 – 3.7)	0.72 ± 0.9	(– 1.5 – 2.3)	1.81 ± 0.9	(-1.5 – 3.7)	<0.0001
	P-value			<0.0001*				
Posterior	Classic	0.99 ± 0.9	(0 – 3.5)	0.83 ± 0.7	(0 – 3.3)	1.19 ± 1.0	(0 – 3.5)	0.0081
	Anatomic	0.22 ± 0.6	(– 1.3 – 2)	0.22 ± 0.6	(– 1.3 –1.4)	0.33 ± 0.7	(– 1.2 – 2)	0.080
	P-value			<0.0001*				
Superior	Classic	3.9 ± 1.6	(0.4 – 7.7)	3.22 ± 1.6	(0.4 – 6.7)	4.72 ± 1.2	(3.4 – 7.7)	0.00038
	Anatomic	2.7 ± 1.5	(0 – 5.7)	2.13 ± 1.4	(0 – 5.7)	3.37 ± 1.5	(1 – 7.5)	0.0057
	P-value			<0.0001*				

*p<0.0001 between Classic Anatomic technique in the global series, in females and in males

Discussion

There is now a consensus on the importance of the restoration of the femoral offset in THA. The anatomical variations of the upper end of the femur have been widely analysed and the Corail® stem, with its wide range of available offsets, allows restoration of femoral offset in most cases.

In contrast, there have been few studies on acetabular offset and this issue is usually neglected. However, this study shows that depending on how the acetabulum is prepared, acetabular offset can change by up to 8.5 mm, which although less than the potential error on the femoral side, none the less is still very significant with respect to global offset and the CRH. To deal with this the surgeon has three options; (1) to decrease the acetabular offset by medialising the CRH and to compensate for this decrease by increasing the offset of the femoral component; (2) to decrease the acetabular offset and not compensate for the medialisation thus reducing global offset; (3) to preserve natural acetabular offset with conservative reaming of the acetabular floor, hoping to preserve the CRH and maintain normal acetabular offset.

A fourth option would be to use lateralised acetabular implants, but high wear and loosening rates have been reported with this type of implant [2].

Most studies that have analysed offset after THA looked at global offset [12]. Dorr studied the CRH shift by making measurements intraoperatively whilst using a navigation system. He reported a 3–6 mm medialisation and a 5 mm superior shift [6]. Sariali, analysed a series of 223 THAs in which the acetabulum had been implanted with minimum reaming; he reported a restoration of the position of the CRH with a mean precision of 0.73 mm in the craniocaudal or longitudinal direction, of 1.2 mm in the mediolateral direction, and 0.05 mm in the anteroposterior direction [13]. In these two studies, the measurements included the correction required to account for the arthritis-induced acquired offset. Likewise, Eggli [7] and Knight [10] report a medialisation of the acetabular cup of 3.4 and 5 mm, respectively, relative to their preoperative x-rays.

The purpose of our implant simulation study was to quantify the shift of the CRH during THA using a non-arthritic healthy hip as a reference and by comparing two surgical techniques. DICOM image analysis using the OsiriX® software eliminated the lack of accuracy linked to x-ray magnification and made it possible to make measurements with an accuracy higher than that of radiographic studies, studies on cadavers, and even those done using navigation [3]. Furthermore, the analysis of healthy hips made it possible to eliminate the alteration caused to CRH by degenerative change. Our objective was not to determine the best technique or the best strategy, but to analyse the anatomic consequences of the two techniques.

The limitations of this study are linked to the uncertainty of the positioning of the simulated prosthetic cup, to the limit of the subchondral bone for the anatomical technique, and to the contact with the acetabular floor for the conventional technique. In vivo reaming depends on the bone density and it is possible that the theoretical positioning does not correspond precisely to the surgical reality. Another weakness concerns the measurement of the posterior overhang of the simulated cup. Indeed, the anteversion was measured from the transverse section scan views, which were perpendicular to the longitudinal axis which does not correspond to the definition of operative anteversion [11]. Also, because our scans commenced below the anterior superior iliac spines we were unable to determine the anterior pelvic plane.

This study shows that the conventional technique of acetabular cup positioning leads to a medialisation greater than 2 mm in 90% of cases, greater than 5 mm in 43% of cases and can go up to 8.5 mm, which cannot be ignored [5, 8]. Global offset can be restored with a compensatory increase in the offset of the femoral stem but this modifies hip kinematics and the impact of this, as compared to the normal situation, is poorly understood [4, 9].

The conservative technique makes it possible to better maintain the CRH which is medialised by 2 mm or less in 82% of the cases. This medialisation only represents 1.5% of the lever arm of the abductors. However, this technique imposes the use of a cup with an increased diameter of 1.2 mm and with a posterior overhang that can reach up to 15 mm. Furthermore, with the anatomical technique, the anteversion of the acetabular cup had to be often increased to avoid anterior overhang which can be a source of iliopsoas impingement. This study was based on simulation and therefore it was not possible to compare the quality of bone anchorage when using these two techniques.

> A more anatomical preparation makes it possible to preserve the acetabular offset and to restore the hip kinematics.
> This in its turn requires caution so as to avoid anterior overhang.

Key Learning Points

> In a THA, the conventional medialisation of the acetabular component, down to the true floor leads to a medialisation of the CRH and a loss of acetabular offset that can reach 8.5 mm.
> The consequences of compensating for this loss of offset by increasing the femoral offset are poorly understood.

References

1. Archbold HA, Mockford B, Molloy D et al (2006) The transverse acetabular ligament: an aid to orientation of the acetabular component during primary total hip replacement. J Bone Joint Surg Br 88:883–886
2. Archibeck MJ, Cummins T, Junick DW et al (2009) Acetabular loosening using an extended offset polyethylene liner. Clin Orthop Relat Res 467:188–193
3. Bonnin M, Saffarini M, Mercier PE et al (2011) Is ATT a reliable landmark for rotational alignment of the tibial component in TKA? J Arthroplasty 26(2):260–267
4. Davey JR, O'Connor DO, Burke DW et al (1993) Femoral component offset: its effect on strain in bone-cement. J Arthroplasty 8(1):23–26
5. Delp SL, Wixson RL, Komattu AV et al (1996) How superior placement of the joint center in hip arthroplasty affects the abductor muscles. Clin Orthop Relat Res Jul(328): 137–146
6. Dorr LD, Malik A, Dastane M et al (2009) Combined anteversion technique for total hip arthroplasty. Clin Orthop Relat Res 467(1):119–127
7. Eggli S, Pisan M, Müller ME (1998) The value of preoperative planning for total hip arthroplasty. J Bone Joint Surg Br 80(3):382–390
8. Kiyama T, Naito M, Shitama H et al (2009) Effect of superior placement of the hip center on abductor muscle strength in total hip arthroplasty. J Arthroplasty 24(2): 240–245
9. Kleemann RU, Heller MO, Stoeckle U et al (2003) THA loading arising from increased femoral anteversion and offset may lead to critical cement stresses. J Orthop Res 21(5):767–774
10. Knight JL, Atwater RD (1992) Preoperative planning for total hip arthroplasty: quantitating its utility and precision. J Arthroplasty 7(1):403–409
11. Murray DW (1993) The definition and measurement of acetabular orientation. J Bone Joint Surg Br 75(2): 228–232
12. Renkawitz T, Schuster T, Grifka J et al (2009) Leg length and offset measures with a pinless femoral reference array during THA. Clin Orthop Relat Res 468(7):1862–1968 [Epub 2009 Sept 19]
13. Sariali E, Mouttet A, Pasquier G et al (2009) Accuracy of reconstruction of the hip using computerised three-dimensional pre-operative planning and a cementless modular neck. J Bone Joint Surg Br 91(3):333–340

8.3 Fixation of Acetabular Cup: Anchorage, Yes, But Not Just Anyhow

Michael M. Morlock and Nicolas Bishop

Uncemented fixation of acetabular cups has become the gold standard for the anchorage of cup components in hip arthroplasty. Press-fitting is universally used to achieve primary stability, which is the prerequisite for bone ingrowth. Hip replacements with larger heads require higher primary stability due to the larger acting moments. This warrants looking in more detail into the mechanism of press-fitting and the consequences of press-fit magnitude and additional screw fixation on micromotion between cup and bone, which is done in this chapter.

Introduction

The long-term loosening rate for cemented acetabular components has been reported to be high and has led to an increased use of non-cemented alternatives. Currently, a revival of cemented all poly cups has occurred due to good published outcomes in young patients [3]. However, these designs do not allow for larger head diameters nor for hard-on-hard bearing articulations and consequently they may not prove to be the best long-term solution for the young and active patient. In this specific group of patients a press-fit uncemented cup with its wider choice of bearing options may offer a better long-term solution. Success of uncemented implants depends on the ingrowth of bone. The ingrowth of bone is dependent on activity-induced micromotion staying below a critical threshold value in the early postoperative period. Micromotion is induced by loading of the hip joint, which is almost impossible to avoid. In vivo measurements indicate that even static activities, such as lying in bed or working against resistance provided by the physiotherapist, create hip joint forces comparable to those occurring during unsupported walking [1]. The findings of Bergmann have challenged the advice of surgeons to patients to avoid full weight bearing and physical activities for the first few weeks after surgery. As a

consequence, today only few surgeons still insist on partial weight bearing following total hip arthroplasty (THA). It would appear that the quality of the initial fixation achieved by the surgeon (referred to as "anchorage" in this paper), the surface characteristics of the implant surface and the quality of the reamed acetabular bony bed are more critical factors in achieving successful bone ingrowth than how the patient loads the implant.

The tendency to use larger head diameters for better function, less dislocation risk and potentially better tribology due to the higher velocity at the interface during movement has introduced some new problems due to the larger friction moments associated with larger diameter heads [8]. This might be one of the reasons for the increased rate of cup loosening observed in hip resurfacing and THA with extra large metal heads [6]. Consequently, the primary stability of the acetabular cup is becoming even more important than in the past.

In order to reduce micromotion and thus facilitate bony ingrowth, various methods of cup fixation have been developed. Both the design of acetabular cups [9] and the surgical procedure used have been shown to influence micromotion in laboratory experiments. These experiments, however, only looked at a few discrete locations at the bone–implant interface and not at the whole interface surface. Given that hip joint loads and pelvic geometry are asymmetric, the extent of the actual micromotion is likely to vary over the entire contact region and consequently investigations may need to look at the whole contact surface and not just a part of it. Another limitation of in vitro experiments is that micromotion is necessarily measured using simplistic axial loading conditions. Such experimental set-ups typically ignore the effects of muscle activity or changes in direction and/or magnitude of loads during a given activity.

Finite element (FE) analysis has been applied to quantify the relative micromotion at the interface between the cup and the bone. These studies have proven useful in demonstrating the importance of friction, dynamic effects and the degree of press-fit interference. In press-fitting, an oversized cup is hammered into an undersized cavity (Fig. 8.11).

The oversizing causes outwards deformation of the bone upon implantation. The resulting elastic recoil induces a compressive stress between the pelvis and periphery of the oversized cup, resulting in a certain amount of stability [9]. Press-fitting has become the

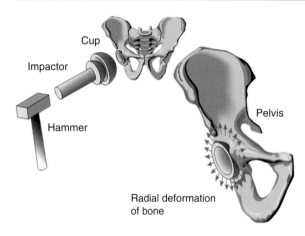

Impactor
Cup
Hammer
Pelvis
Radial deformation
of bone

Fig. 8.11 The procedure of press-fitting

most popular fixation method. The mechanical process involved in cup insertion, the role of press-fit, the use of screws as well as the effect of dynamic activities on micromotion and bone ingrowth have been investigated in detail and are summarised below [11–13].

The Surgical Process of Press-fitting

While the benefits of press-fitting have been reported [7], the lack of bone ingrowth in the polar regions is still a cause for concern. Not only does the presence of a gap imply that less area is available for bone ingrowth, but it also provides the opportunity for the gathering of wear debris. In vivo evidence indicates a link between the lack of bone ingrowth in polar regions and the polar gaps formed during the process of implantation [4]. Although the long-term loosening rates as a result of these polar gaps have yet to be assessed, their presence is nonetheless disconcerting.

The frictional forces at the press-fit cup–bone interface provide postoperative stability. These resistive forces are determined by the friction coefficient and the amount of radial deformation caused by press-fitting [9]. Since cup oversizing causes this compression, large under-reaming, for example by 2 mm, together with a high friction surface are considered desirable for short-term stability of press-fit cups. However, with regard to the former, in vitro studies have recorded greater polar gaps when large interferences are attempted. With regard to the latter, Ries et al. [9] using an FE model, noted that complete seating of a press-fit

cup could not always be achieved with very rough surfaces (friction values higher than 0.15). Thus, although high interference and friction are unquestionably desirable parameters for a perfectly seated cup, such a system may be difficult to implant. With the use of FE analysis, the effects of friction and interference between cup and cavity on the seating of press-fit cups can be investigated systematically [11].

A two-dimensional axisymmetric model of the superior region of a human pelvis was used to simulate the surgical procedure of press-fitting involving repeatedly hitting the cup via an impactor with a mallet. Depending on the momentum of the mallet and the duration of mallet impactor contact, a force is exerted on the cup. Depending on the load duration, friction, interference and bone-stiffness, the cup is driven into the acetabulum. Four load pulses simulating the effect of surgeons' impact blows were applied. Among other findings, when the simulated hammer force is removed, the cup model was found to rebound (Fig. 8.12). Rebounding is resisted by frictional forces and, depending on the friction coefficient and bone deformation, the final position of the cup after total load removal is somewhere between the starting position and the position at peak force. Thus, in addition to a lack of cup penetration into the cavity, this rebounding also plays a significant role on the size of the polar gap. On the one hand, high friction ($\mu = 0.5$) restricts the penetration of the cup during load application, whereas on the other, low friction ($\mu = 0.1$) results in unrestricted rebounding during load removal. In terms of maximising axial pull out force and minimising gaps in the interface, intermediate values of friction ($\mu = 0.2$ and 0.3) give the best results. It has been suggested that the presence of a naturally occurring lubricant (e.g. blood) could reduce high friction values to intermediate values (0.2 and 0.3), which could enhance the seating of press-fit cups (Fig. 8.12).

The two interferences (0.5 and 1.0 mm) modelled resulted in different amounts of cup seating [11]. A larger interference makes it more difficult to fully seat the cup, since the cup gets more easily stuck at the opening of the reamed cavity due to the smaller cavity diameter (in comparison to the cup diameter). Consequently the polar gaps remaining in the 0.5 mm interference model were smaller than those in the 1.0 mm interference model and the contact area between implant and bone was larger with the smaller amount of press-fit.

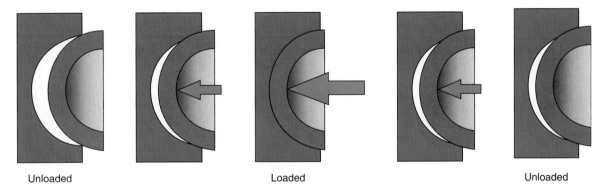

Unloaded   Loaded   Unloaded

Fig. 8.12 Schematic representation of the cup being seated in the cavity during the simulation of a hammer blow. During load application (*arrow*) the cup penetrates into the cavity. During removal of the load the cup bounces back out a small amount

Micromotion Occurring Under Joint and Muscle Loads During Gait

Relative micromotion, the parameter used to quantify the stability between cup and bone during gait, was calculated for a range of fixation methods. This was modelled in an acetabular cavity within a three-dimensional pelvic model (Fig. 8.13). Hemispherical cups of size 1 and 2 mm representing interference fits of 0.5 and 1.5 mm [12] were press-fitted into the cavity. Manual reaming produces cavities about 0.5 mm larger than the reamer size used thereby reducing the nominal interference of 1/2 mm to an effective interference of 0.5/1.5 mm. For comparative purposes, models with exact fit cups, that is line-to-line reaming (with and without screw fixation) were also investigated. The effects of muscle forces on relative micromotion were considered within the model. The models were then subjected to quasistatic joint contact loads occurring during gait [2]. The relative micromotion between the bone in the reamed cavity and the acetabular cup was calculated throughout a gait cycle.

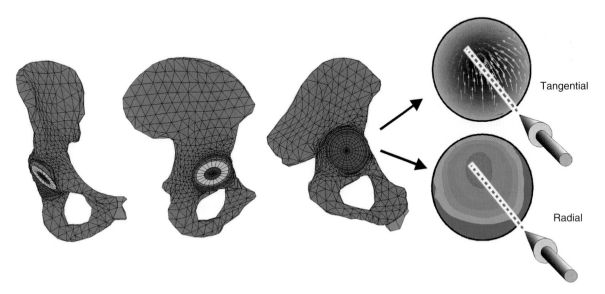

Fig. 8.13 Left: Three-dimensional FE-Model of hemi-pelvis with implanted acetabular cup. Different colours represent the different materials modelled (pink: cortical bone, red: subchondral bone, grey: Titanium, yellow: PE, blue: the acetabular head, green: fixation of the model. *Right*: Projected calculated radial (i.e. normal to the cup surface) and tangential micromotions between cup and bone. The projection was made on a plane normal to the resultant joint force (directed superoposteriorly as indicated by the *arrows*)

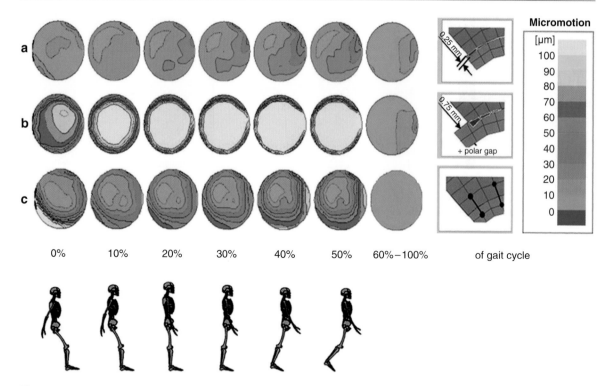

Fig. 8.14 Magnitude of micromotion between cup and bone during seven discrete time instances of one walking cycle for three different press-fit situations: (**a**) 1 mm under-ream corresponding to a 0.5 mm diametral press-fit; (**b**) 2 mm under-ream corresponding to a 1.5 mm diametral press-fit with a 2 mm polar gap; (**c**) line-to-line ream with two superior screws

Patterns of radial micromotion were found to be fairly simplistic. Due to the compressive nature of the loads, gap closing occurs where a gap is present (i.e. in the polar region). In regions of contact (i.e. around the equator), negligible radial micromotions were found. In contrast, the general direction of tangential micromotion followed the direction of the joint force (Fig. 8.13). It also was seen that there is a general tendency for the cup to slide over the adjacent bone. In regions of high external force, i.e. at the periphery in press-fit cases, this sliding is restricted by friction and the adjacent bone moves with the cup. In regions of little or no contact (i.e. in the polar region), the cup slides over the bone. Bone ingrowth most likely depends on the combined radial and tangential micromotions (total micromotion).

Primary stability – when expressed as resistance to micromotion under gait type loading – was found to be better for smaller interferences, that is as reaming approaches line-to-line. These findings imply that press-fit stability is load dependent, whereby a stable press-fit cup during gait may not be necessarily stable during unexpected high or very low joint loads. In the exact fit and 0.5 mm press-fit cases, good cup-bone contact is maintained in the region of the interface perpendicular to the direction of the joint load. Consequently, surface normal loads, in addition to friction, restrict cup-bone movements. In contrast, the polar gaps in the 1.5 mm press-fit case prevent contact in the polar region. Stability is generated almost entirely due to the friction generated at the equator as the high values of micromotions at the pole indicate (Fig. 8.14).

Screw fixation was found to reduce micromotions in the regions of the screws, but their indirect effect was to raise the magnitude of micromotion elsewhere at the interface [7]. Micromotions at the inferior rim indicate gap opening at the periphery, caused by activity of the semimembranosus pulling on the ischium. Even with the addition of an inferior screw, which was slightly anterior to the region of micromotions, gap opening of greater than 30 μm was not prevented. This gap opening could be large enough to allow access of wear debris into the implant–bone interface, leading to eventual osteolysis.

Effects of Different Daily Activities on Long-Term Bony Ingrowth Patterns

The growing trend for a reduced immobilisation period is based on, among other factors, in vivo data of hip joint forces [1]. The relationship between hip joint force and interfacial micromotions has yet to be ascertained. It is commonly found that the direction of hip joint loads when expressed with respect to the femoral side of the joint, does not vary either according to the stage of the cycle or according to the activity under investigation. In contrast, with respect to the direction of loads on the acetabular side, the joint forces vary considerably. Thus, differences in angulation and in magnitude could have an influence on the amount of micromotion occurring at the cup–bone interface. Although, a general description of these forces is available [1], it is noteworthy in this study that activities involving a large amount of hip flexion, such as climbing stairs, result in a large posterior component of force. Whether or not these loads are dangerous to the interface cannot be assessed from the gait cycle alone. The kinematic and kinetic data for six weight bearing activities was obtained, courtesy of Georg Bergmann at the Free University of Berlin [1]. These activities include three different modes of gait (slow, normal and fast) and three other activities (climbing up and down stairs and standing up from a chair). In addition to the patient's activities, it is also likely that the interfacial conditions will change over time. Notably, localised bone ingrowth, which is known to add to local interface stability, could affect the relative micromotions at the cup–bone interface. Thus, whether or not an activity is dangerous depends on the number of weeks after the operation. A model of bony ingrowth was used to estimate the ingrowth behaviour dependent on patient activity and cup interference [13].

Climbing up stairs was found to be the worst activity, most probably due to the larger posterior component of hip force due to the large hip flexion required to negotiate steps. Complete bony ingrowth was predicted in the 0.5 mm press-fit, whereas the ingrowth in the 1.5 mm cases was rather localised close to the rim. Unfortunately, histological patterns of ingrowth for such cups are rare. Of those available, good qualitative agreement was found [4]. The lack of bone ingrowth in the polar region of the 1.5 mm press-fit case is due to the gaps formed, while the lack of ingrowth found in the anterior region of the periphery is the result of

excessive micromotions that occur when walking upstairs. Although not modelled, it was suggested that anterior ingrowth could be achieved if dangerous activities, such as walking upstairs, are avoided in the immediate postoperative period [13].

Conclusions

Anchorage: YES – it is the essential prerequisite for successful bony fixation of uncemented acetabular cups. The anchorage has to be strong enough to withstand the moments and forces occurring during patient activities until sufficient boney ingrowth has been achieved. If primary stability cannot be achieved by press-fit alone, screws may be required. Furthermore, it is hypothesised that by avoiding certain activities, such as stair climbing, in the immediate postoperative period, complete peripheral ingrowth could be achieved. By forming a local seal against wear debris access, such ingrowth might protect the overall interface. Whether patients would comply to the required activity avoidance is an open question. This question could be answered by means of a clinical study. The lack of bony ingrowth at the pole, also a possible source of danger to the interface, can be reduced by using small interferences, that is decreasing the amount of under-reaming. Taking reamer tolerances into account, small nominal interferences always bear the risk of not achieving press-fit at all. However, this should be recognised during the trial insertion and accounted for by using a larger cup diameter.

'The' optimal amount of under-reaming cannot be defined in a single value since the quality of the bone and the diameter of the cup play important roles. The better the bone quality and the smaller the cup diameter, the smaller the interference required. A reamer with a diameter 1 mm smaller than the outer diameter of the cup (producing in average a true diametral press-fit of 0.5 mm) should be a good initial plan for most cases. Using a large press-fit (reamer 2 or 3 mm smaller than the outer diameter of the cup) can cause problems during the seating of the liner, especially if ceramic liners are used [5]. Furthermore, larger head diameters require thinner cups making them even more susceptible to deformation during press-fitting. Cup deformation, however, also has a positive potential. If the cup deforms during press-fitting and this deformation is then corrected by the insertion of the liner, the bone in contact with the cup moves in a radial rather than a shear direction. This has the potential to increase primary stability significantly [10] and might explain the good clinical results for thin press-fit acetabular cups. At the same time, however, it makes liner seating challenging.

References

1. Bergmann G, Rohlmann A, Graichen F (1989) In vivo measurement of hip joint stress. 1. Physical therapy. Z Orthop Ihre Grenzgeb 127(6):672–679
2. Brand RA, Pedersen DR, Davy DT et al (1994) Comparisons of hip force caclculations and measurements in the same patient. J Arthroplasty 9:45–51
3. Busch V, Klarenbeek R, Slooff T et al (2010) Cemented hip designs are a reasonable option in young patients. Clin Orthop Relat Res 468(12):3214–3220. [Epub ahead of print]
4. Cha CW, Shanbhag AS, Hasselman CT et al (1998) Bone in-growth and wear debris distribution around press-fit acetabular components with and without supplementary screw-fixation in a canine cementless total hip arthroplasty (THA) model. Trans ORS 23:373
5. Langdown AJ, Pickard RJ, Hobbs CM et al (2007) Incomplete seating of the liner with the Trident acetabular system: a cause for concern? J Bone Joint Surg Br 89(3):291–295
6. Long WT, Dastane M, Harris MJ et al (2010) Failure of the Durom Metasul acetabular component. Clin Orthop Relat Res 468(2):400–405
7. Morscher E, Bereiter H, Lampert C (1989) Cementless press-fit cups: principles, experimental data and three-year follow-up study. Clin Orthop Relat Res 249:12–20
8. Nassutt R, Wimmer MA, Schneider E et al (2003) The influence of resting periods on friction in the artificial hip. Clin Orthop Relat Res Feb(407):127–138
9. Ries MD, Harbaugh M, Shea JK et al (1997) Effect of cementless acetabular cup geometry on strain distribution and press-fit stability. J Arthroplasty 12:207–212
10. Rothstock S, Uhlenbrock A, Bishop N et al (2010) Primary stability of uncemented femoral resurfacing implants for varying interface parameters and material formulations during walking and stair climbing. J Biomech 43(3): 521–526
11. Spears I, Morlock M, Pfleiderer M et al (1999) The influence of friction and interference on the seating of a press-fit cup: a finite element investigation. J Biomech 32: 1183–1189
12. Spears I, Pfleiderer M, Schneider E et al (2001) The effect of interfacial parameters on cup-bone relative micromotions: a finite element investigation. J Biomech 34(1): 113–120
13. Spears I, Pfleiderer M, Schneider E et al (2000) Inter-facial conditions between a press-fit acetabular cup and bone during daily activities: implications for achieving bone ingrowth. J Biomech 33(11):1471–1477

8.4 Surgical Considerations of Cup Insertion: From Theory to Practice

Tarik Aït Si Selmi and Camdon Fary

Cup insertion is one of the greatest challenges in hip surgery. Even after long periods of training and practice hitting the ideal target every time is not easy. Correct orientation is critical, if we want to minimise instability and wear.

Introduction

From a surgical perspective, anchorage of the cup is more than just cup fixation itself. It is part of the overall surgical process, which includes preoperative work-up, exposure, preparation of the bone bed, trialling and final component insertion. Specific patient problems such as dysplasia, spinal disorder and bone quality are all important considerations. Of course, there will be variations in technique that are surgeon and implant dependent, but nevertheless we can identify three general principles: firstly accurate positioning, secondly effective fixation and thirdly preservation of bone. All three are interdependent.

We will describe our technique for cup insertion. It is important to bear in mind that others may have alternative techniques, but all should respect the three basic principles.

Planning Cup Insertion

Routine planning relies on AP pelvic radiographs and templates, more recently virtual digital templates are being increasingly used. The AP pelvic radiograph is a projection that approximates to reality. Magnification must be taken into account when it comes to sizing (Sect. 3.2). The positioning of the cup will determine the final acetabular joint centre and may differ from the native acetabular joint centre.

The native acetabular centre is the centre of the circle formed by the semilunate cartilage. This cartilage is lateral to the medial acetabular wall where the medial aspect of the cup is usually seated. In the normal native hip the bony acetabulum is relatively

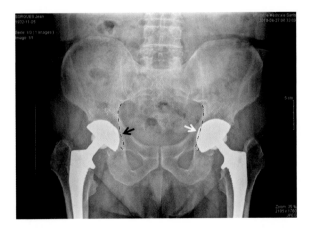

Fig. 8.15 Typical cup position of the right hip with a 45° angle inclination and a short distance to the medial wall (*black arrow*). The lateral aspect of the cup remains slightly uncovered. The left hip shows an excessive medial insertion beyond the medial wall (*white arrow*)

shallow with the labrum providing further depth and head cover, which then approximates to a hemisphere. The apparent acetabular contour (bony contour) is the only available landmark on radiographs and is also the most reliable for assessing the difficulty of gaining adequate cup fixation. If a patient presents with a disruption to normal anatomy because of a subluxed head

or protusio or major medial osteophytes, then the opposite hip, if normal, should be used as the reference to determine the native hip centre.

The cup is templated so as to provide an abduction angle of 45° on the AP pelvis x-ray. The lateral aspect of the cup may not be fully covered by the iliac bone. The medial aspect should sit just lateral to the true floor, although many surgeons will medialise the cup down to the true floor or medial wall of the acetabulum (Fig. 8.15). The cup diameter is determined by the templates that best match these prerequisites. Thus cup position and sizing are dependent on each other. The sizing may also be estimated by templating the head diameter on the lateral x-ray. Normally, our cup sizes will be no more than 4 mm bigger than the original head size.

In dysplastic hips, the cup is usually uncovered laterally. In this situation, the cup overhang can be measured and used as a landmark to ascertain the correct placement. It may also be possible to predict the need for bone grafting. The presence of the osteophytes should be noted because of their potential to cause impingement and dislocation. In protrusio one must anticipate difficult acetabular exposure and potential impingement, if the acetabular joint centre is maintained in its original medialised position (Fig. 8.16).

Fig. 8.16 Major hip protrusio. The cup templating indicates the need for medial grafting of the medial aspect of the acetabulum in order to restore the native hip centre and increase the range of motion (**a**). Postoperative view demonstrating the restitution of the anatomy and the extent of the grafted area (**b**)

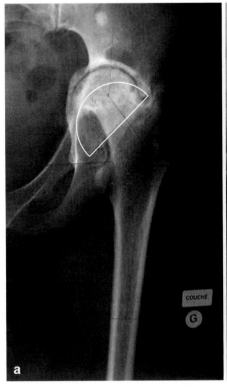

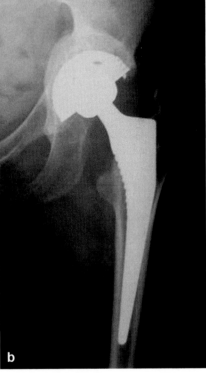

Exposure

We use the posterior approach. The skin incision is usually centred on the tip of the greater trochanter which overlies the acetabulum. In coxa-vara hips or in neck of femur fractures the inexperienced surgeon may expect the acetabulum to be higher and may miss the acetabular contour. This puts the sciatic nerve at risk by exploring too proximally. Moving the leg and hip joint helps to indentify the joint space. Hip dislocation is more challenging in the presence of stiffness due to capsular contraction, ostophytes, heterotopic ossification, protrusio or (often) a combination of these. As well as cutting the posterior and superior capsule, in addition, sometimes part of the anterior capsule may have to be cut in order to permit adequate anterior translation of the femur both for acetabular exposure and to allow adequate removal of superior and anterior osteophytes. This helps prevent groin pain and impingement. A bone hook passed under the neck or a corkscrew fixed in the head-neck junction may be used to aid dislocation. In extreme cases, when it is not possible to dislocate the hip safely, the femoral neck may be cut in situ and the head then removed with a corkscrew. Retractors and/or pins are then inserted in the usual manner to provide a clear view of the entire acetabulum. This includes obtaining good exposure of the transverse acetabular ligament (TAL).

Reaming

Where Shall We Ream?

Reaming provides a bone bed that will accommodate the cup. The direction of reaming can be determined both from the templated radiograph and from intraoperative bony and soft tissue landmarks. At this stage, osteophytes can be removed. If the hemispherical shape of the acetabulum has been retained and there is not much bone to be removed, it is possible to start with a reamer one or two sizes below the templated diameter. In some situations, there is a need to adapt the orientation of the reaming. In dysplastic hips there is often a need to medialise the cup to achieve good coverage and to minimise anterior overhang (Fig. 8.17). When a medial osteophyte is present, the reaming must also address this situation to guard against a lateralised and

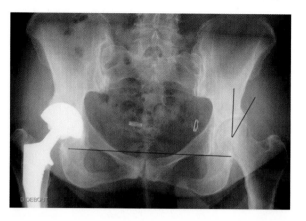

Fig. 8.17 Dysplastic hips. The cup has been inserted medially and proximally (relative to the inter-teardrop line) to achieve good coverage and consistent press-fit. Note the lateral aspect which still remains uncovered

incompletely seated cup. In these situations reaming can begin with a smaller diameter reamer to remove the extra bone. The resulting groove is then used to position successive reamers.

In some instances, a reamer can become stuck within the acetabulum. This happens because the elasticity of the acetabular rim allows the rim to deform thereby admitting the reamer and then allows the rim to return to its original size thereby 'capturing' the reamer. As there are no serrations at the equator of a reamer this may result in a bony ridge just inside the acetabular rim that is smaller than the reamer and may compromise the correct seating of the shell, or worse still, cause a fracture. Excessive medial reaming may also lead to perforation of the medial wall with the risk of a serious vascular injury or poor fixation. A common error is excessive reaming of the posterior wall, which can result in poor fixation. This often occurs due to poor exposure with the reamer handle being levered against the femur, which in turn can produce unintentional increased pressure on the posterior acetabular wall.

How Much Shall We Ream?

The main aim of reaming is to form a bleeding bed of non-sclerotic bone, which allows optimal biological ingrowth. There is no objective way to demonstrate the ideal bone bed. In our experience, removing the cartilage and reaching the subchondral bone is sufficient. Occasionally, in very sclerotic bone, prolonged reaming will result in excessive bone stock removal to form a non-sclerotic bed. Our goal is to minimise the bone loss as we know that our acetabular prosthesis is capable of excellent integration in subchondral bone. Sparing the subchondral bone maintains the physiological bone gradient between soft cancellous bone, hard subchondral bone and the adjacent implant. In hard-on-hard bearings and large cups, as observed in resurfacing, stress shielding has been reported with progressive bone loss at the apex of the cup. Maintaining the physiological transition from soft cancellous bone to hard subchondral bone and using as small a cup as possible is a way to decrease bone-implant stress shielding and to preserve bone stock for revision.

Press-Fit Cups

Press-fit cups achieve sufficient primary stability such that patients can weight bear immediately postoperatively. Press-fit relies on the response of acetabular bone elasticity to a forced deformity. This is obtained by inserting a cup, which is larger than the reamed acetabular bed. Press-fit will vary according to the bone quality. In protrusio, where bone is sclerotic and large circular osteophytes are common, the overall elasticity of the acetabulum is much lower.

Trial cups often have a smooth surface with large windows to visualise cup seating. These factors make the trial more deformable. This may be a reason for the difficulty inserting the definitive cup despite a good press-fit trial.

The cup design, outer geometry and surface finish are other important factors affecting fixation. Additional hydroxyapatite (HA) coating layers are not always included in the cup diameter referred to on the packaging. Maximising bone-implant contact is as important as forming a firm press-fit. Reamer geometry and sharpness are a source of mismatching. The testing technique of the surgeon is also important in assessing the quality of the primary fixation. When trialling, one must remember that testing the fixation with a long handle attached to the cup applies a lever, which far exceeds the physiological conditions on the actual implant, which has a small unconstrained femoral head and a negligible lever arm. However, it must also be recognised that with large metal-on-metal bearings, frictional torque can be quite high under conditions of boundary lubrication.

Successful press-fit has been demonstrated to rely on multiple factors. In our experience, a line-to-line technique is effective and provides adequate fixation through an optimised bone-cup surface contact ratio. When the bone quality is poor or when a large cup is used a +1 mm is sometimes useful. This 'soft-fit' approach prevents incorrect seating and the risk of an overhanging cup edge and/or the risk of fracture. It also contributes to bone preservation.

Cup Insertion

Trial implants of the predicted size are inserted first. The position and contact with the medial wall is assessed. Vigorous attempts to displace the trial cup can compromise the future press-fit and must be avoided. When inserting the trial, care must be taken to avoid compaction of the acetabular cancellous bed.

Cup orientation is of critical importance for hip biomechanics to allow optimal motion and stability. The use of a rimmed liner may compromise the range of motion and may cause impingement (Fig. 8.18). Different landmarks can be used which include bony

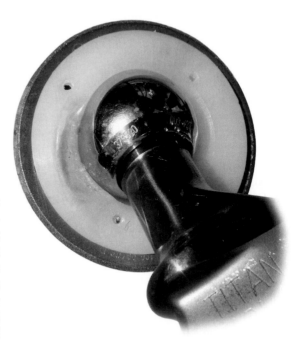

Fig. 8.18 Rimmed liner demonstrating posterior impingement against the neck of the stem and responsible for accelerated polyethylene wear. Note the uncovered aspect of the taper that may also have compromised mobility

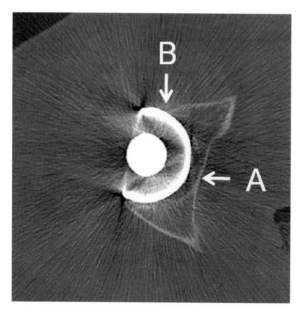

Fig. 8.19 CT-scan of right hip. Iliopsoas impingement related to the poor seating of the cup (*Arrow A*) and subsequent anterior overhanging (*Arrow B*)

Liner Insertion

The anterior and posterior columns of the pelvis envelope the acetabulum with the TAL inferiorly acting as a check rein. When press fit is achieved, the cup is squeezed between the two columns. Thus the cup becomes elliptical with its shortest axis running parallel to the TAL. It is important to be aware of this when inserting either a metal or ceramic liner so as to ensure an even circumferential fit. If this is not done with a ceramic liner, then the leading edge can fracture as it is impacted. Lavage of the shell is also important to remove any debris and blood with its adhesive properties. When inserting the liner, its face must be co-planar with that of the cup. Insertion is then achieved by gently and progressively tapping while maintaining the correct orientation. Any tilt of the shell during this manoeuvre must be recognised and corrected. Seating is then checked by circular palpation with a finger or instrument and confirmed visually. Final impaction can be then performed safely.

anatomy, the labrum or most commonly the TAL (Sect. 8.1). Complete seating is assessed through the polar hole and there must be sufficient anterior coverage to avoid any iliopsoas impingement (Fig. 8.19).

The addition of screws to a cup is routine for some surgeons and provides 'just in case' additional fixation. But additional screw fixation has some drawbacks. If inserted to compensate for a loose cup it can become a source of metallosis and increase the risk of failure. The screw head may overhang, when inappropriately inserted, and compromise liner fixation. Injury to surrounding vessels or nerves has been well documented. In the long term the screws can act as a pathway for the spreading of wear debris away from the cup deep into the pelvic bone and worsen the effect of osteolysis. When screws are broken or damaged, this can make cup removal much more difficult. In our experience, we rarely use screws. When cup stability is compromised we recommend to repeat reaming again with the last reamer or consider the use of a larger cup. If necessary, the screws must be inserted parallel to the radius of the cup, otherwise eccentric forces are created with the subsequent risk of mal-positioning or excessive local peak stresses.

Conclusion

Anchorage of the cup is a technically demanding step. The planning process enables the surgeon to determine the ideal cup position according to the patient-specific anatomy. Reaming must be gradual and limited to preserve bone. Cup fixation requires adequate press-fit and optimal bone implant contact. Cup orientation is critical to the outcome of the total hip replacement and depends on a good fixation technique.

References

1. Debarge R, Lustig S, Neyret P et al (2008) Confrontation of the radiographic preoperative planning with the postoperative data for uncemented total hip arthroplasty. Rev Chir Orthop Reparatrice Appar Mot 94(4):368–375
2. Lavigne M, Siva Rama RK, Ganapathi M et al (2008) A Factors affecting acetabular bone loss during primary hiparthroplasty – a quantitative analysis using computer simulation Clin Biomech 23:577–583
3. Morscher EW (1992) Current status of acetabular fixation in primary total hip arthroplasty. Clin Orthop Relat Res 274:172–193

Direction

9

David Beverland

Content

J.-P. Vidalain et al. (eds.), *The CORAIL® Hip System*,
DOI: 10.1007/978-3-642-18396-6_9, © Springer-Verlag Berlin Heidelberg 2011

9.1 Navigation: Using a Compass for THA

David Beverland and Thomas Kalteis

Correct implant position remains a crucial factor in the determination of outcome and long-term results in total hip arthroplasty (THA). According to recent studies, computer-assisted navigation can significantly increase the reproducibility of implant positioning in THA. The use of navigation as a 'compass' for THA can minimise mal-alignment of the acetabular cup and femoral stem. However, the increased complexity of the surgical procedure, as well as genuine economical constraints, is the main hurdle for the routine use of computer-assisted navigation in THA so far.

Introduction

Without doubt total hip arthroplasty THA is a successful surgical procedure and is generally considered to have an acceptably low complication rate. Improvements in implant design, materials and perioperative management can give excellent long-term results in most cases. Therefore, one might question the necessity to use additional technical aids to:

Reduce the variability of implant positioning
To improve the reproducibility of THA
To decrease complication rate and
To optimise clinical results

Do we need a compass for THA? Or can we be satisfied with our results in THA? Might traditional alignment guides for THA or soft tissue and bony landmarks be accurate enough to orientate the implants correctly or should we consider using modern technical support for THA?

Limitations of Conventional Surgical Technique in Total Hip Arthroplasty

All surgeons, irrespective of how many THAs they do, who critically review their clinical results, will find undesirable examples of cup mal-alignment, incorrect offset and leg length discrepancy. Surgeons often ascribe inappropriate cup abduction or cup anteversion to variations in patients' anatomy, and in reality incorrect implant position rarely causes *early* complications. Therefore, at least on superficial inspection, it would seem that THA is a surgical procedure that forgives mistakes. As a consequence, the inability of conventional surgical technique to achieve consistent ideal component placement has not resulted in any universal concern and has largely been neglected.

Previous studies investigating conventional cup positioning reported a high level of inaccuracy with cup mal-positioning in 42–78% of cases and an undesirable variability in both cup abduction and anteversion: In a multi-centre study, only 27 out of 105 (26%) of the acetabular cups were placed within the 'safe zone' as defined by Lewinnek (1978) [5]. Using CT-scans for evaluation, a range of cup abduction from 23° to 71° (SD $\pm$ 10.1°) and a range of cup anteversion from −23° to 59° (SD $\pm$ 15.0°) was reported [11]. In another study 42% of the acetabular cups were positioned outside the safe zone, despite the use of mechanical alignment guides [3]. In 74 primary THAs, DiGioia et al. (2002) found a range in abduction from 35° to 59° (SD $\pm$ 4.0°) and in anteversion from −26° to 33° (SD $\pm$ 10.0°) [2].

Part of the explanation for this considerable inaccuracy and unreliability of conventional cup placement is the fact that the surgeon has insufficient control of the orientation of the patient's pelvis. Furthermore, even if care is taken to initially position the patient this can significantly change intraoperatively [1]. Also the wide variation in the bony anatomy around the hip joint regularly leads to intraoperative errors in both the depth of placement and orientation of both components. This happens to both experienced and inexperienced surgeons. In reality, most mechanical alignment aids are not orientated with respect to the bony pelvis, but rather are aligned in space and presuppose an ideal, but unfortunately rarely achieved neutral pelvic position on the operating table.

In addition to the alignment of the acetabular component, restoration of leg length as well as femoral offset is important for functional outcome and long-term success in THA. Medialisation of the centre of rotation decreases the moment arm for body weight and increasing the femoral offset lengthens the lever arm for the abductor muscles. Furthermore, marked leg length discrepancy has been associated with abnormal force transmission across the hip joint. However, determining leg length and femoral offset reproducibly and accurately remains a challenge during THA. Minor changes in adduction-abduction, flexion-extension, or internal-external rotation between pre and post-reconstruction measurements can lead to substantial errors in assessing leg length changes intraoperatively and can lead the surgeon to make poor decisions based on this unreliable information. For different conventional measurement methods mean discrepancy in postoperative leg length up to 9 mm has been reported [7]. Leg length discrepancy remains a major reason for litigation.

Computer-Assisted Navigation in THA

The principle of computer-assisted acetabular cup navigation is based on the concept that everything is referenced with respect to the anterior pelvic plane. This greatly simplifies the complexity of pelvic anatomy. This reference plane is defined via four anatomical landmarks – the anterior superior iliac spines (ASIS) and the pubic tubercles. It approximates to the frontal plane of a healthy patient in the standing position. The sagittal plane is defined as being perpendicular to the frontal plane and thus a virtual 3-D coordinate system for cup orientation is created (Fig. 9.1). The position of the acetabular component within this coordinate system can be measured and quantified at any time in the surgical procedure and cup placement is reproducible and independent of both patient position on the operating table and intraoperative movement of the lower extremities and/or the pelvis.

In a similar way, a femoral coordinate system is created by registration of femoral landmarks to navigate stem insertion.

Nowadays, imageless techniques for computer-assisted navigation have squeezed out former image-based techniques. With image-based systems, preoperative imaging, usually in the form of a CT scan, is used to create a 3-D model specific to that individual patient. Then during surgery bony points in and around the patients joint are referenced until the software recognises where it is thus creating a link between the 3-D model and the patient (matching). With imageless systems anatomical landmarks are registered intraoperatively to create a virtual 3-D model without the need for preoperative imaging.

The description of computer-assisted navigation for THA is based on two workflows of imageless

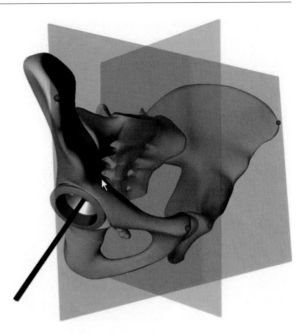

Fig. 9.1 Virtual coordinate system for computer-assisted navigation of the acetabular component (Copyright DePuy-International Limited)

navigation systems (Ci Hip Unlimited, DePuy, Warsaw, USA; VectorVision Hip Unlimited, BrainLAB, Feldkirchen, Germany) that are both used by one of the authors (TK). The surgical procedure is performed either via a mini-invasive anterolateral approach (OCM-approach) or via a direct anterior approach (MicroHip™) and for both the patient is in the lateral decubitus position. Two rigid bodies containing reflective markers are fixed via two 3.5 mm wires; one to the ipsilateral iliac crest and the other to the distal femur. The centre of rotation of the hip is then determined kinematically and the ASIS and pubic tubercles are located by palpation and are registered using a blunt pointer so as to determine the anterior pelvic plane. Additional surface points (epicondyles, malleoli and the piriform fossa) are registered for navigation of the femoral implant. After resection of the femoral head, a cluster of acetabular surface points is acquired to determine the acetabular depth and size. Following the subsequent creation of the virtual model by the navigation system, the operation is continued using cup reamers and cup inserters that are both recalibrated. During acetabular reaming and cup insertion, the cup abduction, anteversion and the centre of cup rotation are displayed in real time on the monitor of the navigation

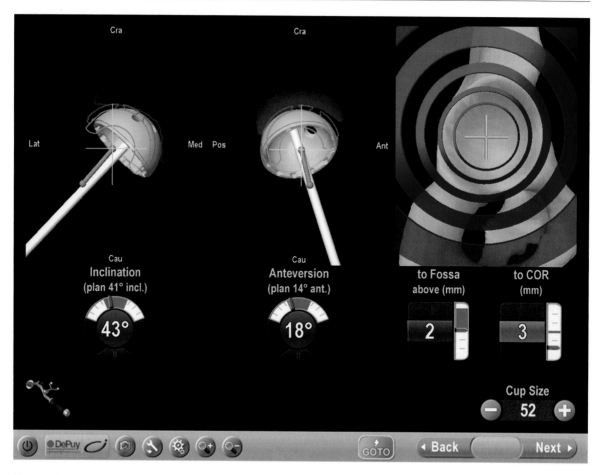

Fig. 9.2 Screenshot displaying cup abduction, cup anteversion and position of centre of rotation (Copyright DePuyInternational Limited)

system (Fig. 9.2). Additionally, computer-assisted femoral stem navigation allows intraoperative measurement of leg length, offset and stem version (Fig. 9.3). Different Corail® stems such as, standard/high offset/coxa vara and/or different head neck lengths can be simulated and measured intraoperatively to achieve optimal reconstruction of the joint centre, offset and leg length. Finally, the range of motion can be controlled and documented.

Clinical Results of Computer-Assisted Navigation in THA

Several studies have shown that the use of computer-assisted navigation can clearly reduce intraoperative inaccuracy in the placement of the acetabular component. In a study published by Paratte et al. (2007) computer-assisted navigation significantly reduced the percentage of acetabular cup outliers according to the criteria described by Lewinnek, from 57% (17/30) in the freehand group to 20% (6/30) in the computer-assisted group [8]. The results are in agreement with the results of one of the author's studies (TK). In a prospective randomised clinical trial, acetabular cups were implanted either conventionally, that is freehand ($n = 30$), or by using CT-based ($n = 30$) or imageless navigation ($n = 30$). The cup position was determined postoperatively on pelvic CT scans. Following conventional freehand acetabular cup placement, only 14/30 cups were within the safe zone as defined by Lewinnek ($40° \pm 10°$ inclination; $15° \pm 10°$ anteversion). In contrast, after computer-assisted navigation,

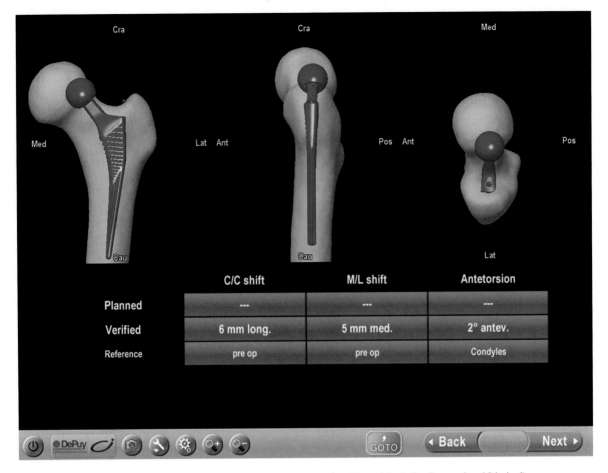

	C/C shift	M/L shift	Antetorsion
Planned	---	---	---
Verified	6 mm long.	5 mm med.	2° antev.
Reference	pre op	pre op	Condyles

Fig. 9.3 Screenshot displaying leg length, femoral offset and stem torsion (Copyright DePuyInternational Limited)

25/30 cups (CT-based navigation) and 28/30 cups (imageless navigation) were within this range (overall $p < 0.001$ when comparing the navigated and non-navigated results). For conventional freehand acetabular cup placement, mean abduction was 43.7° (range: 29–57°; SD ± 7.3°) and mean anteversion was 22.2° (range: 1–53°; SD ± 14.2°). In the case of CT-based acetabular cup placement, mean abduction was 41.6° (range: 34–53°; SD ± 4.0°) and mean anteversion was 10.7° (range: 1–23°; SD ± 5.3). Acetabular cups placed using imageless navigation had a mean abduction of 43.2° (range: 33–50°; SD ± 4.0°) and a mean anteversion of 15.2° (range: 5–25°; SD ± 5.5°) [4].

The decrease in the variation of cup positioning between both navigation methods when compared to conventional freehand surgery is indicated by the lower standard deviation in the navigation groups for anteversion in particular, but also for abduction (Fig.

9.4a, b). Both navigation methods showed a significant reduction in the variation of acetabular cup position compared to conventional freehand THA ($p < 0.001$) [4].

In an anatomic study, Renkawitz et al. (2009) reported very accurate restoration of leg length and offset when using imageless navigation. When they compared the imageless navigation method with a CT-based version values for leg length (LL) and femoral offset (OS) showed a high correlation and mean differences of less than 1 mm (LL, 0.74; SD ± 2.4 mm; OS, 0.89; SD ± 1.8 mm) [10]. Murphy and Ecker (2007) highlighted similar clinical results for leg length restoration in 112 hips. Compared with radiographically measured leg length change, those changes measured intraoperatively based on computer-assisted navigation were very accurate (mean difference: −0.5 mm; range: −5–3.9 mm; SD ± 1.77 mm) [7].

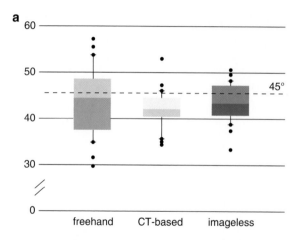
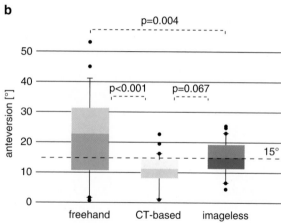

Fig. 9.4 (**a**) Cup abduction following freehand, CT-based navigation and imageless navigation (The boundaries of the boxes indicate the 25th and the 75th percentiles, the lines within the boxes mark the mean values. Whiskers above and below the box indicate the 90th and the 10th percentiles. Overall $p = 0.27$). (**b**) Cup anteversion following freehand, CT-based navigation and imageless navigation (The boundaries of the boxes indicate the 25th and the 75th percentiles, the lines within the boxes mark the mean values. Whiskers above and below the box indicate the 90th and the 10th percentiles. Overall $p < 0.001$) (From Kalteis et al. [4]. Reproduced and adapted with permission and copyright © of the British Editorial Society of Bone and Joint Surgery)

Optional Workflows for Computer-Assisted Navigation in THA

The problem of any 'safe-zone' is that a patient's individual anatomy may not be adequately respected. 'Safe-zones' are the statistical results of clinical, radiological or anatomical studies on varying numbers of patient cohorts, evaluating the incidence of complications after THA. When using any 'safe-zone' as a target for implant positioning, it is not possible to achieve the optimal result for each individual patient.

In an attempt to address the individual variation in patients' anatomy one of the authors (DB) has proposed using soft tissue landmarks or more specifically the transverse acetabular ligament (TAL) to achieve a more individualised acetabular cup orientation. A detailed account is given in Sect. 8.1. The rational of the technique is to align the face of the acetabular component parallel to the TAL, thus in theory re-establishing individual patient anteversion. However, one significant problem with using TAL in some conventional THA approaches is that even if the surgeon can expose it during preparation of the acetabular socket, during cup insertion it is often obscured by instruments or by the acetabular component. In recent software applications for computer-assisted navigation, the so called 'TAL-workflow' has been integrated as an option for navigated cup placement. Before cup

reaming and placement, the orientation of the TAL is registered using the referencing pointer. During cup insertion, the orientation of the TAL is displayed on the navigation screen to guide the surgeon in achieving a patient-specific, anatomy-based orientation of the acetabular component (Fig. 9.5).

A promising development of computer-assisted navigation systems is new software that considers the cup and stem as components of a coupled biomechanical system. This potentially allows the surgeon to find an optimised complementary component orientation. These range-of-motion (ROM)-based workflows require that the femur be prepared first in order to define femoral component anteversion. The acetabular cup positioning is then adapted to achieve an optimal ROM.

Both the TAL workflow and the ROM-based workflow for computer-assisted navigation highlight the advantages of navigation in THA. Computer-assisted navigation should not only be used to place an implant in a strictly fixed position but should also ideally be a technical tool that enables the surgeon to measure intraoperatively patients' individual anatomy and to focus on improved functional outcome. By gathering different data and quantifying the implant positions inside the virtual coordinate system the surgeon can control both cup alignment and stem insertion. Based on this computer-assisted control the surgeon can

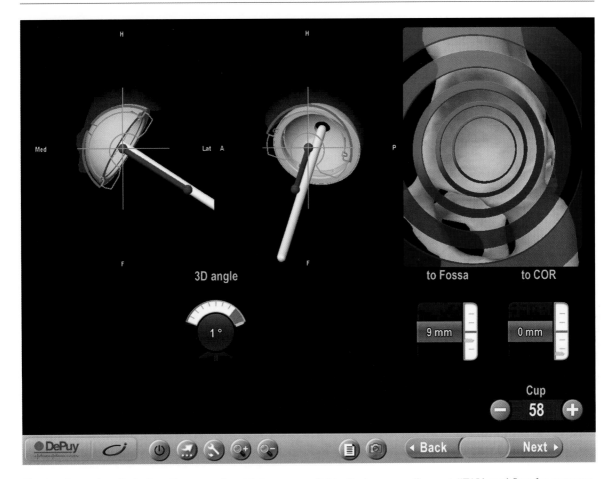

Fig. 9.5 Screenshot displaying alignment of acetabular cup parallel to the transverse ligament ('TAL' workflow for computer-assisted navigation) (Copyright DePuyInternational Limited)

decide intraoperatively whether to place the implants in a standard position or to aim for a more patient-specific implant orientation.

Conclusion

The relationship between implant alignment and complications in THA is well known and accepted. Mal-positioning of the implants in THA can lead to mechanical impingement and recurrent dislocation. Furthermore, leg length inequality is a major source of dysfunction and dissatisfaction after THA. Perhaps, ironically, recent problems with hard on hard bearings have focused the attention of surgeons and engineers alike on tribology and problems relating to wear. It is now more obvious than ever that implant alignment is a major factor determining the extent of wear and damage both in hard-on-soft and hard-on-hard bearing couples. Based on a finite element model and a clinical analysis Patil et al. (2003) underlined the importance of optimising the position of the acetabular component. A 40% increase in mean linear polyethylene wear was seen in cups with an abduction angle of more than 45° [9]. In a retrieval study of revised resurfacing components Morlock et al. (2009) showed a dramatic increase in metal wear rate with cup abduction angles greater than 50° [6]. Also for ceramic-on-ceramic couples, recent reports indicate an increased risk of stripe wear, fracture and squeaking due to surface abrasion related to component mal-position and impingement [12]. Therefore, ensuring correct implant position remains a crucial factor in the determination of outcome and long-term results in THA, despite all the improvements in materials and bearing couples.

Navigation cannot replace the expertise of an experienced surgeon. However, recent publications do suggest that computer-assisted navigation in THA can significantly increase the reproducibility of implant positioning. The use of navigation as a 'compass' for THA can decrease the variability of implant positioning and can therefore minimise mal-alignment of the acetabular cup and femoral stem, incorrect femoral offset and leg length discrepancy. Given this realisation computer-assisted navigation should by now have gained widespread use and global acceptance. However, the surgical procedure increased complexity, as well as genuine economical constraints are the main hurdles for the routine use of computer-assisted navigation in THA. Further research and development is necessary to both simplify the use and reduce the costs of computer-assisted navigation.

References

1. Asayama I, Akiyoshi Y, Naito M et al (2004) Intraoperative pelvic motion in total hip arthroplasty. J Arthroplasty 19:992–997
2. DiGioia AM, Jaramaz B, Plakseychuk AY et al (2002) Comparison of a mechanical acetabular alignment guide with computer placement of the socket. J Arthroplasty 17:359–364
3. Hassan DM, Johnston GH, Dust WN et al (1998) Accuracy of intraoperative assessment of acetabular prosthesis placement. J Arthroplasty 13:80–84
4. Kalteis T, Handel M, Bäthis H et al (2006) Imageless navigation for cup insertion in total hip arthroplasty – is it as accurate as CT-based navigation? J Bone Joint Surg Br 88:163–167
5. Lewinnek GE, Lewis JL, Tarr R et al (1978) Dislocations after total hip replacement arthroplasties. J Bone Joint Surg Am 60:217–220
6. Morlock M, Bishop N, Zustin J et al (2008) Modes of implant failure after hip resurfacing: morphological and wear analysis of 267 retrieval specimens. J Bone Joint Surg Am 90(Suppl 3):89–95
7. Murphy SB, Ecker TM (2007) Evaluation of a new leg length measurement algorithm in hip arthroplasty. Clin Orthop Relat Res 463:85–89
8. Paratte S, Argenson JN (2007) Validation and usefulness of a computer-assisted cup-positioning system in total hip Arthroplasty. A prospective, randomized, controlled study. J Bone Joint Surg Am 89:494–499
9. Patil S, Bergula A, Chen PC et al (2003) Polyethylene wear and acetabular component orientation. J Bone Joint Surg Am 85:56–63
10. Renkawitz T, Schuster T, Herold T et al (2009) Measuring leg length and offset with an imageless navigation system during total hip arthroplasty: is it really accurate? Int J Med Robot 5(2):192–197
11. Saxler G, Marx A, Vandevelde D et al (2004) The accuracy of free-hand cup positioning – a CT based measurement of cup placement in 105 total hip arthroplasties. Int Orthop 28:198–201
12. Walter W, O'Toole G, Walter W et al (2007) Squeaking in ceramic-on-ceramic hips: the importance of acetabular component orientation. J Arthroplasty 22:496–503

Case Studies: Pot-Pourri

Tarik Aït Si Selmi

10

Contents

J.-P. Vidalain et al. (eds.), *The CORAIL® Hip System*,
DOI: 10.1007/978-3-642-18396-6_10, © Springer-Verlag Berlin Heidelberg 2011

Clinical Case 1: The Standard Hip

Laurent Jacquot

Patient Brief History

Left Hip on a 75 –year-old woman who is still very active (hotel manager). Right Total Hip Arthroplasty (THA) in 1998, asymptomatic. She has had pain on the left side for 3 years, with a progressively worsening limp.

Hyaluronic acid injection 6 months previously without any influence on pain.

Patient Relevant Clinical and Radiological Findings

Typical groin pain. Painful Hip with limited ROM (No internal rotation). No Leg length Discrepancy. Patient overweight (BMI: 28). Radiological anterosuperior x-ray narrowing. Osteophytes. Head macrocyst as a consequence of wear.

Conventional morphotype of femoral shape and acetabulum. No dysplasia.

Preoperative X-Ray/Imaging

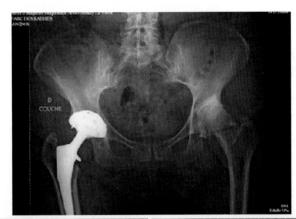

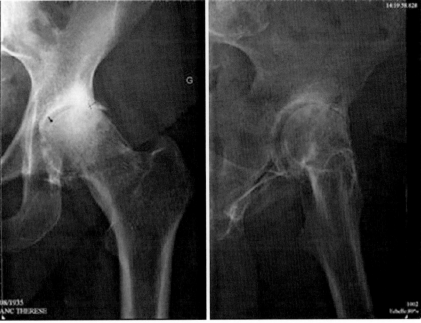

Fig. 10.1 Hip arthritis. Standard anatomy with common 135° CCD angle. Dorr type 2 femurs. Right pelvis tilt due to abduction contracture. Note the small films and truncated images from which no templating can be achieved

Fig. 10.2 Plain lateral and
AP view of the femur
allowing accurate templating.
Head centre and scheduled
neck resection level have
been reported on the films

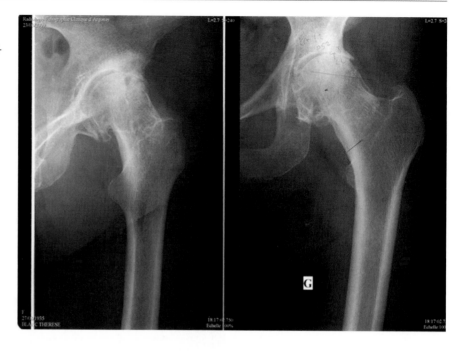

Indication, Strategy and Specific Recommendations

Failure of another medical alternative indicates surgical
treatment for this active woman. The option for the right
side was cementless implant, polyethylene insert and
ceramic head. The right side suggests beginning of wear
because the head is not centralised in the cup. Some
granuloma is observed behind the cup and in zone 7,
related to polyethylene debris reaction. Cementless
option for implants (Corail®/Pinnacle™) confirmed, but
hard-on-hard bearing (Ceramic-on-Ceramic) for friction in order to prevent future wear. Preoperative templating suggests use of a Standard Corail® (size 11, same
as right side), and Pinnacle™ 52 mm cup which enables
the use of a 36 mm ceramic ball.

Postoperative X-Ray/Imaging

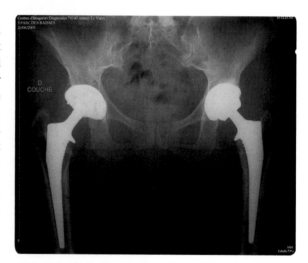

Fig. 10.3 Postoperative AP view: symmetrical hip anatomy.
Cup abduction angle is at 45° and normally anteverted. Note the
restoration of the pelvis horizontal orientation

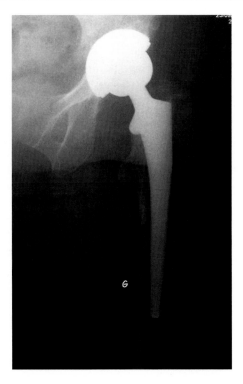

Fig. 10.4 Postoperative lateral view: note the ideal alignment and the absence of cortical contact (cancellous bone sleeve is kept around the stem)

Lessons Learnt/Alternatives

> Despite wear, the right side demonstrates that fixation of stem and cup remains stable at more than 15 years after surgery.
> Poly wear is a recurrent long-term concern with risk of granuloma and loosening, which should be avoided by the use of hard-on-hard bearing.
> In the case of good stem sizing for the first THR, the same size should be planned for the opposing side.
> In this case, we templated the calcar cutting a little bit higher to use a medium neck. The neck length can be adjusted during surgery depending on preoperative findings.

Clinical Case 2: The High Offset Hip

Helge Wangen

Patient Brief History

Fifty-five-year-old man, very active with pain in his right hip. Pain occurs when active during the day but also at night despite taking painkillers.

Patient Relevant Clinical and Radiological Findings

Limited ROM. Lower limb discrepancy, right leg about 10 mm shorter than the left leg.

A high offset hip. Severe osteoarthritis (OA) apparent on x-ray.

Preoperative X-Ray/Imaging

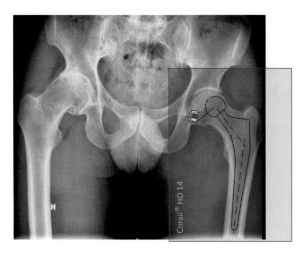

Fig. 10.5 Preoperative AP view. Severe OA. Pelvic tilt due to wear and stiffness. Dorr type 2 femur. Offset in the right hip appears smaller due to fixed external rotation. KHO template is the most appropriate but does not exactly match the patient offset

Indication, Strategy and Specific Recommendations

OA in an active 55-year-old man with a high offset hip. Conservative treatment with physiotherapy and pain-killers are no longer an option to the patient because of the severe pain.

Templating of the hip is important to decide what kind of prosthesis is best to restore the anatomy. Leg discrepancy is related to joint wear. Native leg length and offset restoration will be achieved by templating the opposite (left) hip which is free of OA and well aligned in the AP plane. The picture showing the highest offset is the correct one. Template the cup and try to position the cup in order to restore the original centre of the hip. Place the stem template and determine the right offset and the neck length. Anticipate the appropriate cut level on the x-ray according to your usual intraoperative landmark.

Lessons Learnt/Alternatives

> Do always template.
> The picture/side with the highest offset is the correct one.
> It is important to restore the offset in order to get a good functional outcome without limping.
> Focus on broaching enough laterally proximally to avoid varus of the stem.

Postoperative X-Ray/Imaging

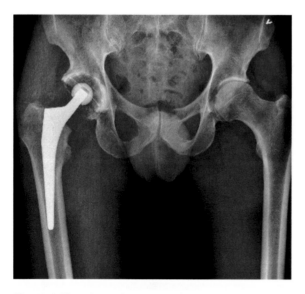

Fig. 10.6 X-ray 3 months postoperative. A cemented cup was used since this is the first choice in Norway. A smaller stem than expected was inserted in some varus. The leg length is corrected and the offset has been restored

Clinical Case 3: The Coxa Vara Hip

Rémi Philippot

Patient Brief History

Sixty-two-year-old male with left hip pain for the past 2 years. Increasing stiffness and limitation of everyday living activities.

Patient Relevant Clinical and Radiological Findings

Clinical examination shows no leg length discrepancy. Limitation of ROM with marked lack of internal rotation. Left Osteoarthritis (OA) with complete joint space narrowing and superior cyst. CCD angle is 123° and an estimated offset is 56 mm. Measurements are from the right hip as it free of OA without fixed deformity.

Preoperative X-Ray/Imaging

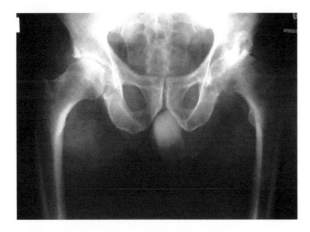

Fig. 10.7 Preoperative x-ray. Note that the left hip is slightly externally rotated (Fixed external rotation deformity), thus the offset is minimised as compared to the right hip

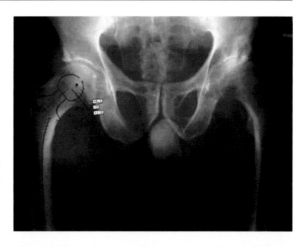

Fig. 10.8 Tempating. According to coxa vara hip morphology a coxa vara (KLA) stem is scheduled. The coxa vara stem features a 125° CCD angle and an increase of 7 mm offset as compared to the standard stem

Indication, Strategy and Specific Recommendations

In coxa vara hip, the quadratus muscle tends to extend its coverage over the neck as compared to other situations where the CCD angle is more opened. It is thus recommended to insist on proximal release of the short rotators to get a clear exposure of the neck before completing the osteotomy.

In coxa vara hip, not only is the neck horizontal but there is a tendency for the whole proximal femur to be bent inwards. In this situation the greater trochanter tends to overhang above the shaft. Thus there is an increased risk for the stem to be inserted in varus, or for the greater trochanter to be detached accidentally. One must insist on careful removal of bony remnants at the junction with the trochanter to allow a straight shaft alignment.

Restoring the native offset is crucial to optimise the gluteus medius function and to balance the capsule length in order to decrease the risk of dislocation. Nevertheless, over-correction of the offset is not recommended. It leads to over-tension of the muscle and capsule, pain and having the sensation of an increased leg length.

With the trial implants in place, it is useful (with any other intraoperative testing maneuver) to assess the capsular tension and length restoration. If over tightened, consider a shorter neck and re-check with the standard offset trial.

The proximal cyst can be grafted with some cancellous bone from the head.

Postoperative X-Ray/Imaging

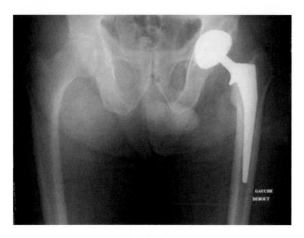

Fig. 10. 9 Postoperative x-ray. Note the restitution of the anatomy including offset, length and hip orientation (symmetrical rotation as of both hips). Note that the stem is slightly aligned in varus

Lessons Learnt/Alternatives

> Coxa vara hip must be addressed by coxa vara stem to restore the offset.
> Guards against the risk of varus alignment due to the proximal bow of the femur
> Over-correction is not well tolerated, clinically. When not sure, do privilege standard stem.

Clinical Case 4: The Valgus Hip

Sébastien Lustig

Patient Brief History

Right Hip of a 51-year-old woman. Primary school teacher. Developed progressive hip pain and disability over many years. Initial limping then subsequent pain and disability affecting her daily activities and her ability to work.

Patient Relevant Clinical and Radiological Findings

Limited internal rotation. Right lower limb 5 mm shorter. Pelvis tilting of 25 mm. Severe coxa valga (CCD angle 155°) with complete loss of joint line superiorly. Moderate dysplasia of the acetabulum.

Preoperative X-Ray/Imaging

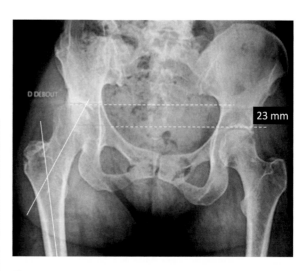

Fig. 10.10 Preoperative AP view. Note the major valgus and leg discrepancy

Fig. 10.11 Preoperative templating. The right hip is planned to keep its native length, thus the templating is not taken from the healthy left hip

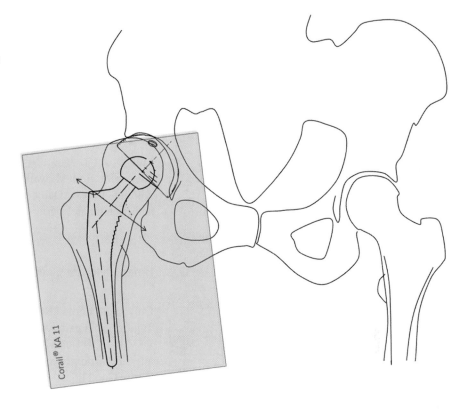

Corail® KA 11

Indication, Strategy and Specific Recommendations

Osteoarthritis with coxa valga and moderate hip dysplasia in a 51-year-old patient. Total Hip Arthroplasty (THA) is the best option as the patient has a superior complete articular cartilage deficiency. Do not template the left (healthy hip), because the hip dysplasia is unilateral and limb length shortening would result in unstable hip joint.

Do template the right (dysplastic) hip. First template the cup and draw the expected hip centre. Place the appropriate sized stem template over the femur to determine the neck length. In this situation we prefer to template a medium (+5) neck to allow the ability to adapt neck length intraoperatively. It is common in these situations to use a short neck (+1.5) to prevent offset increase. To avoid further limb lengthening the level of neck osteotomy is often 2 cm proximal to the lesser trochanter and proximal to the pyriformis fossae.

Beware of a varus tendency of the femoral broach on insertion due to the high level of neck osteotomy

causing lateral bony impingement. Use a canal finder to assess the appropriate direction.

Postoperative X-Ray/Imaging

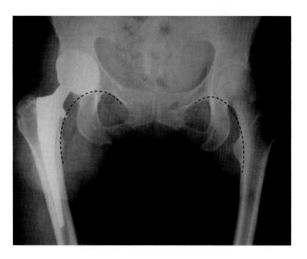

Fig. 10.12 During the planning, do not forget to compensate for limb length shortening secondary to loss of superior joint space. This leads to appropriate reconstruction of the joint including restoration of the leg length

Lessons Learnt/Alternatives

> Focus on preoperative limb length discrepancy and inform patient about it.
> To prevent limb length shortening templating must be from the dysplastic hip.
> Beware of varization of the stem due to the high neck osteotomy. The lateral neck cortical bone impinges on the broaches during introduction into the canal forcing them into varus. This results in an increased offset. This can be countered by the use of a short neck if possible.
> Femoral or acetabular osteotomy is not indicated due to severe superior articular cartilage loss.
> Leg length restoration (shortening) would result in Trendelenburg gate and increased dislocation risk.

Clinical Case 5: The Mild CDH

Hans-Erik Henkus

Patient Brief History

Left hip of a 56-year-old female. Progressive groin pain with limited walking distance. Physiotherapy without success. Daily use of NSAIDs (non-steroidal anti-inflammatory drugs).

Patient Relevant Clinical and Radiological Findings

Only slight limited ROM. No limb length discrepancy. Typical groin pain with rotation.

Mild CDH (left CE: 18°) in both hips. Coxarthrosis left side with slight subluxation of the head of the femur. Good bone stock medial wall.

Preoperative X-Ray/Imaging

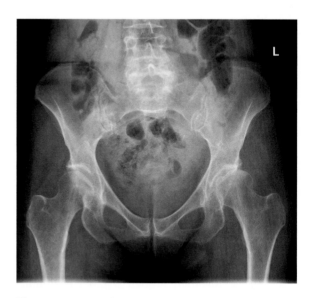

Fig. 10.13 Preoperative AP view

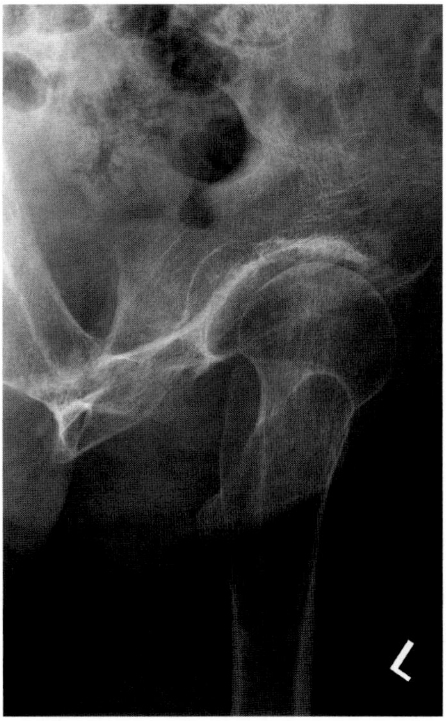

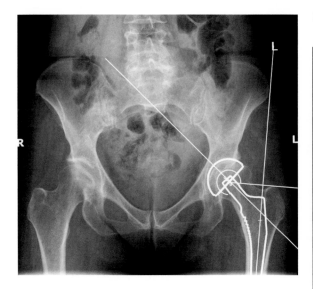

Fig. 10.14 Preoperative lateral view

Indication, Strategy and Specific Recommendations

Coxarthrosis left hip with mild CDH (CE: 18°). Impairment in daily life activities. No success from conservative treatment. Total Hip Arthroplasty (THA) is indicated. Choice of implant was a Corail® stem and Pinnacle™ cup with a ceramic liner. Templating in advance is strongly advised in these cases to anticipate for specific problems. To achieve good seating of the cup in 40° of inclination, allow some medialisation of the centre of rotation. Be aware there is enough bone stock on the medial wall of the acetabulum and decide whether extra bone grafting is necessary. Sometimes screws are necessary to fixate the cup. Medialisation of the centre of the cup must be compensated with the length and CCD angle of the neck to maintain offset and leg length. Templating anticipated for a 52 mm cup. This allows the placement of a 36 mm head.

Surgery was done through a direct anterior approach in supine position. A good press-fit fixation of the cup was accomplished. A size 12 Corail® stem with standard CCD angle and a 5 mm head restored offset and maintained leg length. Direct weight bearing was allowed.

Postoperative X-Ray/Imaging

Fig. 10.15 Preoperative templating

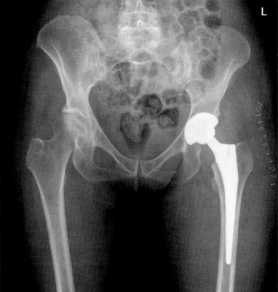

Fig. 10.16 Postoperative x-ray. Excellent planning execution and hip restoration

Lessons Learnt/Alternatives

> Templating is strongly advised to anticipate for specific problems with CDH patients.
> Bone stock of the acetabulum may be insufficient for (press-fit) fixation of the Pinnacle™ cup. Anticipate for the use of screws to fixate the cup.
> Sometimes bone grafting of the acetabulum wall is necessary. When cup and centre of rotation are medialised, care should be taken with the choice of stem to compensate for loss of offset.

Clinical Case 6: The Moderate CDH I

Helge Wangen

Patient Brief History

Forty-seven-year-old man with CDH from Eastern Europe. He was operated on as a child with some kind of osteotomy of the proximal femur on both sides.

Patient Relevant Clinical and Radiological Findings

Limited ROM with right leg fixed in external rotation. Clinically, no limb discrepancy. Severe CDH with Osteoarthritis (OA) apparent on the x-ray.

Preoperative X-Ray/Imaging

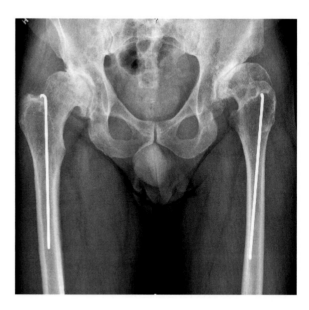

Fig. 10.17 Preoperative x-ray

Indication, Strategy and Specific Recommendations

CDH in an active 47-year-old man. Conservative treatment with physiotherapy and painkillers are no longer an option to the patient because of severe pain especially from the right hip.

Templating of the hip is important to decide what kind of prosthesis is best to restore the anatomy. Template the cup and try to position the cup in order to restore the original centre of the hip. This may also give an indication if additional procedures to achieve enough coverage of the cup are needed. Place the stem template and determine the right offset and neck length.

Postoperative X-Ray/Imaging

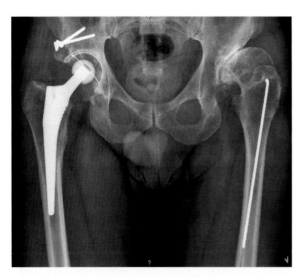

Fig. 10.18 X-ray 3 months postoperative. A cemented cup was used since this is the first choice in Norway. A piece of bone from the femoral head was used to achieve appropriate coverage of the cup. The stem is positioned in some varus. The centre of rotation seems to be restored

Lessons Learnt/Alternatives

> Do always template.
> Try to restore the original centre of rotation of the hip.
> Focus on broaching enough laterally proximally to avoid varus of the stem.

Clinical Case 7: The Moderate CDH II

Vladimir V. Danilyak

Patient Brief History

Left hip. 27-year-old female working as a private secretary with a history of developmental dysplasia of the hip (DDH), Crowe type IV. Open reduction of congenital hip dislocation at 18 months. Mild limping. Pain and progressive disorders after pregnancy and childbirth at the age of 23 years.

Patient Relevant Clinical and Radiological Findings

Marked pain, limited daily activity and work. Moderate limping (walks without support). Positive Trendelenburg sign. LLD of 40 mm (shorter left hip). Limited flexion, abduction and external rotation. Harris hip score: 44, 7. Dislocation and lateralisation of the femoral head (lower type). Proximal femoral valgus. Dorr III type intramedullary canal.

Preoperative X-Ray/Imaging

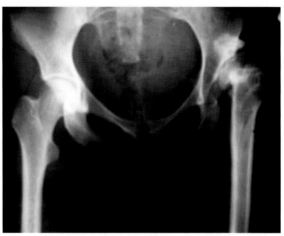

Fig. 10.19 Preoperative AP view

Fig. 10.20 Preoperative templating. Limb lengthening is anticipated from the cup position (Copyright DePuyInternational Limited)

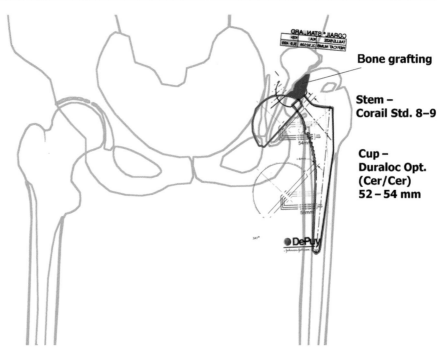

Bone grafting

Stem – Corail Std. 8–9

Cup – Duraloc Opt. (Cer/Cer) 52 – 54 mm

Indication, Strategy and Specific Recommendations

Degenerative disease secondary to DDH. Main goal is cup implantation into the 'natural place'. Do template with orientation on the position of healthy acetabulum. Ceramic-on-ceramic bearing is preferable for a young female. We planned to use big cup (52–54 mm) in order to have thick Biolox®forte insert (preventing of its fracture). In lack of coverage of the cup (less than 70%) remember about possible bone auto grafting. With a 'stove pipe' medullar cavity, valgus stem position is better than varus. Previous scars must be taken into consideration. Inform the patient about high risk of nerve damage.

Postoperative X-Ray/Imaging

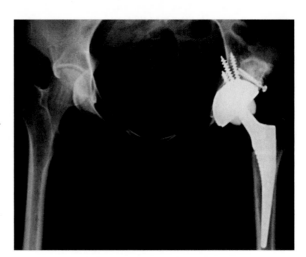

Fig. 10.21 Postoperative view. The cup was inserted in the place of maximum bone stock (point 'of three bones connection' – medial protrusion technique). The length of the left leg was restored. HHS at 12 month is 91, 2

Lessons Learnt/Alternatives

> The main target of a total hip arthroplasty (THA) in the case of arthrosis secondary to DDH is cup implantation in the native acetabular position.
> In a curved stove pipe type intramedullary canal, valgus stem position is preferable.
> Leg length restoration of more than 3/4 cm may lead to nerve root injury.
> Alternative arthrodesis is unacceptable for a young female.

Clinical Case 8: The Severe CDH I

Tim Board

Patient Brief History

Left hip in a 37-year-old female with dysplasia and valgus femur. Presents with increasing pain, Trendelenburg gait and severe osteoarthritis (OA) on x-ray.

Patient Relevant Clinical and Radiological Findings

Previously underwent derotation osteotomy with plate aged 13. No gross evidence of leg length discrepancy. Had no reoperation in the mean time. Willing to recover an active life.

Preoperative X-Ray/Imaging

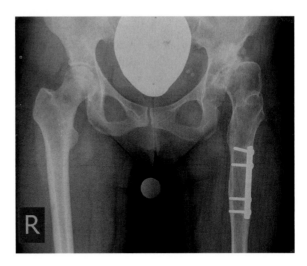

Fig. 10.22 Preoperative AP view. Pelvis tilt due to hip subluxation. Complete joint line narrowing

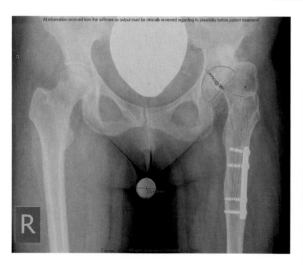

Fig. 10.23 Digital templating. Template has been reported from the healthy hip. Standard stem is the more suitable to restore the native anatomy

Postoperative X-Ray/Imaging

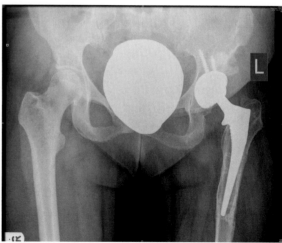

Fig. 10.24 Postoperative x-ray. Excellent clinical result at 1 year. X-rays are satisfactory. Stem is in a degree of valgus and collared implant used. Plate and screws removed without undue trauma to femur, therefore no need to bypass area with a longer stem. Acetabular component a little too steep – could do better!

Indication, Strategy and Specific Recommendations

Pre-existing metalwork does not always need to be removed but CT scan showed screws to be crossing centre of canal and templating showed that the stem would need to bypass at least three of the screws. Consideration given to further rotational osteotomy at the time of total hip arthroplasty (THA) but due to almost vertical neck this becomes unnecessary. Socket appears very dysplastic but templating suggests a standard socket will be adequate.

Lessons Learnt/Alternatives

> Preoperative CT scan will locate the screws in relation to the canal and will measure the neck anteversion.

> Derotation osteotomy is a possibility for valgus, anteverted femora. When valgus is almost vertical this becomes unnecessary.

> Cement can leak from screw holes if performing cemented hip in this situation leading to loss of pressurisation.

> Socket positioning in dysplasia is a trade-off between acceptable inclination angle and bony cover of the cup.

Clinical Case 9: The Severe CDH II

Michel-Henri Fessy

Patient Brief History

Left hip. 32-year-old female. Previous shelf procedure through Hueter approach in childhood. Left leg shortening. Wears a 25 mm lift in the left shoe. Increasing pain and impairment of daily living activities.

Patient Relevant Clinical and Radiological Findings

Clinical LLD of more than 2 cm. Range of motion is partially limited. Previous anterior scar. Preoperative Harris Hip Score of 38. Spine is still flexible. Abductors testing revealed correct muscular strength. Congenital dysplasia of the hip (CDH) Crowe IV. A CT scan was ordered to assess the quality of the acetabulum and the hip version.

Preoperative X-Ray/Imaging

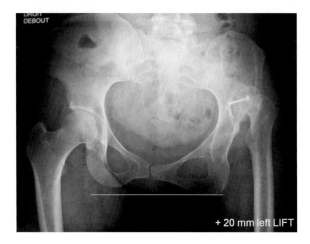

Fig. 10.25 Preoperative AP view. Standing position with a 2 cm left hip compensation. Pelvis is nearly horizontal. Note the typical hypoplasia of the left femur and the dysplastic native acetabulum. Presence of one screw

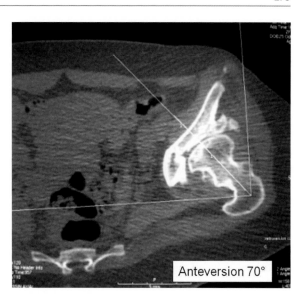

Fig. 10.26 Preoperative CT scan. Major femoral anteversion of 70°. The acetabular cavity was fine (as seen on images taken more distally). The neoarticulation (ilium) is typical very shallow

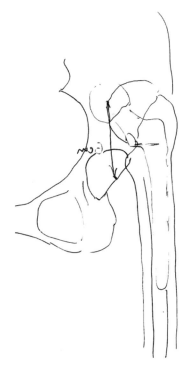

Fig. 10.27 Preoperative templating. A sketch of the hip was drawn from the radiograph to predict the final situation of the femur when put back in the native acetabulum. A lengthening of about 6 cm was expected. The narrow diaphysis could barely accommodate a size 6 dysplasia stem

Indication, Strategy and Specific Recommendations

There is no more room for conservative treatment and a total hip arthroplasty (THA) was an obvious indication. From the templating, the predicted lengthening would have been +6 cm which is far too much (sciatic palsy). The actual LLD being 2.5 cm indicated for a shortening of the femur of about 3.5 cm (6 – 2.5 cm = 3.5 cm) to restore the balance (without a lift) and prevent nerve palsy. The combined correction of the rotation deformity was a second justification for an osteotomy. A size 6 collared stem was selected to adjust the rotation and stabilise the proximal femur after the osteotomy. A small cup was planned and made available at the time of surgery.

A standard posterior approach with a large exposure is our preference. Sciatic nerve must be identified. A comprehensive capsulectomie is required to lower the femur. Neck osteotomy is conducted first in a conservative manner to be able to adjust its height. A 3.5 cm shortening is performed and is temporarily fixed with a clamp. A derotation can be done if there is a need to reorient the greater trochanter to prevent any impingement. Careful broaching and cup preparation was done. A proximal graft from the femoral head was required.

Testing was done with the trial implants. When no further adjustments are required, the osteotomy is fixed using a small plate and screws. Weight bearing was delayed for 45 days. Patient must be informed of prolonged limp after surgery, thus two crutches for 3 months and one crutch for 6 months are indicated.

Postoperative X-Ray/Imaging

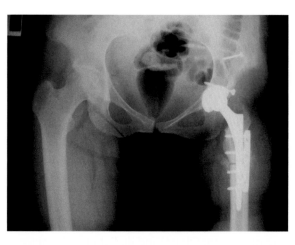

Fig. 10.28 Postoperative AP view after 1 year. The Pelvis is horizontal and the osteotomy is healed. The patient is fine with a Harris Hip Score of 78. Stem 6. Cup 38. Polyethylene liner. Small head (22.2 mm)

Lessons Learnt/Alternatives

> Lengthening of the leg cannot exceed 4 cm.
> Patient must be aware of a higher risk of complication (fracture, nerve palsy…).
> Dysplasia number 6 stem and small cups must be available.
> High hip centre insertion of the cup would result in permanent muscle weakness and fixation would be compromised due to the shallow aspect of the pseudo-acetabulum.

Clinical Case 10: The Stiff Hip

Hans-Erik Henkus

Patient Brief History

Right hip, 43-year-old male patient. High-energy bus trauma march 2009 with acetabular fracture and central protrusion of the hip. Open reduction and fixation through a Kocher-Langenbeck approach. Stent placement for a lesion of the external iliac artery and extensive period in the intensive care unit. One year postoperative, unable to walk unsupported because of extreme pain and severe contracture of the hip joint.

Patient Relevant Clinical and Radiological Findings

Fixed contracture right hip in 50° of flexion and 20° of external rotation. Unable to bear weight. X-ray and CT scan revealed avascular necrosis, residual central protrusion and destruction of the femoral head, extensile surrounding heterotopic ossification (Brooker 4) and a defect (possible non-union) of the medial acetabular wall (see arrow).

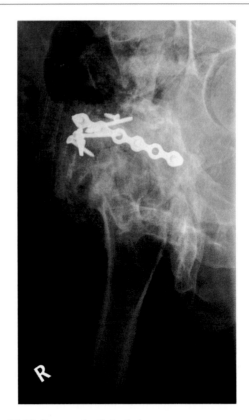

Fig. 10.30 Preoperative Lateral view

Preoperative X-Ray/Imaging

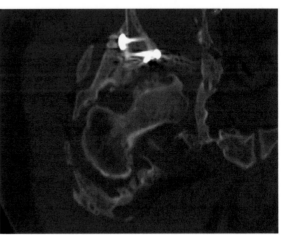

Fig. 10.31 Stiff hip preoperative CT

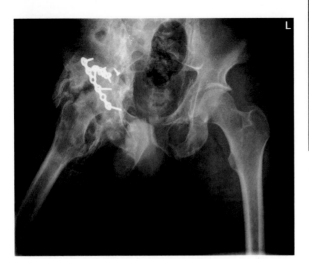

Fig. 10.29 Preoperative AP

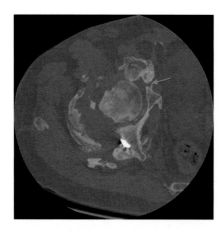

Fig. 10.32 Stiff hip preoperative CT (*arrow*)

Indication, Strategy and Specific Recommendations

Stiff hip with severe flexion; external rotation contracture, avascular necrosis and destruction of femoral head, residual central protrusion with possible nununion of the medial acetabular wall. Severe impairment in daily life.

Preoperative objective: removal of heterotopic bone, reconstruction of acetabular wall and placement of a total hip prosthesis with restoration of the centre of rotation. CT or MR is strongly advised to know the location and extensiveness of the heterotopic bone, its relation with vital structures like the sciatic nerve and to know the quality of the remaining acetabular bone stock.

Choice of implant was a Corail® stem and a double mobility cup (Avantage®, Biomet). This cup was chosen because instability of the implant can be expected after removal of the large amount of heterotopic bone. Templating the opposite side is recommended in these cases to anticipate for specific problems.

Surgery was done in a lateral decubitis position. After removal of heterotopic bone around the tensor muscle, an osteotomy of the greater trochanter was performed leaving the vastus lateralis and gluteus medius muscle attached. This allowed removal of heterotopic bone on the ventral and dorsal side of the hip joint. The sciatic nerve was indentified in advance, but not exposed. After femoral neck osteotomy, the head was removed, allowing access to the heterotopic bone around the psoas tendon. A psoas tenotomy was needed to reduce the flexion contracture completely. The acetabulum showed a central defect but intact and supportive rim. There was a transverse non-union but no instability existed. A titanium cage was placed to

reinforce the medial wall of the acetabulum followed by impaction bone grafting to restore the centre of rotation. A double mobility cup was cemented into place. A size 12 Corail® stem with standard CCD angle and a 5 mm head restored offset and leg length. The osteotomised trochanter was reattached with two standard AO screws. Partial weight bearing was advised for 6 weeks. Meloxicam (15 mg) was given for 2 weeks to prevent new heterotopic bone formation.

Postoperative X-Ray/Imaging

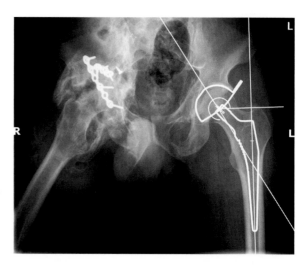

Fig. 10.33 Stiff hip preoperative AP templating

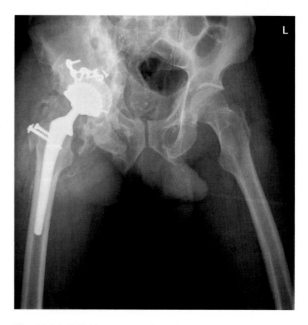

Fig. 10.34 Stiff hip postoperative AP

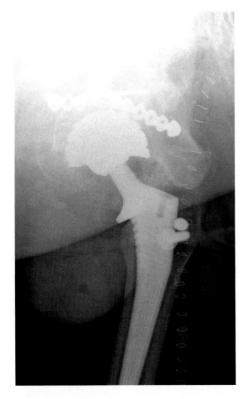

Fig. 10.35 Stiff hip postoperative lateral

Lessons Learnt/Alternatives

> A thorough preoperative work-up is necessary including a CT or MR scan to decide your approach and choice of implant.
> Templates have to be determined from healthy contralateral hip.
> Patient must be informed of increased risk of complications.
> When removing heteroptopic bone, know its relation to vital structures.
> Make a 'what if' plan to be prepared for the worst and have cages, reinforcement rings, (allograft) bone and screws at hand.

Clinical Case 11: The Ankylosed Hip

Jens Boldt

Patient Brief History

Bilateral spontaneous hip fusion/ankylosis following Avascular Necrosis (AVN) of the femoral heads and pelvis 20 years ago. Ex professional volleyball player, 2 m tall, weighing 150 kg. Clinically painful and stiff hip joints for over 15 years, developing increasing lower back pain.

Patient Relevant Clinical and Radiological Findings

Bilateral ankylosed hip joints with 0° of motion. Fusion ended up in a combination of 15° of fixed flexion and 10° of external rotation deformity. Internal hip biomechanics revealed a destruction of both hip centres with 17 mm shortening and 20 mm increased lateral offset on both sides. The femoroacetabular hip joint line is no longer detectable on radiographs.

Preoperative X-Ray/Imaging

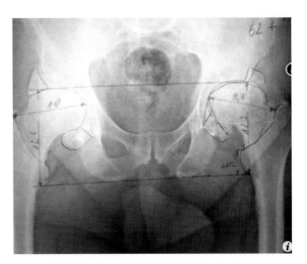

Fig. 10.36 Bilateral hip fusion. Absence of any visible joint line. Fixed external rotation. Preoperative planning and total hip arthroplasty (THA) templating of both hips

Indication, Strategy and Specific Recommendations

Unable to walk normally without severe limping. Significantly reduced activities of daily living. Decreasing groin pain, but increasing lower back pain. Teardrop was the only landmark for templating the acetabulum. The femoral templating was challenging with regard to the correct neck length. A supine position and direct anterolateral modified Hardinge approach was chosen. Hip joint capsule and surrounding muscle groups were extremely contracted and required extensive releases without compromising stability (AL approach). The neck cut was made utilising fluoroscopic image intensifier. The femoral head was fused with the acetabular bone and, therefore, acetabular preparation had to be performed through the femoral neck and head. The smallest acetabular reamer was used to begin with until the teardrop, the transverse acetabular ligament (TAL) and medial wall was reached, again, utilising image intensifying navigation. Increasing acetabular reamer sizes were used until the anterior and posterior columns were detected. The TAL was used for anteversion positioning and the 45° alignment rod for inclination. The femoral preparation revealed soft metaphyseal cancellous bone, which required some additional impaction of autograft from the femoral head reamings. With a 64 mm acetabular implant, a 44 mm metal-on-metal bearing couple was chosen utilising a +5 mm medium neck length. Left hip joint was replaced 6 weeks after the right side. One year follow-up reveals very good scores, pain free mobilisation, very acceptable stable ROM and radiographs showing sound osteointegration of all components. Utilising a 44 mm head size facilitated stable hip joints with very little risk of dislocation.

Postoperative X-Ray/Imaging

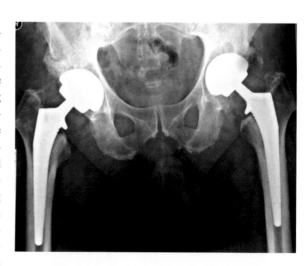

Fig. 10.37 One year postoperative. Sound reconstruction of biomechanics and healing of necrotic and cystic bone areas near the implant interface in both the femur and the acetabulum

Lessons Learnt/Alternatives

> Templating of both hips allow symmetrical restoration of anatomy.

> Extensive capsular joint release to restore motion.

> Hard-on-hard bearing with large (36 or more) is preferable. Mobile bearing cup is an alternative option in older patients.

> Repeat intraoperative imaging to check the cup (stem) positioning

> In childhood diseases and fixed unilateral ankylosis: check the spine flexibility prior to restoring the length, assess gluteus medius function (electromyography, MRI) to get a better view on functional prognosis, inform the patient about prolonged limping, and check the knee joint (typically lateral arthritis in fixed adduction hip ankylosis).

Clinical Case 12: The Obese Patient

Tim Board

Patient Brief History

Fifty-two-year-old female patient with a BMI of 52. Relatively short in stature. Unable to work due to pain in the right hip. Medically well other than obesity.

Patient Relevant Clinical and Radiological Findings

In wheel chair in clinic. Very irritable hip. Significant impingement of adipose tissue around hip makes dislocation a worry postoperatively. Relatively well-preserved joint space but significant peripheral osteophyte formation. Relatively small anatomy.

Preoperative X-Ray/Imaging

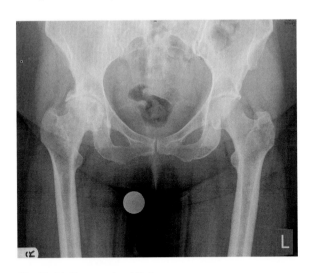

Fig. 10.38 Preoperative AP view

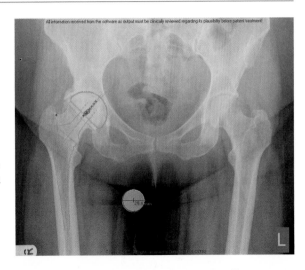

Fig. 10.39 Templating showed a size 48 Pinnacle™ socket and a size 8 Corail® stem confirming the small anatomy

Indication, Strategy and Specific Recommendations

Counselling with regard to potential increased risks of surgery is necessary in this patient group. Positioning of the patient and exposure is of paramount importance in the obese. A sufficiently large incision should be utilised to adequately retract the soft tissues to allow proper component positioning. Careful attention to stability is also necessary and the impingement of the thigh on the abdomen can increase dislocation.

Digital templating systems with marker balls provide accurate templating in obese patients where traditional x-ray magnification may be misleading.

In patients with no shortening of the affected hip and small anatomy, it is relatively easy to lengthen the hip so careful attention is needed to the templated level of neck resection. An intraoperative system of pin and suture was used to accurately re-establish leg length in this case.

Postoperative X-Ray/Imaging

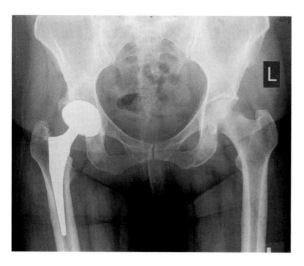

Fig. 10.40 Postoperative x-ray. Despite good exposure, the stem is in slight varus demonstrating the difficulties with these patients. The Corail® stem has been showed to be forgiving in this position. However, the socket alignment is satisfactory and the leg lengths are equal. The templating was accurate and the stability was good

Lessons Learnt/Alternatives

> Preoperative counselling regarding weight loss and increased risk of surgery is appropriate.
> Adequate exposure is paramount (stem alignment and liner insertion).
> Long-term results in the obese are just as satisfactory as the non-obese.
> Beware of incision alignment (skin and fascia).
> Difficult intraoperative testing (risk of lengthening).
> Closure (specific subcutaneous layer drain and stitches).
> Templating is more important in the obese; those with no leg length discrepancy and in small stature patients.

Clinical Case 13: The Septic Hip

Tim Board

Patient Brief History

Left hip in a 47-year-oldmale wagon driver. History of left hip septic arthritis as a child. Previous right distal femoral osteotomy then total knee replacement following childhood trauma. Deteriorating function from left hip with increasing pain and limp.

Patient Relevant Clinical and Radiological Findings

Leg shortening of only 2.5 cm on the left side despite the radiological appearance of much greater discrepancy. This is due to overgrowth of left femur. Galeazzi test preoperatively important to identify source of discrepancy. Acetabular anatomy highly unusual, therefore CT scan is used to ensure adequate bone stock. Templating shows small implants and minimum amount of lengthening achievable.

Preoperative X-Ray/Imaging

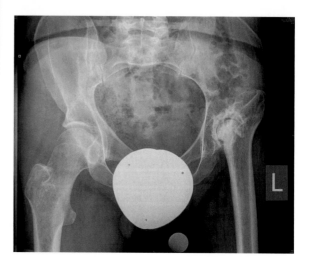

Fig. 10.41 AP view showing head collapse and severe shortening

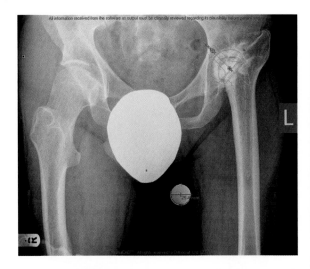

Fig. 10.42 Digital templating using magnification marker is useful in deformities

Indication, Strategy and Specific Recommendations

Risk of re-infection of Total Hip Arthroplasty (THA) following childhood septic arthritis is very low. Cemented implants with extra antibiotics in the cement are not mandatory. In a patient of this age, choice of hard-on-hard ceramic bearings dictates uncemented choice. Standard prophylactic antibiotic cover is all that is required. Microbiological sample sent at time of THA were negative. Risks of over-lengthening explain particularly sciatic nerve injury. Normally not problematic up to 5 cm lengthening.

Postoperative X-Ray/Imaging

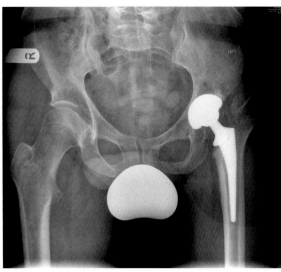

Fig. 10.43 Postoperative control at 2 years. Good postoperative leg lengths (remember the longer femur on the left). Acetabular bone quality was very poor intraoperatively, therefore the patient was kept on protected weight bearing for 6 weeks. Good ingrowth. Patient recovered excellent function and is still a wagon driver

Lessons Learnt/Alternatives

> Uncemented THA following septic arthritis is a good option.
> Microbiological samples should be taken at surgery.
> Leg length discrepancy can sometime be compensated for elsewhere in the limb in conditions present since childhood. Beware of spontaneous overgrowth compensation.
> Excessive lengthening of greater than 5 cm can lead to sciatic nerve palsy.
> Anticipate availability of small implants (notably the cup) in theatre.
> In more recent sepsis, consider two-step procedures (neck resection and samples, then implantation after 2 weeks).

Clinical Case 14: Legg Calve Perthes Disease I

Jean-Claude Cartillier

Patient Brief History

Right hip of a 16-year-old female with severe Legg–Calve–Perthes disease (LCPD).

Previous surgery in her childhood, femoral combined varus and derotation osteotomy. Hardware was already removed. Painful hip with limited daily activities and a major Trendelenburg limp.

Patient Relevant Clinical and Radiological Findings

Coxa plana with typical femoral head. Narrow femoral canal due to morphology and previous surgery. No pelvic tilt (bilateral disease) but bilateral shortening (from intra-articular origin) with collapsed head and lack of offset as observed in typical LCPD. Excessive post-osteotomy external rotation (lesser trochanter appears to be very apparent on AP view).

Preoperative X-Ray/Imaging

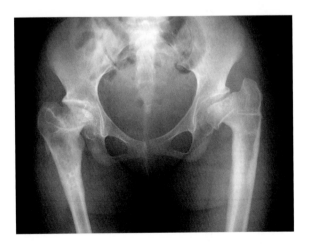

Fig. 10.44 Preoperativee x-ray. Bilateral LCPD with typical aspect of 'coxa plana'. Femoral heads are deformed, partially destroyed and shifted downwards. The joint lines are partially narrowed

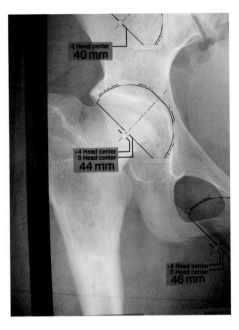

Fig. 10.45 Cup templating. The head cup is pointed as being the new (implant) hip centre

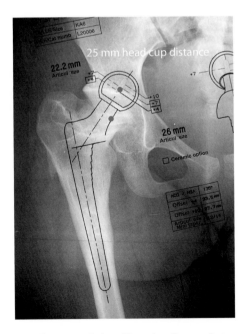

Fig. 10.46 Stem templating. Note the distance between the head centre and the cup centre of about 25 mm which determines the future increase in leg length

Indication, Strategy and Specific Recommendations

Goal: restoration of normal anatomy with appropriate offset to provide the gluteus medius with an optimal lever arm. No major acetabular deformity but a rather small diameter. Standard templating, Cup 44, Stem 6 (Dysplastic type) is scheduled. Rotation can be adjusted intraoperatively thanks to the horizontal design of the collar according to cup orientation and impingement testing. Ceramic-on-ceramic bearing has been selected in this very young patient. Patient and family must be aware of the postoperative lengthening and the need for a temporary lift until left hip surgery is to be performed. Request the specific dysplasia tray (Contact your reps).

Careful approach and capsular release will allow offset restoration. Head resection is then performed. Following acetabular preparation the trial cup must be used and temporarily left in place. Careful shaft alignment is achieved with the use of a curette or a canal finder. A careful and progressive broaching (specific size 6 broach) with an estimated anteversion of 15° must be achieved. Insertion of the Corail® size 6 trial then follows. Intraoperative testing confirms the appropriate anteversion that provides an optimal range of motion and the absence of any impingement. Final implant selection featured: press-fit cup 44, ceramic 28 liner, ceramic head 28 + 1.5 (short neck) and 6A Corail® stem. Postoperative regimen: Immediate weight bearing, two crutches for 1 month.

Postoperative X-Ray/Imaging

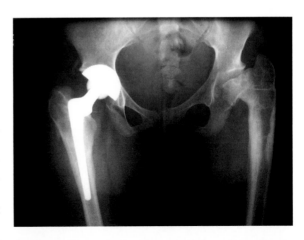

Fig. 10.47 Postoperative x-ray. Restoration of the anatomy including offset has been achieved. Shelton line is harmonious. Lengthening of 25 mm as expected

Lessons Learnt/Alternatives

› LCPD features typical onset of deformity from childhood.
› Be aware of possible rotation issues from previous surgery.
› Forecast specific implants when out of standard range (Dysplastic stem, small cup diameter).
› Clearly inform patient about limb length discrepancy when expected.
› Do consider reliable hard-on-hard bearing in young patients.
› In unilateral disease restoration of the exact limb, length is not always suited (check spinal deformity and its reducibility through clinical examination and/or bending films).

Clinical Case 15: The Legg Calve Perthes Disease II

Jean-Charles Rollier

Preoperative X-Ray/Imaging

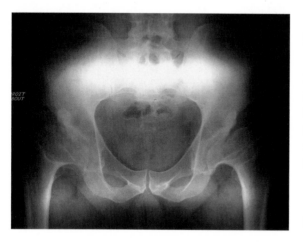

Fig. 10.48 Preoperative radiograph. Typical LCPD aspect. Bilateral osteoarthritis with coxa plana and acetabular dysplasia. No limb discrepancy

Patient Brief History

Bilateral hip disease in a 36-year-old male. Occupation – Chemist. Limitation of daily activities. Patient presents with a bilateral osteoarthritis secondary to a Legg Calve Perthes Disease (LCPD) when he was 5-years old. No previous surgery.

Patient Relevant Clinical and Radiological Findings

Bilateral hip pain and stiffness. No ability to walk more than half an hour or to stand for a long time. Limited range of motion as follows: flexion is 70°, abduction 10°, lack of extension 10°. Gluteus medius muscle evaluation is good. No apparent leg length discrepancy.

Indication, Strategy and Specific Recommendations

In young patients, conservative treatment must be discussed. Femoral osteotomy does not apply here

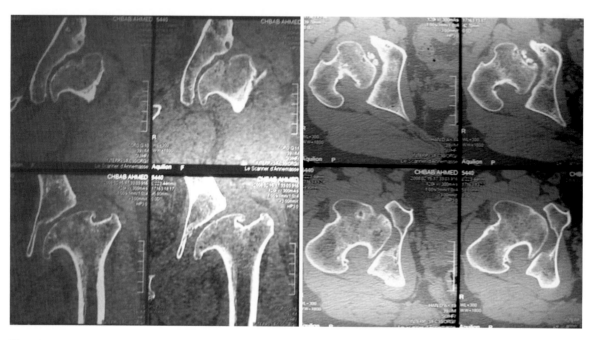

Fig. 10.49 Preoperative CT scan confirms the extent of acetabular dysplasia with limited coverage of both anterior and posterior walls. One can anticipate medial insertion of the cup to achieve a stable primary fixation

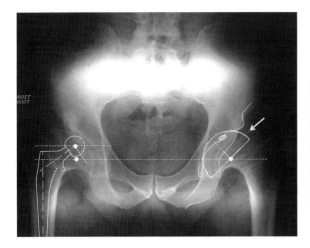

Fig. 10.50 Preoperative templating. Cup planning shows uncovered superior and lateral aspect of the shell (*left arrow*) and subsequent need for bone grafting. Restoration of muscular lever arm without excessive lengthening is best achieved with the use of a coxa vara stem (right hip template)

Postoperative X-Ray/Imaging

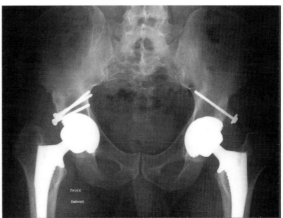

Fig. 10.51 Postoperative view. One can notice a short femoral cut just above the lower trochanter. No pelvis tilt. Medial placement of both cups provided a good coverage and fair fixation. Acetabular bone grafts were performed in order to augment the acetabular bone stock

because of the head deformity combined with acetabular dysplasia. Total hip arthroplasty (THA) appeared to be the best solution in an active patient.

From the preoperative work-up we did anticipate the need for additional bone grafting and medial placement of the cup. Coxa vara stem appeared to be the best solution to maintain the offset with an acceptable lengthening. Ceramic-on-ceramic bearing was selected.

Left hip was done first with a resulting 20 mm leg over length as anticipated. A temporary 15 mm lift was used in the right shoe. Right hip was operated on 4 month later. In both hips partial weight bearing was observed during 45 days.

Lessons Learnt/Alternatives

> Preoperative CT-Scan is recommended in difficult primary hips.
> Limb lengthening must be anticipated and discussed with the patient.
> Ceramic-on-ceramic bearing is the best option in young and active patients.
> Bilateral hip replacement is an alternative option.

Clinical Case 16: The Paget's Disease

Scott Brumby

Patient Brief History

Right hip in a 77 year old female. Complains about activity pain and walking distance gradually reducing. Medically and biochemically stable Paget's disease.

Patient Relevant Clinical and Radiological Findings

Relatively old patient with reduced function despite appropriate conservative treatment. Absence of leg length discrepancy. Limited range of motion. Good general health condition.

Preoperative X-Ray/Imaging

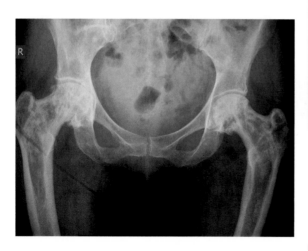

Fig. 10.52 Preoperative AP radiograph. Typical aspect of Paget's disease. Sclerotic bone. Proximal bow of both femurs combined with coxa vara

Indication, Strategy and Specific Recommendations

Preoperative Endocrine review is mandatory. Avoid surgery within 3 months of intravenous bisphos-

phonates infusion. Templating indicates the need for a coxa vara stem. Lateral radiographs do not show significant deformity.

Standard posterior approach is with no particularity. Box chisel must be available to achieve a good alignment of the stem and the use of appropriately sized stem. Identify a calcar crack and wire the femur if any. Need for end cutting reamers for acetabular preparation (sclerotic bone). Be prepared for additional fixation using screws. Anticipate greater than expected blood loss from femoral canal in conjunction with the anaesthetist. Inform patient about specific complications such as bleeding.

Postoperative X-Ray/Imaging

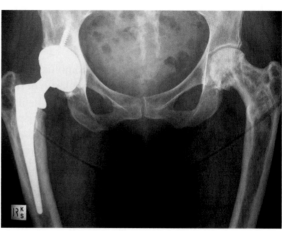

Fig. 10.53 Postoperative AP view. Excellent restitution of the overall anatomy. Appropriate sizing and cup orientation sizing. Note the cup slightly inserted in varus

Lessons Learnt/Alternatives

> Screw fixation of acetabular component to improve initial fixation of sclerotic hard bone.
> May not achieve an initial press-fit.
> Collared stem to obtain greater rotational stability and minimise subsidence as osteointegration may be slow.

Clinical Case 17: The Benign Tumour

Jean-Claude Cartillier

Patient Brief History

Right hip. 75-year-old male. Chronic dysplastic cyst and developed severe osteoarthritis (OA). Leg length discrepancy of 30 mm. Stiff hip. Progressively increasing pain and disability.

Patient Relevant Clinical and Radiological Findings

Right hip OA with complete joint line narrowing. Major bone cyst in the proximal femur and greater trochanter area resulting in proximal varus deformity (progressive frontal bow).

Preoperative X-Ray/Imaging

Indication, Strategy and Specific Recommendations

Two challenges must be addressed. The anatomic challenge consists in realigning the femur through catheterisation of the curved canal; to achieve consistent primary fixation of the stem and to restore the leg length. The biological challenge is the anticipated difficult proximal integration in absence of good cancellous bone bed. There is thus, a need for reaching more distal untouched bone to provide reliable osteointegration.

Cup placement and templating will determine the hip centre. Revision Corail® has been selected to achieve appropriate fixation. An extended proximal trochanterotomy is anticipated. The head will be kept for grafting at the calcar level to fill up the defect and restore adequate bone stock. Correction of length discrepancy is by positioning the stem, proximally 30 mm above the head centre as determined by the centre of the cup. Templating: threaded cup 56 (Spirofit™), Stem Corail® Revision (KAR™ 18) Long Neck.

Posterior approach recommended, facilitating femoral access. Trochanterotomy is oblique and at least 2 cm below the inferior aspect of the cyst to reach normal bone area. Biopsy samples will be

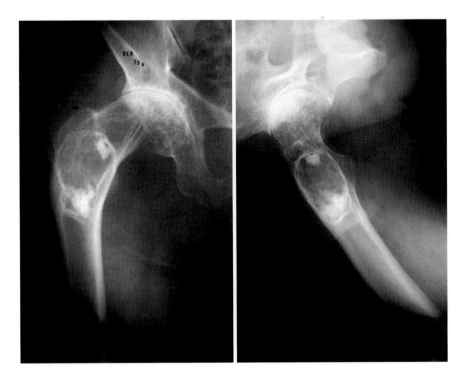

Fig. 10.54 Preoperative AP and lateral view showing the extensive metaphysis void along with a major inwards bending of the proximal femur

Fig. 10.55 Preoperative templating. The Corail® Revision template is placed at the level to compensate the LLD. Lateral view templating is crucial especially with longer stems

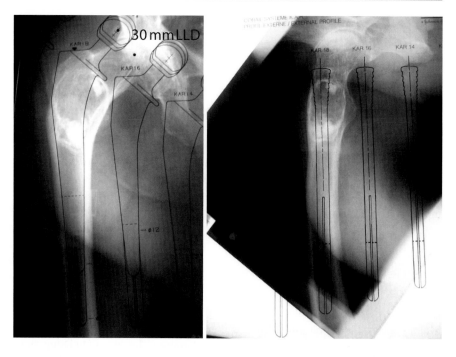

taken. Delicate manipulation and anterior shifting of the flap is needed to allow complete removal of the cyst and facilitate distal femoral reaming and broaching. Trial implant (size 18) is placed to check length and primary stability. Finally, revision Corail® 18 is inserted. Grafting of the calcar area and fixation of the flap around the stem was done using five wires. A +8.5 head is selected. Final checking has shown good mobility, stability, limb length restoration and solid fixation of the femoral flap. Postoperative regimen consisted in a non-weight bearing period of 45 days.

Postoperative X-Ray/Imaging

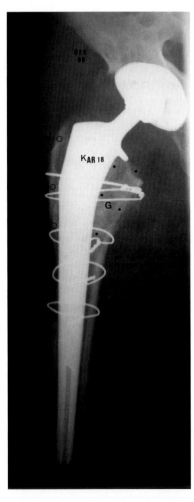

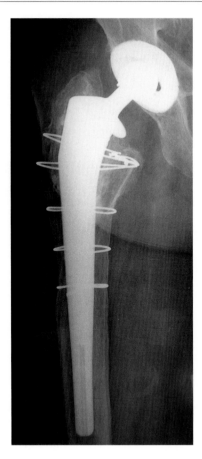

Fig. 10.57 Postoperative x-ray after 6 years. Excellent result after 6 years with maintaining of bone stock and integration

Fig. 10.56 Postoperative view after 3 months. Restoration of the anatomy including offset and leg length. Complete healing of the femoral flap. Total osteointegration of the stem. No stress shielding because of extended integration along the stem from proximal to distal. Note the restoration of the calcar bone stock

Lessons Learnt/Alternatives

› Consider longer stem when proximal bone fixation is compromised (biological challenge).

› Consider a femoral flap osteotomy in maligned femur or other deformity (anatomical challenge).

Clinical Case 18: The Malignant Tumour

Jens Boldt

Preoperative X-Ray/Imaging

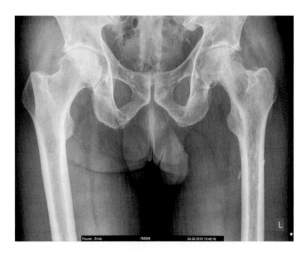

Fig. 10.58 Lung adenocarcinoma with femoral head and lesser trochanter metastasis of the left hip joint. Collapse of the femoral head and severe groin pain

Patient Brief History

Primary adenocarcinoma of the lungs detected coincidentally following a routine chest X-rays during preparation for Total Hip Arthroplasty (THA) surgery. Pelvic radiographs revealed a collapsed femoral head and pathological mineralisation of the proximal femur. Groin pain and mobilisation deteriorated rapidly and after femoral collapse.

Patient Relevant Clinical and Radiological Findings

The cancer team opted for chemotherapy and early THA. Removing the proximal femur and implanting a tumour prosthesis was not felt necessary due to the various reasons.

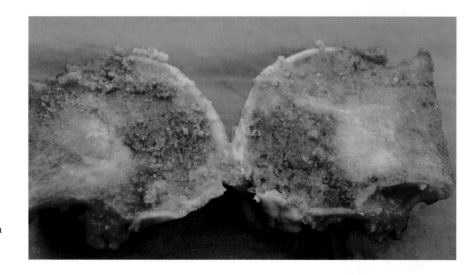

Fig. 10.59 Macroscopic examination of the head. Primary lung cancer and secondary adenocarcinoma metastasis of the femoral head

Indication, Strategy and Specific Recommendations

Following clearance from the cancer team, the indication for primary THA was given and templating performed. Intraoperatively, multiple specimens from soft tissues, bone tissues and reamings were taken for histological review. A primary Corail® and Pinnacle™ THA with ceramic-on-ceramic bearings was implanted. Histology revealed that the only metastasis involvement was found in the lesser trochanter. The proper dignity and entity from the tumour was obtained (adenocarcinoma) and chemotherapy as well as radiotherapy was followed 6 weeks after THA. Lessons learnt include, in particular, a very careful look at preoperative radiographs. In retrospect, the pathological bone changes can be detected within the femur. Secondly, a tumour prosthesis was not necessary in this particular case. Thirdly, preoperative planning together with the cancer team is strongly recommended. Fully HA coating of the Corail® stem provides rapid osteointegration, which was very favourable in this case.

Lessons Learnt/Alternatives

> Management of malignant tumours of the bones must be discussed in conjunction with cancer specialist team.
> First decision is related to complete or partial (palliative) tumour resection according to tumour type, size, extension.
> Patient and family information regarding procedure and expectations is crucial.
> Preoperative irradiation or patient's general condition may increase the complication rate.
> Resection of the proximal aspect of the femur and use of long stem with distal interlocking screws fixation (Reef® stem), combined with mobile bearing cup or constrained liner.

Postoperative X-Ray/Imaging

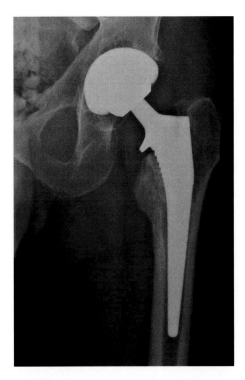

Fig. 10.60 Five months postoperatively. Well-integrated Corail® stem. No changes in position, no subsidence, and no osteolysis. Questionable mineralisation changes in the lesser trochanter. Patient is pain free and well mobilised. Continued cancer treatment

Clinical Case 19: The Neck of Femur Fracture (NOF)

Tarik Aït Si Selmi

Patient Brief History

This 75-year-old woman fell on her right side in the street. Patient had immediate intense groin pain while the leg was slightly shortened and externally rotated. She was unable to walk. X-rays were taken in the Emergency Department.

Patient Relevant Clinical and Radiological Findings

Active patient, living on her own. Enjoyed any outdoor recreational activities. Had no previous history of either hip problems, nor any articular concerns, and is in good general condition.

Preoperative X-Ray/Imaging

Indication, Strategy and Specific Recommendations

Displacement is not obvious but the head is in varus with a posterior tilt. In this situation, the mechanical conditions are not suitable for a conservative option. In addition, any attempt to get a reduction would compromise the healing process. With the patient being 75 years old, but still active, we moved to a total hip arthroplasty (THA).

Planning was done on the contralateral healthy side to restore the anatomy. A mobile bearing cup was selected to prevent the risk of dislocation and facilitate the postoperative rehabilitation as the patient will have no restriction advices.

During approach, one must remember that the greater trochanter appears to be higher relative to the head than expected. When looking for the neck one must achieve careful blunt dissection starting from the femur in a slight downwards direction as opposed to routine hip approach. Pulling the leg down before incision can be helpful. Capsule must be widely opened to facilitate head removal. Head must be kept available as grafting may be necessary. The remaining neck must be cut according to preoperative templating. Careful progressive broaching must be started after clearing off any neck remnants at the trochanteric junction to prevent varus insertion. Calcar planner must be used to

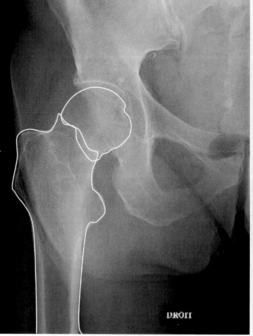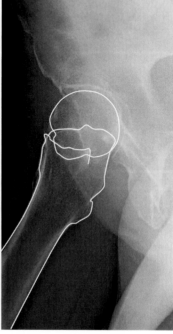

Fig. 10.61 Preoperative AP and lateral views. Note the medial and posterior shift of the head that was not clearly seen at a first glance by the emergency fellow

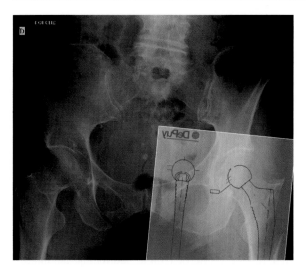

Fig. 10.62 Templating is set from the left hip. A standard stem is appropriate. Level of the cut is determined (Copyright DePuyInternational Limited)

accommodate the collar. Cup preparation is not specific. The use of collared stem is recommended in fragile environment. Identify any crack before and after stem insertion. Do wire the proximal femur if any crack. Be careful while getting the hip back in place while torsion effort may provoke or propagate any unrecognised calcar crack.

Preoperative X-Ray/Imaging

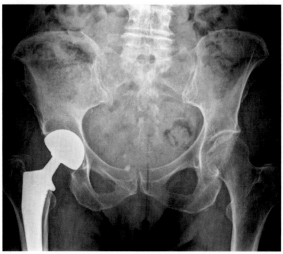

Fig. 10.64 Postoperative 6 month x-ray. Harmonious restoration of the anatomy. Note that calcar cut is rather low related to neck fracture level. +5 mm neck was used to restore the length

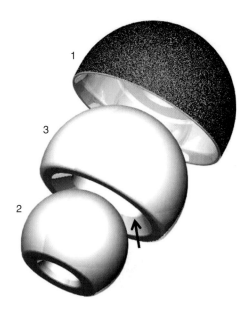

Fig. 10.63 The mobile-bearing cup comes in three parts. The cup is a press-fit implant of which the inner contour is spherical and highly polished (*1*). The standard 28 mm head (*2*) is clipped into the spherical PE liner (*3*) through the inner lip of the liner (*arrow*) which is slightly smaller than the head. The liner is mobile in the metal shell in extreme movements when the neck contacts its contour. Its large diameter allows enhanced ROM with outstanding stability

Lessons Learnt/Alternatives

> Try to template the NOF patient with a correct AP view of both hips.
> Use preferably a collared version of the Corail® stem.
> Favour THA in patients that are still active.
> Use a mobile bearing cup to guard against dislocation.

Clinical Case 20: Total Hip Arthroplasty (THA) After Neck Fixation

Tarik Aït Si Selmi

Preoperative X-Ray/Imaging

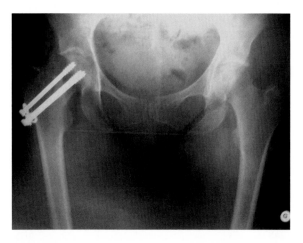

Fig. 10.65 Preoperative x-ray showing medialised and shortened right hip

Patient Brief History

Right hip in 57-year-old retired woman with history of neck of femur fracture 3 years ago. Had ORIF with cannulated screws. Developed progressive right hip shortening, limping, then subsequent disability affecting her daily activities. Use of 10 mm right lift did not improve the patient.

Patient Relevant Clinical and Radiological Findings

Limited ROM. Lower limb discrepancy 10 mm shorter right hip. Pelvis tilt of 10 mm. Shortening due to neck malunion. Hardware present. No evidence of joint line narrowing.

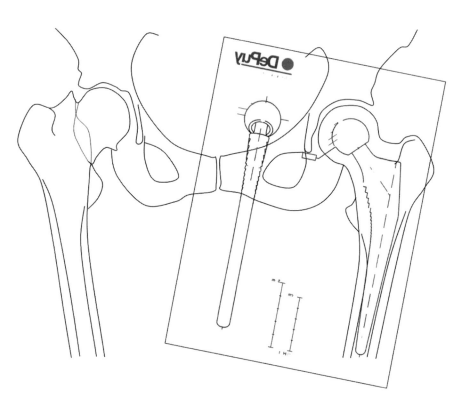

Fig. 10.66 Templating the healthy hip. Standard stem is appropriate (Copyright DePuyInternational Limited)

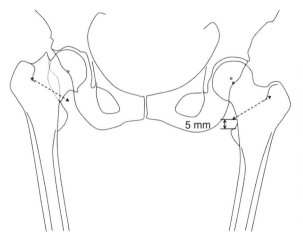

Fig. 10.67 Planning recorded on right hip with a neck osteotomy of 5 mm above the lesser trochanter (Copyright DePuyInternational Limited)

Postoperative X-Ray/Imaging

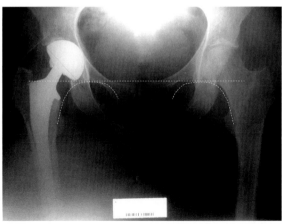

Fig. 10.68 Postoperative x-ray showing symmetrical restoration of the hip

Indication, Strategy and Specific Recommendations

Neck malunion in 57-year-old patient. THA appears to be the best option. Compensation with lift was not successful. Template the left (healthy hip) and the cup. Draw the expected hip centre. Place the expected stem template and determine the neck length. Use preferably medium (+5 mm) neck in order to be able to adapt intraoperatively. Make sure you get the appropriate screw driver to take the screws (and washer) off.

Use the previous incision as much as possible. Record the planned neck osteotomy. Beware of varus tendency due to previous canal obturation. Use a canal finder if needed to assess the appropriate direction.

Lessons Learnt/Alternatives

> Template have to be determined from healthy contralateral hip
> Patient must be informed of increased risk of complication in repeated surgery
> Beware of possible malalignment of the stem (varus)
> Alternative conservative option such as neck osteotomy is not suitable because of high risk of subsequent non-union

Clinical Case 21: Total Hip Arthroplasty (THA) After Proximal Femoral Osteotomy I

Laurent Jacquot

Patient Brief History

Left Hip on a 70-year-old male. Femoral osteotomy 30 years ago. Leg length discrepancy 40 mm. Major limping for a long time. Farmer still active but concerned about pain and stiffness.

Patient Relevant Clinical and Radiological Findings

Increasing pain for the last past 3 years. Fixed deformity with 10° of internal rotation. Hip osteoarthritis (OA) with joint narrowing. Malunion secondary to proximal varus femoral osteotomy.

Preoperative X-Ray/Imaging

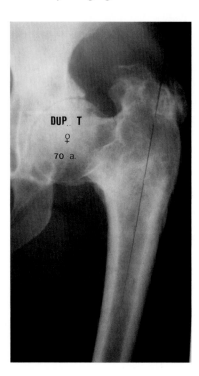

Fig. 10.69 Varus deformity of the proximal femur, with 40 mm of shortening (Extra-articular deformity)

Indication, Strategy and Specific Recommendations

The patient is ready for surgery due to stiffness and pain.

Surgical options are: osteotomy before THA, Osteotomy and THA in the same setting, customised stem or conventional stem. Templating is crucial before surgery, on anteroposterior and lateral view. The option was to use a standard stem because there was no deformity on the lateral view, and it was possible to plane a straight stem, with an acceptable varus positioning. Cup templating had no particularity. A standard neck osteotomy 5 mm above the lesser trochanter was planned. Insertion of the stem would necessarily be in varus because of the greater trochanter overhanging above the shaft. Varus insertion of the stem allows restoring the offset while moving the tip of the trochanter off the pelvis (preventing impingement) and restoring better gluteux medius lever arm. Head size and neck length were difficult to schedule preoperatively because of the uncertainty of the final position of the stem. Femoral broaching must be guided carefully to avoid any lateral shaft fracture or false route.

Postoperative X-Ray/Imaging

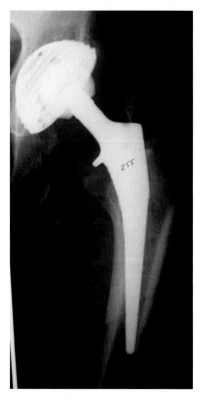

Fig. 10.70 X-ray after 19 years of implantation, showing limited poly wear, but no loosening, no lucent line, no cortical reaction. The patient is doing extremely well without any complaints

Lessons Learnt/Alternatives

> THA after femoral osteotomy requires a careful clinical and radiological planning including predicted varus positioning when it does not increase the resulting offset too much.

> Limited femoral malunion can be addressed with a conventional stem

> Varus positioning is sustainable with a fully HA coated stem which allows long-term fixation without bone reaction.

> Corail® stem is somewhat forgiving even in obvious malalignment, without any clinical or radiological backdrops.

> Straight alignment of the stem would have been possible with the addition of a trochanterotomy and subsequent challenging reattachment in repeated surgery.

> Customised stem is an option, having in mind that final insertion is sometimes hazy since prediction of canal matching remains uncertain. Bone quality and stem insertion is rather unpredictable in previously fractured or osteotomised bone.

> Combined osteotomy of the proximal femur is a technically challenging option but it is recommended in extreme deformities or in malunion combining malalignment and torsional deformity.

Clinical Case 22: Total Hip Arthroplasty (THA) After Proximal Femoral Osteotomy II

Markus C. Michel

Patient Brief History

Forty-seven-year-old male. Intertochanteric osteotomy at the age of 21 the left followed by the right at the age of 24. The hardware was removed on the left side by the age of 23, on the right side 2 years later. Ongoing hip pain since he was 14 years. After surgery, he was never pain free. The last 6 years has developed increasing pain with progressive inability to walk. At the time of intervention, maximal walking distance of less than 200 m, severe pain at night.

Patient Relevant Clinical and Radiological Findings

Reduced and extremely painful ROM, similar in both hips. Deformity of both heads, reduced and irregular joint space. Discrepancy of CCD angle between the two hips. Sclerotic zones on two levels in both hips.

Preoperative X-Ray/Imaging

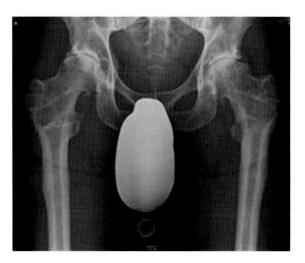

Fig. 10.71 X-rays calibrated with spherical marker. Severe osteoarthritis (OA). Narrow femurs and sclerotic cortical formations within both necks and femoral canals

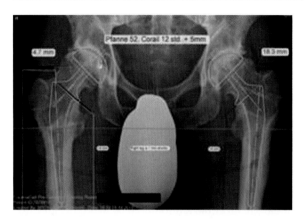

Fig. 10.72 Templating of both hips using Trauma Cad Software

Indication, Strategy and Specific Recommendations

Indication for THA was given by the pain level of the patient, loss of life quality, reduced ROM and the destruction of the joints.

For templating Trauma Cad software was used, calibrated in our institution. The templating was performed using a standard protocol, where first the centre of rotation is restored, before offset and length. Because of the different CCD angle the positioning of the implants is different from the right to the left hip, in order to restore leg length.

Because a direct anterior approach was used (MicroHip®), the distance from the tip of the greater trochanter to the implant was measured on both sides, to be used as landmarks during the surgery. During the intervention, we followed the DAA (MicroHip®) procedure in lateral decubitus position, without traction table. Even if the osteotomy and the removal of the hardware was done through a lateral approach, our experience shows that it is a rehabilitation advantage to use an anterior approach in order to minimise the soft tissue trauma.

Implantation technique had to be adapted especially with regard to the sclerotic zones. To open up the medullary canal a chisel should be used. Also to ream the partially sclerotic medullary canal it is recommended to use a canal reamer in order to fit the stem perfectly.

Postoperative X-Ray/Imaging

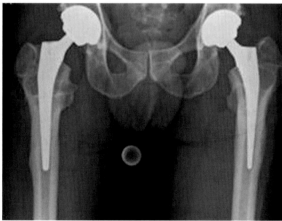

Fig. 10.73 Postoperative control: Centre of rotation as well as leg length in both hips has been reconstructed following the templating. Note that the left hip implants are smaller. At 3 months after surgery the patient was pain free and able to walk for more than 2 h

Lessons Learnt/Alternatives

> In this specific condition templating of both hips is crucial. It is not possible to apply the templating from one side to the other.
> This type of surgery, specifically using a DAA should only be performed by experienced surgeons.
> The implantation technique for the Corail® stem has to be adapted. Nevertheless it is crucial to attempt rotational stability as well as adequate compaction of the trabecular bone even in these circumstances.

Clinical Case 23: Total Hip Arthroplasty (THA) After Fibular Strut Graft

Tom Hogervorst

Patient Brief History

Both hips of a 26-year-old male with treatment for testicular carcinoma with surgery and chemotherapy including prednisolone regimen to treat side effects. In a few months time he developed avascular necrosis of the femoral heads. He had a treatment with forage and placement of fibula strut graft on the left side. He developed pain in both hips that severely limited his daily activities and work as a technical draughtsman.

Patient Relevant Clinical and Radiological Findings

Limited ROM with pain on straight leg raising and on rotation. No limb length discrepancy. Avascular necrosis (Ficat 4) with head collapse and coxarthrosis.

Preoperative X-Ray/Imaging

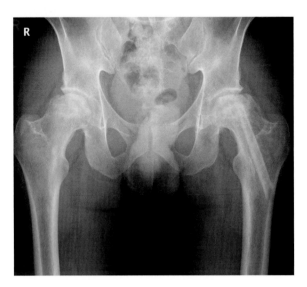

Fig. 10.74 Preoperative AP view

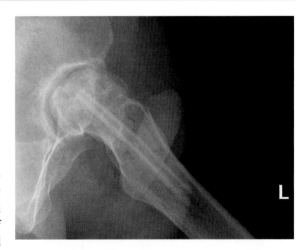

Fig. 10.75 Preoperative lateral view

Indication, Strategy and Specific Recommendations

Young patient with bilateral coxarthrosis. There are no signs of recurrence of his testicular carcinoma. In our view, there are no other options other than a bilateral THA. Resurfacing is not attractive with collapse of the femoral heads. We feel the bearing couple with the least amount of wear is indicated in a young person, that is ceramic–ceramic. We chose a Corail® stem and Pinnacle™ cup with 36 mm femoral heads. In consultation with the patient, we planned bilateral hip arthroplasty with direct anterior supine approach in a single operative session. We anticipated difficulties with stem placement on the left side due to the fibular strut graft, and therefore planned use of fluoroscopy.

Postoperative X-Ray/Imaging

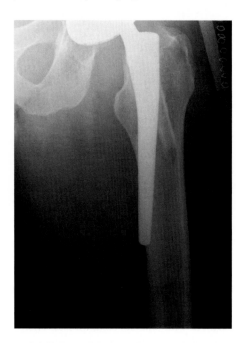

Fig. 10.76 Initial postoperative radiograph showing a mediodorsal false route noted. Fluoroscopy was not available at the time of surgery. Prompt revision of the stem, with fluoroscopy, was without further difficulty

Lessons Learnt/Alternatives

> Do not accept violation of your operative plan by equipment failure.
> Fluoroscopic control and use of a canal finder can be very useful in cases with altered femoral morphology.
> Bilateral THA in one session is a good option if done in consultation with the patient.

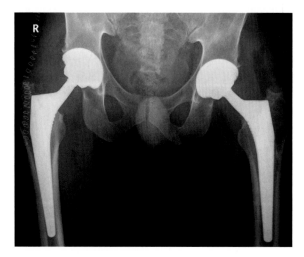

Fig. 10.77 Postoperative control

Clinical Case 24: Total Hip Arthroplasty (THA) After Resurfacing

Tom Hogervorst

Patient Brief History

Left hip. 55-year-old male with fairly strenuous work in agriculture. Hip resurfacing, in 2007, for coxarthrosis done with trochanteric osteotomy (Ganz approach). Hip has never been without problems since. After 2 years, pain in and around the hip developed and he describes a feeling that something blocks in the hip.

Patient Relevant Clinical and Radiological Findings

Limited ROM. No limb length discrepancy. Two screws in healed trochanter. Extremely steep cup with high anteversion. No clear signs of loosening or neck narrowing.

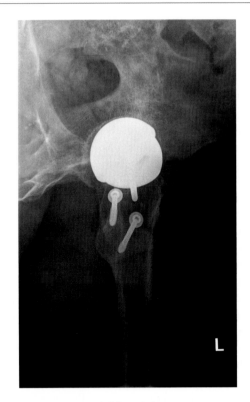

Fig. 10.79 Preoperative left lateral view

Preoperative X-Ray/Imaging

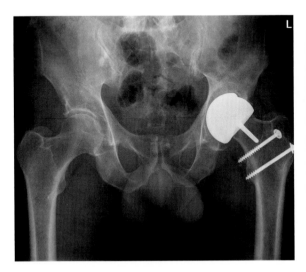

Fig. 10.78 Preoperative AP view

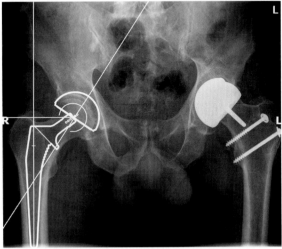

Fig. 10.80 Preoperative templating

Indication, Strategy and Specific Recommendations

Cup malposition of resurfacing in 55-year-old patient. Edge loading generates high wear and may lead to pseudotumour and soft tissue damage. THA appears to be the best option with change to bearing couple other than metal-on-metal.

Template the right (healthy hip) to get best information on neck offset. Template the cup and anticipate a larger size to prevent a high position of the cup in the superior area of the 60 mm resurfacing cup. Draw the expected hip centre. Place the expected stem template. Use coxa vara (CCD 126°) and long or extra long (+12 mm) neck in order to recreate the high offset of this hip. Make sure you get the appropriate screw driver to take the screws (and washer) off.

We used the previous (lateral) incision but did anterior (Huetter) approach to the hip, giving us optimal control of cup position and leg-length. The femoral neck osteotomy can pass just below the pin of the femoral head. Remove the cup with curved and flexible osteotomes. Ream to a larger size, making sure not to create a high hip centre. 66 mm size Pinnacle™ cup was placed here. Use a canal finder in the femur if needed to assess the appropriate direction.

Lessons Learnt/Alternatives

> Templating is best done on healthy contralateral hip.
> Revision of resurfacing is supposed to be easy, but cup problems may compromise result.
> Re-revision rate after revision of resurfacing is high.
> Patient must be informed of increased risk of complications in revision surgery.
> Alternative may be cup revision only, but femoral head is likely out-of-round due to edge loading and bearing issues may persist.

Postoperative X-Ray/Imaging

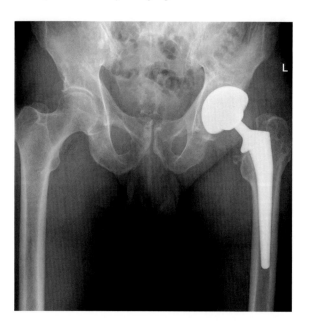

Fig. 10.81 Postoperative AP view. Restoration of the anatomy has been achieved. Cup inclination and orientation is optimal

Clinical Case 25: Total Hip Arthroplasty (THA) After THA

Tim Board

Patient Brief History

This 51-year-old rheumatoid patient had already undergone revision surgery with application of a posterior lip augmentation device (PLAD) to treat recurrent dislocation. Unfortunately, this was not successful and she presented with recurrent instability of the hip.

Patient Relevant Clinical and Radiological Findings

Patient in a hip brace, very anxious when out of the brace. Severely limited quality of life due to problem, therefore surgical solution required. Trochanteric nonunion pre-existing. Recurrent instability despite PLAD indicates other factors such as socket wear, PLAD malposition. Due to monoblock stem this will require revision to enable a large head prosthesis to be used. Due to the patient's relatively young age and the good quality of the metaphyseal/diaphyseal bone, a long revision stem is not thought necessary.

Preoperative X-Ray/Imaging

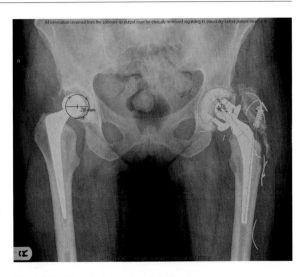

Fig. 10.83 Templating using digital software

Indication, Strategy and Specific Recommendations

Surgical plan was removal of all components without further osteotomy. Templating showed no significant leg length discrepancy and a good calcar despite the bone loss laterally. A DeltaMotion™ socket was used which allows a ceramic-on-ceramic large bearing to be used to treat the recurrent dislocation. A collared Corail® stem was used after removal of all cement. If there was any intraoperative concern about axial or rotational stability of the stem then a Corail® revision stem would have been used. The trochanteric nonunion was found to be a fibrous union and was left.

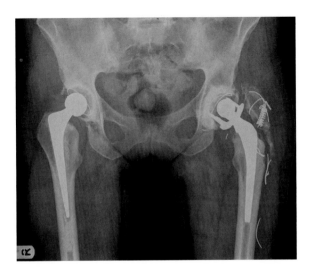

Fig. 10.82 Preoperative AP view

Postoperative X-Ray/Imaging

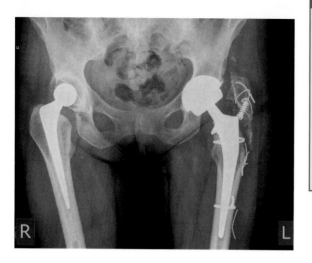

Fig. 10.84 Postoperative x-rays show good bone preservation in this potentially difficult revision case. Clinical outcome shows no further dislocations. Collared implant is a must in revision uncemented short stems

Lessons Learnt/Alternatives

› Conversion to large head prosthesis is a good option for recurrent dislocation.
› Modern large ceramic bearing surfaces allow a durable bearing option for this young patient.
› Always use a collared implant for revision surgery with a short stem.
› Bone preservation and conservative revision option is paramount in the younger patients undergoing revision hip surgery.

Hip arthritis is one of the most disabling diseases in the world. The World Health Organisation (WHO) estimates half a million total hip replacements per annum in 2030. Health care systems around the world differ but all have a common need to spend limited resources wisely. There is an intrinsic conflict between science and economy. The stakeholders include: patients, surgeons, hospitals, payers and manufactures. In the UK, the Primary Care Trust defines the tariff for a hip replacement and all other medical procedures. Piers Yates states that the Corail® stem is more expensive than the cemented Exeter stem, but cheaper than the cemented C-stem, when taking all costs involved into account. High performance total hip replacements are usually most expensive, for example a Corail® stem, a cementless press-fit cup and a ceramic on ceramic articulation. However, approximately 1,500 USD can be saved when using an early discharge programme and in the longer term much greater savings can be made with the reduced costs for repeat revision surgery for all reasons. The newest and the most expensive implants are not necessarily the best. The whole package of a total hip arthroplasty (THA) procedure must be taken into account and valued against expensive implants. Regular follow-up is mandatory for future decision taking.

Introduction

Total hip replacement is one of the most rewarding operations that we perform in Orthopaedics today. Sir John Charnley started this era of total hip replacements in the UK and the success of the operation has led to increasing demands for the surgery. The WHO has stated that 40% of over 70-year-olds suffer from osteoarthritis. It is the most common cause of chronic disability in the world. It is estimated by the year 2030 that 500,000 joints per year will be implanted [1]. The number of total hip replacement will rise as will the number of different total hip implants available. Research and development bring new implants to the market offering new options in joint replacement surgery. Mostly they are more expensive than their predecessors. The combination of increasing demand and the increasing costs per unit means that the overall economic burden of hip replacements is significant.

There is, however, a limited pot of cash available for medicine in general and hip replacements in this particular example. Health care systems around the world differ but all have a common need to spend limited resources wisely. No country health economic pot is bottomless. There is an intrinsic conflict in the system where science and economics meet. In some cases science may win, in some cases economics may win but virtually always a compromise is necessary. This chapter looks at the different influences that come to bear on any health system when managing the hip replacement market. The stakeholders include: patients, surgeons, hospitals, payers and manufactures.

The patient profile is changing. Patients when deciding on hip replacements are less concerned with quantity of life rather than quality of life. They tend to ask for their surgery at an earlier stage of the disease, expect to regain full activity after surgery, and expect

J.-P. Vidalain et al. (eds.), *The CORAIL® Hip System*,
DOI: 10.1007/978-3-642-18396-6_11, © Springer-Verlag Berlin Heidelberg 2011

to live for a long time. They will often be well read in the available options and often will expect to have input into the choice of hip replacement that they are given. Their requests are based on scientific and marketing information and not on cost.

The surgeon's main focus will be on providing for his patient the best hip replacement he can. His decision will be made on the experience of his training, his experience with a particular implant and from reviewing scientific data from his peers. His decision, however, will also be influenced by patient demands and manufacturers' marketing. Last, but not least, his decision will also be influenced by his hospital management team who will be looking at the economic factors.

In the UK, the hospital provides the environment in which hip replacements are carried out. The hospital management relies on the funding for these procedures from the Primary Care Trust. The hospital management is in a difficult position. The money that the hospital is given per case (the tariff) is provided by the Primary Care Trust but the level is dictated by the government. The tariff is therefore fixed primarily by the type of operation the patient has, but also by the fitness of the patient. The hospital has to balance the demands of the surgeon with the demands of the Primary Care Trust to provide the best possible treatment for the population it serves.

In the UK the Primary Care Trust provides the funding at a tariff dictated by the government. The Primary Care Trust has to fund all aspects of medical service provided by the hospital and allocate funds to try and achieve the optimum balance. In the case of hip replacements it can be difficult for the Primary Care Trust to make a reasonable evaluation. Their budgets are short term when many of the decisions on the type of hip replacement a patient should have and the funding of it is a long-term argument.

The manufacturers are constantly trying to improve on design and spent 'millions' in research and development. Products quickly come to market and often appear attractive to surgeons as they offer improvements. However, hip replacements need to perform well in a patient for a long time before conclusions on longevity can be drawn.

If asked, each of the stakeholders would state their aim to be able to give the best possible medical care to each individual patient. If however they were asked to then list the criteria on which their decisions were made, each stakeholder may have similar criteria but different priorities. Some of these criteria are scientific based and some are economic based. There has to be a compromise between the two. In the UK health economy, this compromise is between the hospital management and the surgeon.

The Warwick Hospital Experience

Warwick Hospital is known as a District General Hospital. It covers a catchment area of approximately 290,000 people and its Orthopaedic Consultant body is at this time ten, of which three surgeons are involved primarily in hip replacement surgery. Warwick does approximately 400 hip replacements per year. The hospital's experience of managing this compromise has been a rewarding one for everybody working in the area. In 2001, the clinicians were concerned about the results of the cemented hip that they were using and looked for other options. The Corail® was chosen in view of its long-term results, the variations it offered in terms of neck length, offset and bearings and lastly, the good experience in the hands of the clinicians. It was more expensive than the predecessor that had been used and this expense had to be tackled. There were three ways in which this was done.

Firstly, the cost of the prosthesis: Piers Yates wrote an article for the *Journal of Arthroplasty* in 2006 [4] that looked at the relative costs of cemented and uncemented THAs. He found that the cost of the Corail® hip was more expensive than its cemented counterparts. He then valued the other items used in the operating theatre to achieve a well-fixed cemented stem. This involved the cost of the cement, a pulse lavage, the mixing set, extra gloves, a femoral stem brush, a cement restrictor, a femoral pressuriser and the sterilisation of additional trays. In contrast, the extra costs for implanting a Corail® stem is nothing. He found that the Corail® stem became a more viable proposition being more expensive than the Exeter cemented stem, but cheaper than the C-stem. In 2009, a similar assessment was carried out in Warwick Hospital and the difference between the Corail® and the Exeter system was around 90 USD.

Warwick Hospital is a high volume user of the Corail® stem, but the costs of the Corail® is not dependent upon Warwick only. The Warwick Hospital is part of a larger consortium that covers the West Midlands in England. This consortium buys in high volume from the suppliers so that the cost of the implant is the same for any hospital within the consortium, irrespective of the numbers of cases performed.

The cost of the Corail® femoral implant is just one part of the hip joint. Three further parts are needed: a modular head, an acetabular cup and an acetabular liner. All these attract additional costs. It is in this area that the greatest compromise in choice of implant has to be made. If one takes 28 mm and 36 mm heads diameters as examples, the cheapest combination used with a femoral implant would be a 28 mm metal head with a cemented polyethylene socket. This would cost approximately two thirds of the femoral Corail® implant. Using an acetabular porous in-grown cup with a 28 metal head and a polyethylene liner would cost approximately 120% of the femoral implant. This same bearing, but in a 36 mm head, raises the cost to approximately 140% of the femoral implant. Using more advanced bearings with a 36 mm ceramic on ceramic combination will raise the bearing and cup costs to approximately 200% of the femoral implant cost. In conclusion, there is a significant saving to be made using the cheaper implant.

Many surgeons find it easy to decide on whether a cheaper or more expensive version should be used when the patient is at one end of the spectrum or the other, that is a young and active patient compared to an elderly, less active patient. There is a large grey area in the middle where surgeons will differ in choosing a cheaper or more expensive option. There are two arguments put forward in determining whether the more advanced, more expensive bearings should be used versus a cheaper option. One is in terms of wear. The more advanced bearings are harder wearing and potentially will last longer. This is a potential long-term benefit and can be difficult to justify when economic budgets are made on a yearly basis. The second argument however is more immediate. Stability in hip joints is an issue, particularly if a posterior approach to the hip joint is used. Dislocation of the hip will often manifest itself in the first 6 months after hip replacement. Larger diameter heads dislocate significantly less than smaller diameter heads. Dislocation is a problem for the patient, the surgeon and the hospital. Sanchez-Sotelo et al. [2] showed that the cost of relocating a dislocated hip prosthesis is approximately 20% of the cost of the primary hip. The cost of revision

surgery for a dislocated hip prosthesis was on average 148% of the cost of a primary hip replacement. The hospital's financial burden is significant. For the surgeon, dislocation is disappointing and depressing. To the patient, dislocation is extremely distressing. It destroys their confidence in the hip and significantly affects the perceived success of the hip replacement. At one end of the spectrum for the hospital it is an expensive complication but for the patient the ability to prevent dislocation is priceless. Warwick Hospital, in 2006, embarked on a policy of using a 36 diameter head whenever it was possible. The version of the acetabular implant is always placed according to the transverse acetabular ligament and the posterior capsule is repaired whenever possible. Compared to a previous cohort of patients, using this policy has reduced the dislocation rate at Warwick from 1.8% to 0%.

Another factor to be put into the economic melting pot is how the choice of implant can influence the whole procedure. In Warwick Hospital, the Corail® stem became the catalyst for change in the patient's journey through a hip replacement. This developed following the experience in the operating theatre, when using the Corail® stem produced a fast surgery with a stable construct. The patients' rehabilitation became quicker. This was formalised so that patients could sit from day one, use crutches for 3 weeks and progress their activities as fast as their pain will permit. Their only longer-term advice is to remain sleeping on their back for the first 6 weeks. It was because of this more rapid rehabilitation that Warwick introduced in 2005 an early discharge programme [3]. The important factor in the discharge programme is that 95% of all patients are accepted onto the programme. On the day of discharge a nurse will visit the patient in their house and subsequently on each day a nurse or physiotherapist will visit until they are safe and able to manage themselves. This is normally a further two visits. The plan for early discharge starts at the preoperative assessment when patients are given a lecture by the nurses and physiotherapist involved with the early discharge about what will be expected of them and how the programme will work. About 85% of patients go home by day 3. The patients are settled in on their first visit, the wound is managed and physiotherapy is given as necessary. The patients have welcomed the early discharge and an audit shows that there are very few re-admissions for orthopaedic or related medical problems. As a cost-saving exercise, it has been a huge

Fig. 11.1 Warwick orthopaedics tariff versus costs:
x-axis shows cost in pounds
sterling, *y*-axis total cost of
hip and knee replacement. *Red*
equal tariff cost and *blue* local
costs. The *green bars* refer to
numbers of patients seen

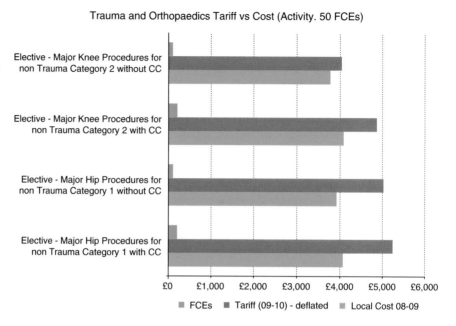

benefit for the hospital. The savings made from reduced bed days, a reduction of the number of hospital beds needed to run the service and an increased number of hip replacements done must be offset by the cost of running the service.

The management of Warwick Hospital has supported the Orthopaedic department and total hip replacement costs now approximately 80% of tariff cost. In real terms, this means that each hip replacement carried out in Warwick brings over 1,500 USD worth of profit into the hospital (Fig. 11.1).

The experience of Warwick Hospital shows that by collaboration between clinicians and managers it is possible for science and economics to come together in a productive way. It means that managers must accept that not the cheapest prosthesis gives the cheapest result but also the surgeons must understand that if they are using more expensive prostheses, at a local level, the service can be seen to benefit from the change.

Money Does Not Buy Happiness

If we return to the stakeholders, the patients and clinicians can be tempted by the manufacturers into believing that the newest range of implants available must be the best. Usually, they are not only the newest, but the most expensive. In the same way that the newest wine

is not always the best, this applies to hip replacements as well. As this book is written the metal on metal issues, which is really a problem of XL heads on more conventional implants, is testament to this. The extent of the crisis and the financial burden of it is not yet fully understood. It is however important to stress that in deciding which compromises should be made in hospitals, it is essential to understand the success of the operation. This requires appropriate measuring of outcomes. Evidence-based decisions must put a scientific basis behind economic decisions that are made, and it is vital that clinicians within hospitals maintain adequate data on regularly followed-up patients and that this information is kept locally and fed into national joint registries which can then guide all stakeholders along the right path.

Conclusions

In looking to the future, there is no doubt that hard decisions will have to be made in all areas including THA. The newest and the most expensive implants are not always the best, and compromises may have to be made. It is only with regular follow-up that outcomes can be measured and then assessed in terms of performance and cost of the whole package, and not just the cost of the prosthetic implant.

References

1. Kurtz S et al (2007) Projections of primary and revision hip and knee arthroplasty in the United States from 2005 to 2030. J Bone Joint Surg Am 89:780–785
2. Sanchez-Sotelo J (2006) Hospital cost of dislocation after primary total hip arthroplasty. J Bone Joint Surg Am 88(2):290–294
3. Thomas G et al (2008) Early discharge after hip arthroplasty with home support: experience at a UK District Hospital. Hip Int 18(4):294–300
4. Yates P et al (2005) The relative costs of cemented and uncemented total hip arthroplasties. J Arthroplasty 21(1): 102–105

The history of total hip arthroplasty (THA) in the former USSR was led by a single orthopaedic surgeon, namely, Professor K. M. Sivash. It was the first hip implant made from titanium and it was designed for cementless implantation. DePuy established an Instructional Course coupled with an Integrated Extensive Visitation for orthopaedic surgeons in St. Petersburg, Russia. The course has three modules and aims to spread knowledge and expertise on THA, both in theory and practice. This professional education programme improved the standards on THA in different parts of Russia.

metaphyseal stem area were designed for bone integration. The acetabular cup implant included sharp screw threads with increasing diameter from the pole to the equator and was designed for rigid primary fixation as well as bone integration (Fig. 12.1). The first report was probably published by the author in Western Europe and occurred in the Swiss journal Reconstruction Surgery and Traumatology in 1969. Individual reports about this device, mostly studies of failed total joints, were also published in European and American journals in the 1980s. The device was exported and used in Europe and the USA.

Introduction

The history of total hip arthroplasty (THA) in the former Soviet Union Republics started in 1956, when Professor Konstantin M. Sivash, chief of the Orthopaedic Department in the Central Institute of Trauma and Orthopaedics (CITO), Moscow, Russia designed and developed his own hip joint endoprosthesis [4, 5]. It was the first THA, with parts made of titanium. The use of titanium in this device was due to the vast experience with this metal that existed in the Soviet aerospace and military industry. The whole total hip joint was made from metal: the shaft component was made from titanium and the rest of the device was made initially from stainless steel, later on from cobalt chrome alloys. The Sivash prosthesis had a linked design with all parts casted from titanium alloy with a pre-manufactured hinged metal on metal bearing surface. The tapered stem was made of polished titanium with a round cross section. Two windows in the proximal

The Sivash Hip Prosthesis

The surgical technique of the Sivash hip prosthesis is very difficult and highly demanding for the surgeon, simply due to the fact that the implant comes in an already hinged and pre-assembled piece. There is no way to implant this device other than performing a major invasive trochanteric osteotomy. The stem is impacted first and the acetabular component is screwed in afterwards utilising a punch and hammer followed by wire reattachment of the greater trochanter at the end of the procedure.

One has to appreciate that in the 1970s and decades thereafter, hip replacement surgery was not a standard surgical procedure in the USSR. Excision arthroplasty and arthrodesis was more commonly performed for osteoarthritis and Avascular Necrosis (AVN) of the hip joint. When the Sivash prosthesis was introduced, very few centres within Russia were able to perform (and afford) this type of hip surgery. A mere total of 10,000

J.-P. Vidalain et al. (eds.), *The CORAIL® Hip System*,
DOI: 10.1007/978-3-642-18396-6_12, © Springer-Verlag Berlin Heidelberg 2011

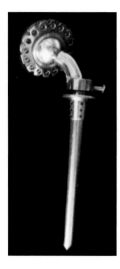

Fig. 12.1 Sivash MoM linked total hip prosthesis with proximal modular sleeve (Copyright DePuyInternational Limited)

Sivash prostheses were implanted in a 25-year period. Scientific reports in terms of peer-reviewed papers were not common practice in Russia and, therefore, literature on Sivash THA is very limited. The largest series implanted in one institution includes about 500 Sivash THA, however, without any peer reviewed reports.

In 1967, Dr. Sivash modified his original stem and added a modular sleeve. In 1971, a US surgical device company obtained licensing rights for the Sivash hip prosthesis. The design was then improved including a distal stem coronal slot, eight flutes, a calcar spout and ZTT calcars. The implant was renamed to S-ROM® (Sivash Range of Motion) and has remained essentially unchanged since 1985 [6].

The destiny of Sivash prosthesis in Russia was less favourable. At the beginning of the 1970s the cobalt chromium content of the alloy was replaced by titanium alloy even within the bearing components. As a result of this, high metal wear, toxic synovitis and early aseptic loosening increased dramatically. This led to a decreased popularity and the implant was virtually eliminated from clinical use.

Total Joint Replacement in the USSR

Dramatic and relevant changes of the political, economic and social system of the USSR in 1989 marked an introduction of total joint arthroplasty into the health care system. The opening of the borders and subsequent broad information exchange promoted the first appearance of international implant manufacturers on the Russian market. A limited number of specialists gained fellowships in leading clinics and institutions across Europe and the USA. Modern operating room technology and anaesthetic equipment was delivered in several hospitals across Moscow and other regional institutions.

At the same time, local companies began manufacturing modern hip prostheses and compulsory administrative distribution of these products among the region. Some manufactures began to replicate old-fashioned prostheses or those that ran out of patents. Samples, drafts and pictures were used to accomplish that goal. However, poor quality of local high molecular polyethylene, various ceramics, and lack of experience in production technologies led, at times, to catastrophic wear and its clinical consequences. Also the use of titanium alloy heads instead of Co-Cr-Mo alloys had significant impact on poor clinical outcomes. Estimated 10-year survivorship data was under 30% and early revision surgery was often required after 1 year of implantation due to high metal wear, osteolysis, and aseptic loosening. Twenty years ago the author of this chapter was a high volume THA surgeon and scientifically involved in numerous local Russian publications on 'home-made hip prostheses.' His papers eluded the problematic issues of local prosthetic design and poor manufacturing quality. More than 400 generic copies of the 'Universal' total hip prostheses (original implant designed by Biomet, USA) were implanted in the Hospital of Emergency Care, N.V. Soloviov in Yaroslavl, Russia. However, early failure and catastrophic clinical results led to considerable frustration and disappointment to the effect that the author of this chapter decided to discontinue the use of these prosthetic implants. In 1999, last attempts were made to manufacture copies from a Swiss acetabular component (Bionit 2, Matthys) utilising a Russian titanium stem and a locally manufactured ceramic head. The clinical results were devastating and included numerous ceramic head fractures. Ten years ago, the author and his team of total joint surgeons decided to exchange local implants with well-performing hip prostheses that have excellent long-term survivorship and reported proven data. Their choice fell towards the Corail® stem and the universal Pinnacle™ cups (DePuy).

Combined Efforts and Initiative from Government and Surgeons

In 2006, the Government of the Russian Federation initiated a project of national development. The content of this large project included significant improvements in the fields of healthcare, education, housing, pension and others. One particular objective emphasised the use of advanced technology in medical care. In the orthopaedic field, this meant access to modern total joint implants and improved surgical techniques for the Russian population.

The Russian Government's efforts to make hip replacement surgery available to the public are challenged by economic constraints and high costs of foreign implants. An in-depth analysis by the author listed all costs involved when performing a THA procedure. This included medicines, materials, equipment, instruments, surgeon's fee, staff reimbursement, operating room, intensive care, physical therapy, public utilities, and taxes. The costs for the implant swallowed more than 75% of the overall expenses [1, 2]. When comparing this data to a similar THA procedure performed in the USA, the proportion of implant costs are between 25% and 35% (Figs. 12.2 and 12.3). The reasons for this significant difference and the high implant costs in the USSR include, amongst others, a generally low level of income and low insurance compensation.

The approximate reimbursement, which public hospitals receive from the government for a total hip procedure is approximately 4,000 USD per THA case. In addition to these restrictions, the Ministry of Health regulates the number of THA procedures per annum. In 2010, there were 18,000 quotas for total joint replacements, including other joints than the hip. The Russian government succeeds in constantly building new public clinics in which total joint procedures can be performed. Particularly, the more remote areas benefit from these actions. The specific type of implant is

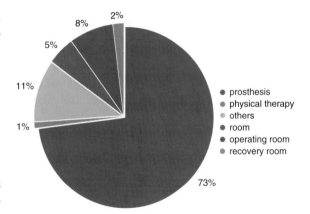

Fig. 12.2 Implant costs for THA in the Clinical Emergency Hospital, Yaroslavl, Russia

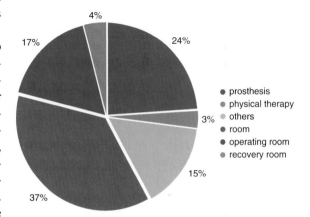

Fig. 12.3 Implant costs for THA in Lahey Clinic, Burlington, MA, USA

generally chosen (and then purchased) during official state auctions and contests.

The challenges for reconstructive joint surgeons within Russia are multiple and one main issue is the fact that most patients live remotely from hospitals. This impedes everything for both the surgeon and the patient/relatives, from the first consultation to their discharge from the hospital. The surgeon usually does not see his patients for follow-up, unless there are obvious problems after THA surgery. Proper follow-up data in THA are therefore not available. Usually, the surgeon cannot simply implant the prosthesis of his choice, even if the patient would be willing to compensate for a better prosthesis. Senior health officials decide the type of prosthetic implant that is available to orthopaedic surgeons. Often the entire system is exchanged by more economic implants from different providers. This has implications on both the quality of surgery and any future revision that may be required.

Professional Education Programme in Russia

Surgeons across Russia highlight the importance of professional education, specific surgical training and on-site support during hip replacement surgery. In order to provide good standards in THA, surgeons should be trained in courses, in operating theatre, and if applicable on cadavers. In an ideal setup, the surgeon then performs THA surgery in his institution together with an experienced surgeon from abroad. Historically, Russian orthopaedic surgeons have more access to trauma surgery than total joint reconstructive surgery. Estimated figures reveal data that there are only 400 orthopaedic surgeons, who perform on average 30 or less total joint replacements per annum. The overall number of THA in Russia was 23,000 hip replacements in 2009. This counts for approximately 20% of the demand.

Orthopaedic opinion leaders at the *Russian Scientific Institute of Traumatology and Orthopaedics* named after Professor R. R. Vreden, St. Petersburg, Russia, have created a surgical learning centre in collaboration with DePuy [3]. The goal was to train and educate orthopaedic surgeons with different experience levels in Russia and Russian speaking countries in order to improve the quality of surgical technique skills and to help feed the high demand of total hip replacements in Russia. The project was named 'Peter the Great' in honour of the founder of St. Petersburg. The first course took place at the above mentioned institute under the supervision of the author, a senior orthopaedic surgeon with a special interest in total hip arthroplasty surgery.

The course is divided into three modules: basic, advanced and experienced. Each module is tailored to fit the specific problems of each country with regard to medical issues, economy, demography and morbidity. Hip joint pathologies in Russia differ from other European countries in many aspects such as untreated arthritis, nutritive toxic AVN, high levels of genetically caused developmental dysplasia of the hip (DDH), and all types of commonly performed non-implant osteotomy surgeries.

The basic course is designed for traumatologists, residents and low volume orthopaedic surgeons, who perform less than 20 arthroplasty procedures per annum. The programme includes lectures on general hip anatomy, hip biomechanics, indication for hip replacement surgery, hip approaches, implant classifications, preoperative planning, post-operative treatment, rehabilitation and potential complications. Finally, the concepts of specific hip arthroplasty are demonstrated when utilising the Corail® and Pinnacle™ systems (DePuy).

The advanced course is tailored for more experienced orthopaedic surgeons with a volume of 50 THAs per annum. The content of this module includes the following topics: abnormal hip biomechanics, pearls of surgical techniques, complex primary hip arthroplasties, non-complex revision THA cases, tribology, implant selection and management of complications.

The expert course is designed for high volume orthopaedic surgeons, who perform more than 100 THA procedures per annum. The participant should be affiliated to an institution with a scientific set-up, allowing for in-depth analysis of THA indications, results, complications and follow-up. This module contains complex primary hip cases, revision situations and management of bone defects. One particular part of this module is to learn from poorly performed THA and complications that were performed by the participants themselves.

The experienced course runs over 2 days and includes numerous lectures, workshops on plastic bones and, for the first time in Russia, cadaver sessions. This is very unique because, in general, cadaver courses face strong criticism as well as ethical and religious issues in Russia. However, cadaver sessions allow surgical approaches and implantation of a real hip prosthesis and, therefore, represent the best learning media without doing harm to a human. Furthermore, it comes closest to real surgery and can be repeated several times on one single corpse. These valuable learning effects and improved surgical skills are immediately transferred to the trainees' home set-up.

After each course the participant receives a certificate of attendance, which is authorised by the *Russian Scientific Institute of Traumatology and Orthopaedics*.

All delegates have the opportunity to attend a further 2-week extended visitation in one of the faculty's hospital in order to practice in the operating room under the supervision of a core faculty member. After this fellowship, the attendee can communicate directly with his mentor via e-mail in order to pose questions or comments on THA cases.

Conclusion

The first *Russian Modular THA* course held in St. Petersburg was highly successful and will continue to teach THA procedures to orthopaedic surgeons across Russia. DePuy has announced to further sponsor this professional education programme and to spread this experience to other developing countries.

> **Key Learning Points**
>
> › Professional education for orthopaedic surgeons in Russia
> › Benefits of cadaver courses on THA are available in St. Petersburg, Russia
> › Advantages of THA learning centres
> › Improvements of THA procedures across Russia
> › History of total hip replacement in the former USSR

References

1. Barber TC, Healy WL (1993) The hospital cost of total hip arthroplasty. A comparison between 1981 and 1990. J Bone Joint Surg Am 75:321–325
2. Healy WL, Iorio R, Lemos JM et al (2000) Single price/case purchasing in orthopaedic surgery: experience at the Lahey clinic. J Bone Joint Surg Am 82(5):607–609
3. Pshenisnov KP, Danilyak VV, Panchenko KI (1994) The fate of free, pedicled and free vascularised cancellous iliac bone grafts and the effect on the healing of femoral osteotomy: an experimental study. J Reconstr Microsurg 10(6):393–401
4. Sivash KM (1965) A new method of alloplasty of the hip joint in ankylosing spondylathritis. Khirurgiia Moskau 41(6):112–117
5. Sivash KM (1969) Development of alloplasty of the hip joint during the past 15 years. Ortop Travmatol Protez 30(11): 28–33
6. Spitzer AL (2005) The S-ROM cementless femoral stem: history and literature review. Orthopaedics 28(9 Suppl): s1117–1124

Educational Programme from Europe to Asia Pacific: Travelling the Seven Seas

13

Jens Boldt

The purpose of a travelling surgeon is to offer peer to peer support to improve surgical skills to a level where any orthopaedic surgeon is capable of safely performing a total hip arthroplasty (THA). The Corail® Hip System requires few instruments, is relatively easy to implant and has forgiving features when implanted in a less than optimal manner. By using this hip system, surgeons across the globe are able to perform a safe and successful THA, without the necessity of being a high volume surgeon. THA is best taught face-to-face in a one-to-one surgeon environment. This type of training programme was developed less than 10 years ago by the co-author, who is an orthopaedic surgeon himself and responsible for professional education within DePuy. Professional education can also reach a wider audience via live surgery with simultaneous video and audio conferencing. The challenge is to bring the surgical skills required for safe THA into remote and developing areas in Europe, the Middle East and Asia Pacific. One key objective of DePuy's professional educational programme is the desire to improve surgical skills, to enhance the survivorship of THA and to increase the overall quality of life and safety of patients (Fig. 13.1).

Introduction

As this book was being written, the Bone and Joint Decade (2000–2010) was just on its way out. It was a decade of worldwide development of musculoskeletal medicine. It brought together industry, governments, health professionals and patients who continue to focus on further research, education and services in musculoskeletal diseases. The challenges included an ageing population suffering increasingly from chronic degenerative diseases. The health system focused on cost-effectiveness, patient outcomes and patient involvement. As far as THA was concerned, orthopaedic surgeons created a more sustainable and outcome-orientated procedure. Professional education and research fellowships were supported by the implant manufactures and evolved from didactic lectures into inter-professional training. This was not only achieved within developed countries, but also in developing areas across the world. DePuy was amongst the first to make a significant investment in this type of professional education. With these programmes, an increasing number of surgeons quickly gained access to the skills and tools required for modern THA, which has enabled them to benefit their local communities. In contrast, only a limited number of specialists gained fellowships in leading clinics and institutions across Europe or the USA.

Professional education and training is a well-known and cost-effective practice in medical education [2]. The practice of orthopaedics provides excellent opportunities for inter-professional training. One aspect of DePuy's professional education programme is the travelling surgeon. This person travels and educates hip arthroplasty surgeons in their own country within their own environment in both theory and practice. Insufficient access to this type of education, inferior equipment and low volume THA are thought to contribute to the poor outcomes that are often observed following THA in many developing countries. The standard of THA being achieved in the bigger centres

J.-P. Vidalain et al. (eds.), *The CORAIL® Hip System*,
DOI: 10.1007/978-3-642-18396-6_13, © Springer-Verlag Berlin Heidelberg 2011

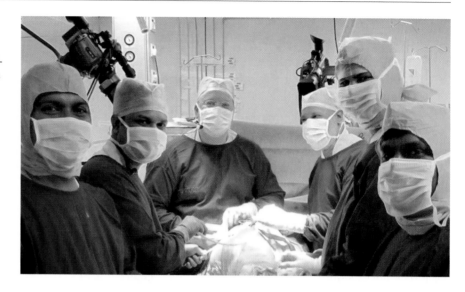

Fig. 13.1 Live surgery in Aurangabad, India. A THA procedure is wired to a moderator, who is communicating with both the surgeon and the audience

and capitals across the Middle East and Asia Pacific is excellent. However, more remote areas in India and the Middle East face the triple challenge of low volume, sparse inter-professional education and often difficult hip pathologies. The type of hip pathology mostly seen in the Middle East and Asia differs from that seen in European countries. They often present late, and as a result the disease process tends to be more advanced. There is also a high prevalence of genetically induced hip dysplasia and ankylosis [1, 4] (Fig. 13.2).

DePuy's Initiative and Professional Education Programme

In the year 2000, DePuy launched multiple professional educational programmes and initiatives in all fields of orthopaedic services. In the emerging economies and developing countries, the travelling surgeon idea was first put into practice in Russia. DePuy's professional education efforts extended then to other European countries, the Middle East and Asia Pacific, and included various scientific meetings and learning centres run by experienced surgeons. Orthopaedic surgeons in remote and less developed parts of the world benefited from access to well-established hip prosthesis optimised surgical technique and appropriate instruments. Most important of all, the travelling surgeon could teach and assist with THA on-site using

the local set-up of the learning surgeon. The education programme included lectures on general hip anatomy, hip biomechanics, indications for hip replacement surgery, hip approaches, preoperative planning, postoperative treatment and the potential complications. The concepts of specific hip arthroplasty are

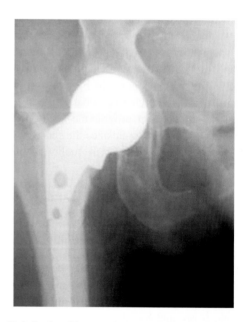

Fig. 13.2 Broken hip stem in a cementless hemiarthroplasty 3 years following surgery for a fractured neck of femur. Surgery performed in Chandigarh, India. Specific instruments for metal stem extraction are usually unavailable. Successful revision hip replacement took place in the summer of 2010

demonstrated with the use of the Corail® and Pinnacle™ hip systems (DePuy). All surgeons have the opportunity to attend further learning centres in Europe or Asia, when needed.

The organisation and the professionalism of this education method were unique at that time. Both authors of this chapter travelled extensively across the globe for professional education and will continue to do so. Over fifty countries were visited and hundreds of THA procedures were performed in a one-to-one environment. Live surgeries with video and audio conferencing were also performed in order to bring education on THA to a larger audience. Invariably, the host surgeon has benefited from the visit of a travelling surgeon both in terms of an improvement in surgical technique as well their general knowledge and understanding of THA.

Remote areas benefit particularly from this type of educational programme. The challenges for THA surgeons in developing countries in the Middle East and in Asia are multiple and some have already been alluded to. In addition, economic constraints reduce the overall number of hip prostheses that can be implanted despite the need being much higher. The vast majority of people in developing countries simply cannot afford a THA. In India, for instance, the estimated unmet need for THA is thought to be between five and ten million! However, only a fraction of those can afford the procedure. Although about half a million patients in India could potentially afford hip replacement, they do not undergo surgery because THA is not considered to be a long lasting and safe procedure when performed in remote areas of India. Discerning patients who can afford it usually go to the larger cities such as Mumbai, New Delhi or Chennai. There they can have their THAs performed by highly experienced surgeons, who have usually trained in Europe or the USA.

In combination with our educational programme, it is our ambition to provide a total hip system, which is easy to perform, easy to teach and utilises few instruments. We feel that the Corail® stem and Pinnacle™ cup in combination with DePuy's travelling surgeons meet these criteria. The travelling surgeons demonstrate that good clinical outcome can be achieved following THA for those who need it most. Professional education in less developed areas are very well received and appreciated not only by the orthopaedic surgeons, but also by the patients, local politicians and media.

For us, the reward for being a travelling surgeon is being able to help our host surgeon colleagues achieve an educational and confidence level, which enables them to safely and reproducibly perform THA, for their own and their patients benefit (Fig. 13.3).

A further goal was to train and educate orthopaedic surgeons with different experience levels across all developing countries. This helped to improve the

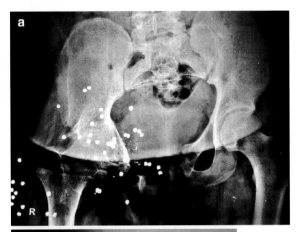
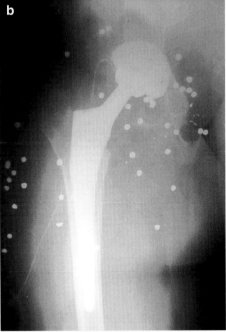

Fig. 13.3 (**a, b**) Traumatic hip joint ankylosis following gunshot injury 21 years ago. Example of a challenging and difficult THA in a small and remote hospital near Jalandar, India. The senior surgeon performs less than 20 THAs per annum. Preoperative and postoperative radiographs showing a successful THA using a Corail® stem and Pinnacle™ cup

quality of surgical technique and to meet the high demand for THA in those countries.

Discussion

In general, the quality of orthopaedic training provided in Asia Pacific is on an equal level to that in Europe. However, socio-economic challenges and little access to modern technology are common obstacles particularly in more remote areas. Travelling surgeons reported satisfactory experiences with inter-professional orthopaedic training. Professional supervision and live surgery may be regarded as essential ingredients in helping less experienced surgeons to learn effectively within their own authentic clinical setting. Orthopaedic surgery offers extensive educational opportunities for surgeons. DePuy's educational programme includes exposure to all aspects of hip replacement, both scientifically and practically. The aim of DePuy and the travelling surgeons is to enable the provision of high quality and safe patient care through professional education.

There is a group of travelling surgeons, who are frequently involved in this type of professional education and who share their experience on a regular basis. This improves both the quality and consistency of professional surgical education. All relevant safety and quality parameters were considered while travelling the classic seven seas: Black Sea, Caspian Sea, Mediterranean Sea, Persian Gulf, Red Sea, Adriatic Sea and Indian Ocean. The travelling surgeon is faced with multiple challenges while performing his duties: cultural and religious differences, language barriers, difficult logistics, lack of surgical instruments and operating room facilities. All of this demands high concentration (and at times exhaustion) for everyone involved [5] (Fig. 13.4).

Orthopaedic surgeons in developing countries are facing multiple challenges with regard to THA. On the one hand volume is low due to financial constraints and on the other hand hip pathology has often reached an advanced state by the time the patient presents to his surgeon [1, 4]. There is, for example a high number of genetically predisposed hip ankylosis in vast rural areas in India. As a result, orthopaedic surgeons in remote areas often face difficult cases as well as political pressure in terms of planned governmental restrictions in allowing total joint replacement in low-volume hip practices. If only high volume centres are allowed to perform joint replacements, then the vast majority of poor people across the Middle East and Asia Pacific will not have access to care [3]. Voluntary efforts from manufacturing companies such as DePuy and well-trained joint surgeons have been very successful and should be highlighted as an example of inter-professional education in developing countries.

Europe	Middle East	Asia Pacific
England	Lebanon	India
Ireland	Saudi Arabia	China
Germany	Oman	Hong Kong
Switzerland	Bahrain	Malaysia
Austria	UA Emirates	Australia
Spain	Qatar	New Zealand
Italy		
Slovenia		
Greece		
Estonia		
Latvia		
Russia		

Fig. 13.4 Continents and countries visited for professional education and THA one-to-one surgery. Most countries were visited multiple times to meet their demands

Conclusion

DePuy will continue to offer professional education programmes, including those that involve the use of travelling hip surgeons. This type of education is superior to conventional arthroplasty courses or learning centres, and has proven to be very successful. Ideally, surgeons are taught in specific hip courses and learning centres first in order to gain theoretical and practical knowledge with regard to the Corail® and Pinnacle™ hip system. Following this, the participants can then be visited at their own hospital by a travelling surgeon who can perform THA with them. This type of education has been shown to be one of the most efficient and effective tools available, and thousands of patients have benefited from it. In summary, travelling surgeons have helped to improve surgical technique skills for orthopaedic surgeons from Europe to Asia Pacific, and have enhanced the quality of life of numerous patients.

Professional education, one-to-one peer-to-peer support in THA, live surgery with simultaneous video and audio conferencing, improvement of surgical skills, enhancement of THA survivorship, increase of the overall quality of life and safety of patients.

References

1. Bhan S, Eachempati KK, Malhotra R (2008) Primary cementless total hip arthroplasty for bony ankylosis in patients with ankylosing spondylitis. J Arthroplasty 23(6):859–866
2. Hansen TB, Jacobsen F, Larsen K (2010) Cost effective inter-professional training: an evaluation of a training unit in Denmark. J Interprof Care 23(3):234–241
3. Losina E, Barrett J, Baron JA et al (2004) Utilization of low-volume hospitals for total hip replacement. Arthritis Rheum 51(5):836–842
4. Mirdad T (2002) Incidence and pattern of congenital dislocation of the hip in Aseer region of Saudi Arabia. West Afr J Med 21(3):218–222
5. Woolson ST, Kang MN (2007) A comparison of the results of total hip and knee arthroplasty performed on a teaching service or a private practice service. J Bone Joint Surg Am 89(3):601–607

Glossary of Terms and Abbreviations, Trademarks

Total Hip Arthroplasty (THA)
Developmental Dysplasia of the Hip (DDH)
Direct Anterior Approach (DAA)
Hydroxyapatite (HA)
X-ray
Intraoperative
Postoperative
Preoperative
Offset

Trademarks

Corail®
Corail® Hip System
Corail® femoral stem
Corail® Stem
Corail® Revision Stem
Corail® AMT – Articul/eze® Mini-Taper
KAR™
KAR™ stem
Pinnacle™ Acetabular Cup System
Charnley®
Titan
Reef®
Articuleze®
Solution System™
S-ROM®
Control Cable™

Biostop®
Cemvac®
CMW®
Ceramax™
Smartmix™
Biolox®
Biolox® Delta
Biolox® Forte
BHP™ (Zimmer)
Smartset®
Spirofit™
AML® Total Hip System
PROfx™
HANA™
Siemens® Sensation
OsiriX® software
BHP™ (Zimmer)
Alloclassic®
MicroHip™
Ultima
Ultamet®
Marathon™
Wroblewski
Elite Plus
Ogee® Cup
DePuy
DePuy International Ltd
ARTRO Group
Corail® International Faculty

J.-P. Vidalain et al. (eds.), *The CORAIL® Hip System*,
DOI: 10.1007/978-3-642-18396-6, © Springer-Verlag Berlin Heidelberg 2011

Postscript

Total Hip Arthroplasty (THA) was born more than 40 years ago! Since the time of the very first implantations performed by Sir John Charnley, significant and even remarkable improvements have been achieved resulting from an increased understanding of the interrelations between biomaterials, biomechanics and bone biology. The introduction to orthopaedics of hydroxyapatite (HA) about 25 years ago has given rise to a considerable number of studies and publications, helping us improve our knowledge of bioactive ceramics.

In the mid-1980s, the ARTRO Group joined the circle of pioneers, which included Ronald Furlong, Freidrich Osborn, and Rudolph Geesink, who all believed in the use of hydroxyapatite. Since this took place a few decades ago, the group can now justifiably claim with pride to have the richest and longest-standing clinical experience of the use of hydroxyapatite in France. The Corail® prosthesis is now distributed worldwide and is considered to be the leading implant in this specific field of hip replacement. Throughout the decades, many orthopaedic surgeons from outstanding universities and institutes, as well as surgeons from smaller and less prestigious hospitals, joined the original group of developers to share their experiences and insights. Our purpose in producing this book was to gather all this knowledge and experience and present it in one place. From the beginning, we wanted this book to be a forum, open to all users of the Corail® system, whether they were daring early adopters or part of the later majority and we wanted the testimonies to be a benefit to younger and less experienced surgeons. In other words we wanted this book to be a guide, a user manual, part of a real educational program. Over the past few years, we have become very aware of the necessity to share our knowledge through learning centres and workshops taking place several times a year in our clinics and hospitals. One purpose of the book was to provide practical guidance and to answer some of the most frequently asked questions. The Corail® system is no longer limited to the sphere of its inventors. It is open to everyone, enriched by the significant contribution made by some of you, but belonging to all. Because of the wide use of the Corail®, system we wanted to preserve the original heritage and to try to prevent unintentional misuse. This was one of the objectives of this book.

We began the book (Part I) by describing the major stages in the development of the Corail® prosthesis and the main principles that constituted the specifications and requirements submitted to the engineers. At that time, this innovating and original multidisciplinary work brought together a team of surgeons, biologists, engineers and scientists – all working towards the same goal. Driven on by our common spirit and aspirations, we continually evolved the Corail® system to improve and enlarge the original range of implants. This collaboration contributed to the effectiveness and success of our project!

The book continues on with a more practical outlook of the system. Most newly converted users of the Corail® system find it simple. The stem is easy to use. The implantation procedure is straightforward and the Corail® prosthesis probably forgives many small mistakes. However, for a successful implantation, some basic rules and principles must be strictly observed. For this reason, these practical chapters are authored by the original designers. We wanted to transmit the core knowledge and our original message to the new generation of users. We hope this practical advice will help resolve difficulties and will prevent errors and misuse. The system is also simple for the patient, since the postoperative management is generally complication free. Immediate, full weight bearing is allowed. There is no significant pain, and return to normal activity can commence after a short rehabilitation period. Despite the absence of HA coating–related complications, some complications may occur which require the use of a product-specific strategy. Therefore, we have also provided advice on how to manage such problems in the last section of this practical part.

The long-term results provided concrete evidence of the Corail® prosthesis' good performance. To ensure objectivity, the studies were performed by independent evaluators renowned for their methodology and critical sharpness. Survival analysis is the most reliable method for evaluating long-term performance of arthroplasties. Today, even the greatest sceptics admit that the survival of the Corail® prosthesis is impressive and this is true whatever endpoint is used, be it implant revision or radiographic criteria. These results were so positive that the Corail® prosthesis compares well with 'historical' models considered as 'gold standards'. We reported, among other things, the data collected from different national arthroplasty registers, which showed an estimated survival rate of 95% at 15 years with stable and long-term radiographic fixation. The importance of restoring the physiological and anatomical parameters of the hip is well-established. All these parameters, including hip centre of rotation, length of the lever arm of the abductor muscles, leg length equalization and range of motion, are determining factors in implant stability, mobility and wear. The Corail® range of implants mimics the natural hip and provides the patient with an artificial joint that he will 'forget'.

HA coating has proven to be a reliable method for implant fixation and this technology is part of the current orthopaedic arsenal. It is now admitted that bioactive fixation allows greater leeway in the positioning of the stem. Primary stability will always be a key factor for a successful implant, but due to the HA technology, it is not as detrimental as with other non-cemented implants, particularly those with porous metal coating.

Therefore, no prior selection criteria are imposed in terms of surgical indications. Osseointegration was achieved whatever the age, the aetiology or the amount of bone stock. Successful outcomes have been regularly reported in challenging situations such as in very young and active patients, in old osteoporotic patients and even in complex revision procedures in which the bone was sclerotic. Even infection was not a contraindication, provided appropriate systemic and local treatments are applied. In all cases primary stability is essential and must be achieved intra-operatively. This means that the hip system must include a range of situation-specific options. This is what the Corail® system does. Our philosophy is bone stock conservation, preservation and reconstruction, whenever necessary. Therefore, according to our golden rule, femoral stems should be as short as possible, but as long as necessary.

The following part (Part II) of the book could be entitled 'ABC', where A is for 'Approaches', B for 'Bearings' and C for 'Cups'! The Corail® prosthesis can be implanted using any conventional surgical approach and any minimally invasive approach, which preserve peri-articular soft tissues. Individual approaches were described by a user of that approach, but to facilitate the comparison of these approaches, they are all described using an identical framework. Also, we did not forget that total hip arthroplasty includes management of the acetabulum. The Corail® system is compatible with all commonly available bearing combinations. Modern joint surfaces commonly make use of hard-on-hard bearings, but advanced polyethylene bearings are also widely used. Tribology has made continuous progress in the laboratory, but in practice these improvements have advantages and disadvantages, which make the choice of bearing couple more difficult. At the time of publishing, the ARTRO Group recommends the use of large, ceramic-on-ceramic bearings (femoral head size 32 mm or larger) in those patients where life expectancy or activity level is a consideration to avoid wear-related problems.

We included a part (Part III) on case studies to give the reader some practical advice. These case studies cover a wide range of hip surgery pathology. They were the subject of exciting and impassioned debates during our meetings and they probably represent the most original and innovative part of the book.

We concluded the book (Part IV) with a look into the future. We included a variety of subjects such as medico-economic and educational considerations. We are all aware of the current worldwide economic situation from which the practice of medicine is not immune. Our objective must therefore be to provide high-quality products at the best possible quality–price ratio. Plasma-sprayed HA coating is an advanced biotechnology and it does incur an additional cost. However, this extra cost is probably not significant, since, although non-cemented hip arthroplasty is still perceived to be the more expensive option, all reliable studies confirm that the cost of both cemented and non-cemented THA is statistically identical when taking into account the total cost of the procedures.

The authors wished to celebrate this 25th anniversary by means of an original idea: a series of 25 consecutive patients with no selection criteria, managed in 25 different centres. The follow-up period was 12 months.

The assessment results of each study were recorded on a customized data sheet which included questions targeted for a 1 year study. Statistical analysis was carried out by an external team.

The chapters in the book were intended to be short and didactic. Probably some authors would have preferred to write longer pieces, but from a practical point of view and to keep the book to a manageable size, this was not possible. We therefore used illustrations to reduce the number of words. Images can speak better than words!

For the same reason, the bibliographical references given at the end of each chapter were also limited in number. We hope these references will be a valuable tool to assist in future research. Electronic publishing of this book will allow regular content update and expansion (www.spingerlink.com).

The editorial process was the following: the editorial board defined the contents of the book and the titles of the chapters. The ARTRO Group acted as a facilitator. The authors wrote the manuscripts and these manuscripts were received from all over the world: Europe, United States, and Australia. The manuscripts were reviewed by a reading committee, but the overall meaning of each chapter was not changed. Finally the manuscripts were gathered together, so as to obtain a coherent document, easy to read and easy to consult. As editors of this book, we would like to extend our sincerest thanks to all those who so generously contributed to this project and lent their expertise and experience. Their contributions have made the completion of this book possible.

The ARTRO Group has already participated in two works. Each one made an important contribution to the history of hydroxyapatite. In 1995, under the aegis of the SOFCOT, Pr Jacques Duparc, J.A Epinette and R.G.T. Geesink, published a book describing the experience of bioactive coated implant developers and entitled *Hydroxyapatite Coated Hip and Knee Arthroplasty*. (Cahiers d'Enseignement de la SOFCOT N°51. Expansion Scientifique Française. 1995). In 2004, J.A Epinette and M.T. Manley published a reference work considered as a 'bible' in the field of hydroxyapatite coating: *Fifteen Years of Clinical Experience with Hydroxyapatite Coatings in Joint Arthroplasty* (Spinger-Verlag France. 2004). These books have certainly contributed to the worldwide acceptance and success of the bioactive fixation concept. For a long time, our youthfulness and lack of hindsight were criticized. But was it really a fault? Now we have grown up, we can provide clinical series with sufficiently long follow-up times that very few current prostheses can match. The quality of the clinical and radiographic outcomes and the excellent survival has not changed and the nightmare scenarios predicted by some 'doomsters' did not occur. On the contrary, independent studies conducted with unquestionable objectivity, impartiality and rigour have supported the preliminary work done by those directly involved in the development of the Corail® system.

It is hazardous to predict the future. Today, we feel highly satisfied and enthusiastic about the technology of HA-coated implants and especially about the Corail® system. This 25-year-old technology has withstood the test of time, resulting in the development of a new 'gold standard'. Most users tell us, 'Please, don't give in to commercial and marketing pressures and please change the original Corail® prosthesis as little as possible.' According to popular wisdom, one should never change a winning team. However, we cannot deny that further advances are possible. HA coatings will almost certainly improve with the development of new methods of application, new morphologies and new chemical compositions. Also there may be advances in bone growth stimulation and in the prevention and management of infection. Some of these advances, after careful evaluation and taking into account financial considerations, may result in real improvements. Yes, even in orthopaedics, progress is never-ending!

Annecy le Vieux, France   Jean-Pierre Vidalain

List of Illustration Ownership

The following figures are published with the kind permission of the respective owner:

Figures 2.1–2.7, 2.10, 2.11, 2.15, 2.17, 2.19, 2.22–2.33, 2.35, 3.1–3.7, 3.10–3.18, 4.8, 5.3–5.8, 5.10, 5.14, 5.19–5.24, 5.26, 5.30, 6.8–6.11, 6.21, 8.4, 8.7, 9.1–9.3, 9.5, 10.20, 10.62, 10.66, 10.67, 12.1 – ©DePuyInternational Limited

Figure 3.31 reproduced with permission from SLACK Incorporated

Figure 4.26 reproduced with permission from Norwegian Arthroplasty Register, 2009 Annual Report, p. 20, Fig. 5

Figure 4.27 reproduced with permission from Norwegian Arthroplasty Register, 2009 Annual Report, p. 30, Fig. 23

Figures 4.28, 4.29, 8.5, 9.4 reproduced with permission and copyright of the ©British Editorial Society of Bone and Joint Surgery

Figure 6.20 reproduced with permission from Journal of Bone and Joint Surgery

Figures 6.23–6.26 ©Urban & Vogel

Figure 8.2 reproduced with permission from Wolters Kluwer Health

Index

Printing and Binding: Stürtz GmbH, Würzburg